T0263093

Orthopedics

Editor

GEORGE G.A. PUJALTE

PRIMARY CARE: CLINICS IN OFFICE PRACTICE

www.primarycare.theclinics.com

Consulting Editor
JOEL J. HEIDELBAUGH

December 2013 • Volume 40 • Number 4

ELSEVIER

1600 John F. Kennedy Boulevard • Suite 1800 • Philadelphia, Pennsylvania, 19103-2899

http://www.theclinics.com

PRIMARY CARE: CLINICS IN OFFICE PRACTICE Volume 40, Number 4
December 2013 ISSN 0095-4543, ISBN-13: 978-0-323-26122-7

Editor: Yonah Korngold

Primary Care: Clinics in Office Practice (ISSN: 0095–4543) is published quarterly by Elsevier Inc., 360 Park Avenue South, New York, NY 10010-1710. Months of issue are March, June, September, and December. Periodicals postage paid at New York, NY and additional mailing offices. Subscription prices are $216.00 per year (US individuals), $353.00 (US institutions), $108.00 (US students), $264.00 (Canadian individuals), $415.00 (Canadian institutions), $169.00 (Canadian students), $329.00 (international individuals), $415.00 (international institutions), and $169.00 (international students). Foreign air speed delivery is included in all *Clinics* subscription prices. All prices are subject to change without notice. POSTMASTER: Send address changes to *Primary Care: Clinics in Office Practice*, Elsevier Periodicals Customer Service, 11830 Westline Industrial Drive, St. Louis, MO 63146. Customer Service Health Sciences Division, Subscription Customer Service, 3251 Riverport Lane, Maryland Heights, MO 63043. **Customer Service: 1-800-654-2452 (U.S. and Canada); 314-447-8871 (outside U.S. and Canada). Fax: 314-447-8029. E-mail: journalscustomerservice-usa@elsevier.com (for print support); journalsonlinesupport-usa@elsevier.com (for online support).**

Reprints. For copies of 100 or more, of articles in this publication, please contact the Commercial Reprints Department, Elsevier Inc., 360 Park Avenue South, New York, NY 10010-1710. Tel. 212-633-3874; Fax: 212-633-3820; E-mail: reprints@elsevier.com.

Primary Care: Clinics in Office Practice is covered in *MEDLINE/PubMed (Index Medicus)* and *EMBASE/ Excerpta Medica, Current Contents/Clinical Medicine, and ISI/BIOMED.*

Printed and bound by CPI Group (UK) Ltd, Croydon, CR0 4YY

Transferred to digital print 2012

Contributors

CONSULTING EDITOR

JOEL J. HEIDELBAUGH, MD, FAAFP, FACG
Clinical Associate Professor, Departments of Family Medicine and Urology, Clerkship Director, University of Michigan Medical School, Ann Arbor; Ypsilanti Health Center, Ypsilanti, Michigan

EDITOR

GEORGE G.A. PUJALTE, MD, CAQSM
Assistant Professor, Division of Sports Medicine, Departments of Family and Community Medicine, and Orthopaedics and Rehabilitation, Penn State Milton S. Hershey Medical Center, Hershey, Pennsylvania

AUTHORS

ANDREA L. AAGESEN, DO, MS
Clinical Instructor, Department of Physical Medicine and Rehabilitation, University of Michigan Health Systems, Ann Arbor, Michigan

STEPHANIE ASHBAUGH, MD
Assistant Professor, Department of Family and Community Medicine, Penn State Milton S. Hershey Medical Center, Penn State Hershey Medical Group, Harrisburg, Pennsylvania

AMBA AYLOO, MD
Chief Resident, Family Medicine Residency Program, Department of Family Medicine, Mount Sinai Hospital, Chicago, Illinois

BRENDEN J. BALCIK, MD
Resident Physician, Department of Emergency Medicine, Robert C. Byrd Health Sciences Center, School of Medicine, West Virginia University, Morgantown, West Virginia

GREGORY BILLY, MD
Assistant Professor, Department of Orthopaedics and Rehabilitation, Penn State Orthopaedics, State College, Pennsylvania

VIVIANE BISHAY, MD
Department of Family Medicine, Mount Sinai Hospital, Chicago, Illinois

JASON CROOKHAM, DO, CAQSM
Fortius Sport and Health, Burnaby, British of Columbia, Canada

TERESA CVENGROS, MD, CAQSM
Attending Physician, Family Medicine Residency Program, Department of Family Medicine, Mount Sinai Hospital, Chicago, Illinois

ERIC E. FLORANDA, MD
Staff Neurologist, The Center for Neuroscience, Calvert Memorial Hospital, Chesapeake Neurology Associates, Prince Frederick, Maryland

ROBERT A. GALLO, MD
Assistant Professor, Department of Orthopedics, Bone and Joint Institute, Milton S. Hershey Medical Center, Pennsylvania State University College of Medicine, Hershey, Pennsylvania

KATHRYN GLOYER, MD, CAQSM
Assistant Professor, Department of Family and Community Medicine, Penn State Milton S. Hershey Medical Center, Hershey; Department of Orthopaedics and Rehabilitation, Penn State Orthopaedics, State College, Pennsylvania

BRET C. JACOBS, DO, MA
Assistant Professor, Departments of Family and Community Medicine, and Orthopaedics and Rehabilitation, Penn State Milton S. Hershey Medical Center, Hershey, Pennsylvania

JULIE ANN JARDELEZA, RN, BSN
Staff Nurse, Medical/Surgical Unit, Penn State Milton S. Hershey Medical Center, Hershey, Pennsylvania

MUHAMMAD NAUSHERWAN KHAN, MD
Resident Physician, Department of Family and Community Medicine, Penn State Milton S. Hershey Medical Center, Penn State Hershey Medical Group, Harrisburg, Pennsylvania

WILLIAM KRANTZ, MD
Assistant Professor, Department of Radiology, Robert C. Byrd Health Sciences Center, School of Medicine, West Virginia University, Morgantown, West Virginia

SCOTT A. LYNCH, MD
Associate Professor, Bone and Joint Institute, Penn State Hershey, Penn State College of Medicine, Hershey, Pennsylvania

MICHAEL A. MALONE, MD, ABIHM
Assistant Professor, Department of Family and Community Medicine, Penn State Milton S. Hershey Medical Center, Hershey, Pennsylvania

SRIMANNARAYANA MARELLA, MD
Resident, Family Medicine Residency Program, Department of Family Medicine, Mount Sinai Hospital, Chicago, Illinois

MAGED MELEK, MD, MBCH
Chief Resident, Department of Family Medicine, Mount Sinai Hospital, Chicago, Illinois

AARON J. MONSEAU, MD
Assistant Professor, Departments of Emergency Medicine and Orthopedics, Robert C. Byrd Health Sciences Center, School of Medicine, West Virginia University, Morgantown, West Virginia

CAYCE A. ONKS, DO, MS, ATC
Assistant Professor, Departments of Family and Community Medicine, and Orthopaedics and Rehabilitation, Penn State Milton S. Hershey Medical Center, Hershey, Pennsylvania

SEAN M. OSER, MD, MPH
Assistant Professor, Department of Family and Community Medicine, Penn State Milton S. Hershey Medical Center, Hershey, Pennsylvania

TAMARA K. OSER, MD
Assistant Professor, Department of Family and Community Medicine, Penn State Milton S. Hershey Medical Center, Hershey, Pennsylvania

JAIME PEDRAZA, MD
Sports Medicine Fellow, Department of Family Medicine, University of Michigan Health System, Ann Arbor, Michigan

MATTHEW L. SILVIS, MD
Associate Professor, Departments of Family and Community Medicine, and Orthopedics and Rehabilitation, Director, Primary Care Sports Medicine, Penn State Milton S. Hershey Medical Center, Hershey, Pennsylvania

PARMINDER SINGH NIZRAN, MD
Resident Physician, Department of Family and Community Medicine, Penn State Milton S. Hershey Medical Center, Penn State College of Medicine, Hershey, Pennsylvania

RAFAELANI L. TARUC-UY, MD
Resident, Family Medicine Program, Department of Family Medicine, Mount Sinai Hospital Chicago, Chicago, Illinois

Contents

in the case of sternoclavicular joint dislocations. Often, nonoperative management is indicated but, occasionally, surgical intervention is required. Due to the high incidence of clavicle injuries, it is paramount that the primary care physician be able to recognize, diagnose, and manage these injuries.

Nerve entrapment syndromes in the upper extremity are being recognized with increasing frequency. Prompt and correct diagnosis of these injuries is important. This article is a review of the common entrapment nerve injuries seen in the upper extremity. Each of these clinical syndromes is discussed independently, reviewing the anatomy, compression sites, patient presentation (history and examination), the role of additional diagnostic studies, and management.

Many patients suffering from pain and dysfunction attributable to musculoskeletal conditions will use some form of complementary and alternative medicine (CAM). Unfortunately, there is a paucity of both the quantity and quality of CAM treatments for specific musculoskeletal conditions. Many CAM treatments are used for a variety of musculoskeletal conditions, but may be more commonly used for specific conditions. This article addresses the use of CAM for specific musculoskeletal conditions, followed by a review of other CAM treatments and their potential indications for a multitude of conditions, based on the current medical literature and traditional use.

Exercise is universally recognized as a key feature for maintaining good health. Likewise, lack of physical activity is a major risk factor for chronic disease and disability, an especially important fact considering our rapidly aging population. Biking and running are frequently recommended as forms of exercise. As more individuals participate in running-related and cycling-related activities, physicians must be increasingly aware of the common injuries encountered in these pursuits. This review focuses on the evaluation and management of common running-related and cycling-related injuries.

Musculoskeletal injections are a common procedure in primary care and sports medicine but can be intimidating for some clinicians. This article addresses current evidence for corticosteroid injections, and common injection indications and techniques, namely knee, subacromial bursa, glenohumeral joint, lateral epicondyle, de Quervain tenosynovitis, and greater

PRIMARY CARE:
CLINICS IN OFFICE PRACTICE

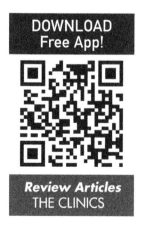

Foreword

Office Orthopedics: From Diagnosis and Treatment to Prevention and Motivation

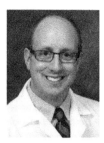

Joel J. Heidelbaugh, MD, FAAFP, FACG
Consulting Editor

As I stated in the foreword for the "Sports Medicine" issue of *Primary Care: Clinics in Office Practice* published this past June 2013, musculoskeletal complaints and injuries continue to rank as some of the most commonly encountered presenting complaints in primary care practices. Educational training in allopathic medical schools, nursing schools, and physician assistant programs often falls short of providing the necessary tools for appropriate cost-effective diagnosis and management of these conditions, while postgraduate residency training attempts to fill these gaps in knowledge. Moreover, our practices are riddled with the same nonsepcific and poor advice that we give to our patients on a daily basis: "exercise more." Yet, as we all know, this advice lacks the assessment of a given patient's motivation, as well as details on *how* to advise them to exercise.

This issue of *Primary Care: Clinics in Office Practice* commences with two very important articles dedicated to the preparticipation physical examination and strategies for writing an exercise prescription. The first of these topics holds special interest for me, since as I write this foreword at the end of August, our office can't meet the demand for back-to-school and "sports physicals." What I always find interesting about sports physical forms is the lack of continuity from one form to the next, as most are quite generic, lack evidence-based screening recommendations, and omit many key provisions of wellness and health care germane to adolescents. The concept of how to write an exercise prescription has been around for decades, but most primary care clinicians still struggle with how to actually accomplish this on a sustained basis for patients. Perhaps as clinicians become more and more accountable for their patients' outcome measurements for chronic diseases, we can use this information to both of our advantages.

Prim Care Clin Office Pract 40 (2013) xiii–xiv
http://dx.doi.org/10.1016/j.pop.2013.09.002
0095-4543/13/$ – see front matter © 2013 Published by Elsevier Inc.

primarycare.theclinics.com

While there is often a great degree of overlap in what we categorize as "office ortho-pedics" and "sports medicine," most primary care clinicians still struggle with feeling confident that they can appropriately diagnose and manage common orthopedic complaints without the obligatory referral to an orthopedic surgeon, a physical thera-pist, or a physiatrist. In the past decades this notion has greatly escalated the cost of caring for these patients, much of which centers on radiographic imaging, a sizeable portion of which is not always necessary.

This issue of *Primary Care: Clinics in Office Practice* runs the gamut from articles that focus on specific injuries including those to the chest wall, clavicle, rotator cuff, and upper extremity nerve entrapment, to the evidence-based diagnosis and treatment for the common disorders of osteoarthritis and cervical radiculopathy. It also contains articles dedicated to giving our patients guidance on orthotics and appropriate foot-wear, something commonly overlooked in our practices. An increasing number of patients request "alternative" and holistic approaches to healing their musculoskeletal complaints. In an era whereby physical therapy and other "standard" treatment modalities often require long wait times for evaluation and substantial co-pays, other options including yoga, Pilates, meditation, and tai chi provide the option of patient-directed and cost-effective healing alternatives with high patient satisfaction. Also impressive is an article dedicated to injection therapy, since in most cases, primary care clinicians can perform in-office joint and intramuscular injections with similar skill and outcomes as specialists after appropriate training.

I would like to offer my gratitude to Dr Pujalte and his authors for compiling a top-notch primer on orthopedics for the primary care clinician. While providing outstanding manuscripts based on current and salient literature, what will set this issue of *Primary Care: Clinics in Office Practice* apart from other orthopedics textbooks and compila-tions is its attention toward cost-effective provisions of care and tenets of motivation that we can use to improve the physical fitness and well-being of our patients.

Joel J. Heidelbaugh, MD, FAAFP, FACG
Departments of Family Medicine and Urology
Department of Family Medicine
University of Michigan Medical School
Ann Arbor, MI, 48109 USA

Ypsilanti Health Center
200 Arnet Suite 200
Ypsilanti, MI 48198, USA

E-mail address:
jheidel@umich.edu

Preface

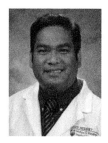

George G.A. Pujalte, MD, CAQSM
Editor

Thank you for choosing this resource in your efforts to provide quality care to your patients. We edited this issue to expand on nonoperative and primary care sports medicine topics that are typically not well covered in other orthopedics books. Authors involved in relevant fields have banded together to produce this volume, with the objective of presenting the latest evidence for both old and new treatments. As such, this issue covers emerging treatments as well as evidence regarding well-known approaches to various musculoskeletal and sports medicine–related conditions, even the controversial ones. We feel that it is important to always consider the plethora of patient treatments available in view of continuing research and not fall into the trap of repeating approaches over and over again without reevaluation. It is also important to have a resource that succinctly summarizes useful information and does not dive too deeply into specifics that may be useful for basic scientists but not necessarily for clinicians. We hope that the reader will closely examine the references listed under each topic—they might help with the design or formulation of additional studies, whenever they appear to be needed. This issue intends to educate the clinician reader, in practical terms, as to what conditions he or she needs to consider when presented with musculoskeletal conditions or sports medicine–related conditions "fresh from the street," so to speak. The issue specifies evidence behind imaging and additional lab testing that may help to determine the appropriate evidence-based therapy. Lastly, this issue discusses emerging treatments, which, despite limited evidence, are bound to be encountered in the real world by physicians who take care of athletes and active individuals. The main difficulty we had was sifting through the existing body of

Prim Care Clin Office Pract 40 (2013) xv–xvi
http://dx.doi.org/10.1016/j.pop.2013.09.001
0095-4543/13/$ – see front matter

knowledge. We made every effort to select the strongest evidence for the practical knowledge, and we hope that this is evident in the articles within.

Our thanks once again—and enjoy.

George G.A. Pujalte, MD, CAQSM
Division of Sports Medicine
Departments of Family and Community Medicine, and
Orthopaedics and Rehabilitation
H154
Penn State Milton S. Hershey Medical Center
500 University Drive, Hershey, PA 17033, USA

E-mail address:
gpujalte@hmc.psu.edu

The Preparticipation Physical Examination

Jaime Pedraza, MD[a],*, Julie Ann Jardeleza, RN, BSN[b]

KEYWORDS

- Preparticipation physical examination • Clearance • Safety
- Sports participation guideline • Athlete screening

KEY POINTS

- The main goal of the preparticipation physical examination (PPE) is to ensure the safe practice of sports by athletes and the identification of conditions that may put the athlete at higher risk of injury or disability, or that may be life-threatening.
- The PPE is meant to be an adjunct to the routine medical examinations by a primary care provider, not a replacement for them.
- The medical history portion of the PPE is the single most important part of the process.
- The role of health care professionals should be to ensure the safe participation of athletes, notwithstanding the pressures surrounding sports, such as scholarships and the potential for a professional career. The goal should be to get an overall assessment of the participant's health.

INTRODUCTION

Physical activity and participation in sports are important parts of health and development. Their practice is encouraged as a means of becoming physically fit and to develop skills that may be applicable beyond sports and into real life situations. It is also of extreme importance to encourage activity in the adolescent population, especially in the United States, where there is a staggering rate of childhood obesity.[1]

In the United States, the number of adolescents practicing sports continues to increase every year, reaching millions across the country.[2] Children are being introduced to organized sports, on the other hand, at younger and younger ages, and, although discouraged,[3] specialization in sports is still sometimes seen at an early age.

The preparticipation physical examination (PPE) is a tool used at different ages and at different levels of competition. Its main goal is to ensure the safe practice of sports

Disclosures: The authors have nothing to disclose and no conflicts of interest.
[a] Department of Family Medicine, University of Michigan Health System, 1500 East Medical Center Drive, SPC 5239, Ann Arbor, MI 48197, USA; [b] Medical/Surgical Unit, Penn State Milton S. Hershey Medical Center, 1500 University Park Drive, Hershey, PA 17036, USA
* Corresponding author.
E-mail address: jpedraza@orthonc.com

by athletes and the identification of conditions that may put the athlete at higher risk of injury or disability, or that may be life-threatening. It investigates past medical history, family history, and includes a medical, as well as, a musculoskeletal physical examination. Routine cardiac, laboratory, and pulmonary screening tests, as suggested by the Preparticipation Physical Evaluation monograph, are currently not recommended as part of the PPE due to the lack of evidence supporting their utility.[4]

Presently, states regulate who can perform the PPE. It is recommended, however, that a physician be ultimately responsible for the examination.[5] The development and utilization of a standardized form or questionnaire for the examination would allow gathering the health information needed. The form or questionnaire could be used by practitioners without an MD or DO degree in the states where this is permitted.[4]

As physicians evaluating athletes, the goal of the PPE is to ensure their safe involvement in sports and to also ensure the safety of those around them, not to exclude them, or to limit their participation in sports activities.

There are different ways in which the PPE can be performed. Two common models are the office-based model and the station-based model.[4] Both have significant advantages and should be encouraged.

The office-based model promotes physician–patient relationship and continuity of care. It allows the physician to focus in sport-specific screening, such as injury prevention, and the development of an individualized program. It also allows time and privacy for addressing more sensitive issues such as sexual practices, alcohol use, drug use, and other at-risk behaviors.[4]

The station-based model allows the participation of specialized personnel (athletic trainers, coaches, and medical volunteers) in the examination of a large number of athletes. Stations for height, weight, vital signs, vision testing, and physical examination are set up,[4] making for an efficient and cost-effective process. With this type of screening, athletes of similar ages can be compared, making the identification of musculoskeletal pathology, such as ligamentous laxity or similar issues, easier.[6] Additionally, it provides an excellent opportunity to introduce resources available to the athletes, such as nutritional education and emotional support, among other things. On the other hand, considering the time the athlete spends with the physician, the station-based model makes it difficult to identify some sensitive problems such as female athlete triad and psychosocial issues, and follow-up of issues found during the examination may become difficult. Additionally, it can be overwhelming if the number and the capacity of the personnel involved are not adequate for the number of athletes to be examined.[4,7]

There is no specific guideline as to when the PPE should be performed. However, it is suggested that the PPE be done several weeks prior to the athlete's involvement in any kind of practice, training, or conditioning.[4,6] Performing the examination at least 6 weeks before training allows adequate time for any problems that may have been uncovered during the examination to be addressed, and for the athlete to get clearance before the beginning of the season. If the athlete was found to be fit for activity, it is still his/her responsibility to notify the athletic trainer, physician, and/or coach of any illness or injuries that may have happened between the PPE and the beginning of practice.[6,7]

In terms of frequency, some authors suggest that the preparticipation examination be performed every school year, while others recommend it be done prior to every sport season, or when the athlete moves from 1 school level to another. There are schools that do a complete and thorough examination at an athlete's first entry in a sport activity, and then perform annual physical examinations and updates on any new medical issues. The ideal frequency may differ depending on the school's specific requirements, and on the athletes and parents.[4,7]

The PPE is meant to be an adjunct to the routine medical examinations by a primary care provider, not a replacement for them. Having said that, it is also important to understand and to know that for many student athletes, the PPE may be their only interaction with a health care professional. Thus, every effort must be made by the examiner to identify and address any potential issues that could be easily overlooked, such as high-risk behaviors.

This article is meant to touch on what the authors believe are the most important aspects of the PPE. It is not meant to be a comprehensive review or guideline. The recently updated monograph: "PPE: Preparticipation Physical Evaluation" in its fourth edition,[4] is an excellent resource put together by the American Academy of Family Physicians (AAFP), American Academy of Pediatrics (AAP), American College of Sports Medicine (ACSM), American Medical Society for Sports Medicine (ACSM), American Orthopaedic Society for Sports Medicine (AOSSM), and the American Osteopathic Academy of Sports Medicine (AOASM).

HISTORY

The medical history portion of the PPE is the single-most important part of the process. History alone has been shown to lead to the diagnosis of most medical and musculoskeletal conditions during the PPE process.[8] It is, however, important to be able to gather accurate information. Ideally, the history portion of the PPE should be completed by the athletes and parents. The history-taking questionnaire suggested by the authors of the PPE monograph is simple, self-explanatory, and a thorough screening tool. There are, however, several other different forms put together by different organizations that can be used. Some state athletic associations have forms that can be found on their Web sites, such as the one used by the Pennsylvania Interscholastic Athletic Association (PIAA), which can be found at: http://www.piaa.org/news/details.aspx?ID=2570. Regardless of the source, any positive response in the history should trigger follow-up questions to try to clarify the issue.

Cardiovascular

This part of the history is extremely important, considering that most of the fatalities in young athletes during sports participation occur as a consequence of cardiac pathology.[9] History of exercise-induced syncope or near-syncope, chest pain, lightheadedness, shortness of breath, and seizures are considered red flags and may indicate an underlying cardiac problem such as arrhythmia, valvular disease, and hypertrophic cardiomyopathy, among other things.[7] It is also important to consider ischemic heart disease as part of the differential diagnosis and ask questions to differentiate it from other potential causes, such as hypoglycemia and asthma. A past medical history of hypertension, high cholesterol, Kawasaki disease, a heart murmur, or a heart infection should be documented. It is also important to note any family history of sudden death before the age of 50. Some forms of cardiac pathology can be hereditary, such as Marfan syndrome and hypertrophic cardiomyopathy.[4] In addition, any prior electrocardiography (ECG/EKG) or echocardiogram testing, the reason for the testing, and its outcome, should be documented.

Central Nervous System

Awareness about concussion and its long-term effects continues to increase day by day. A history of prior concussions or head/neck injuries and the inclusion of the length and severity of symptoms should be obtained. This may help identify athletes who should be counseled about risks of further injury. A history of frequent headaches or seizures should be documented, as well as a history of peripheral symptoms, such as those caused by stingers, burners, or cervical cord neuropraxia.[4]

General

The overall health of the athlete should be assessed. The history should include past illnesses, hospitalizations, surgeries, and current medical problems. Additionally, it is important to know if the patient has been restricted from sports participation in the past. If so, the cause of the restriction should be determined. The outcome of any work-up should be obtained. A list of medications, either over-the-counter or prescription, as well as a list of supplements used by the athlete should also be included. In addition, a list of medications may help identify conditions inadvertently not mentioned in other parts of the questionnaire. For instance, if the athlete is on Lisinopril, this may mean that he or she is actually hypertensive, even though he or she may have forgotten to mention this in the pertinent part of the questionnaire.

Pulmonary System

Asthma and exercise-induced bronchospasm are the most common pulmonary conditions among athletes.[10] A history of shortness of breath, coughing, or wheezing, during, or after exercise, should raise the suspicion that an athlete has asthma. A prior history of asthma, or inhaler use, should also be documented.

Dermatologic Conditions

A history of rashes, sores, or skin infections is important, because they are common causes of temporary restriction to play.[11] They also require proper diagnosis and treatment before a decision to return to play can be made. The National Collegiate Athletic Association (NCAA) has published a handout with specific guidelines on how to manage skin conditions and details return-to-play decisions for athletes with skin infections (http://www.ncaapublications.com/productdownloads/MD12.pdf).

Musculoskeletal Concerns

In this part, a history of prior injury, loss of playing time, joint pain or swelling, and fractures, as well as the use of orthotics or other assistive devices, should be documented and evaluated. It should also help examiners focus on areas that may benefit from the development of a rehabilitation protocol or an injury prevention program. For example, a potential soccer player with laxity of ankle ligaments may benefit from a strengthening protocol prior to his or her involvement in practice in order to prevent injury.

The Female Athlete

Special attention should be given to a female athlete with a history of injuries, fractures, or stress fractures.[4] Questions regarding eating habits, the athlete's concerns about weight, as well as a history of eating disorders, should be included.[4] A menstrual history should be obtained, including regularity, frequency, and history of amenorrhea, as female athletes with menstrual dysfunction tend to have longer interruption of training due to musculoskeletal conditions than those with regular cycles.[12]

Other

Other important areas of history are the absence of a paired organ, heat illness, sickle cell trait or disease, and eye disorders. Identification of any of these problems is important in order to counsel the athlete on the use of protective equipment and educate those with conditions that may predispose them to injuries or illness.[4] For example, an athlete who has only 1 functional eye should be advised against participating in a sport involving projectiles, as this puts him or her at risk of losing the functional eye. A history of immunizations should also be obtained. A history of alcohol, tobacco, or drug use, and psychological problems, such as anxiety or generalized stress, may be indicators of more serious problems and should be further investigated.[7]

PHYSICAL EXAMINATION

The physical examination portion of the PPE should focus on the areas that are most important for the safe practice of sports, as well as the areas that may have raised any red flags during the history-taking portion of the examination.

Vital Signs

Height, weight, pulse, and blood pressure should all be obtained. Height and weight give a general assessment of nutritional status. Concerns regarding potential for eating disorders should be further investigated. Special consideration should be given to blood pressure, because elevation of blood pressure has been found to be the most frequent medical abnormality during the PPE.[13]

Cardiovascular

Auscultation for heart murmurs
The heart should be auscultated in the supine position, with the athlete doing the Valsalva maneuver, and in the standing position. Murmurs are common in the adolescent, and special attention should be given to murmur changes in different positions. A murmur of hypertrophic cardiomyopathy will be louder with the patient standing and will be softer with squatting. Innocent murmurs, on the other hand, will increase with squatting and decrease with the Valsalva maneuver and while standing.[7] This is because there is decreased venous return to the heart while standing and during the Valsalva maneuver, which leads to a decrease in the size of the left ventricle and stroke volume. Conversely, blood volume and stroke volume are increased in the left ventricle from the increased venous return while squatting.[4]

Palpation of pulses
Femoral pulses should be palpated concurrently with the radial pulses to evaluate for aortic coarctation. A delay in the pulse sensation at the femoral level compared with the radial artery should raise a concern for aortic coarctation.

Examination for stigmata of Marfan syndrome
Marfan syndrome is associated with mitral valve prolapse, aortic root dilatation, or dissection. As such, stigmata of the syndrome should be deliberately assessed. Some of the physical examination findings include arachnodactyly, arm span greater than height, a high-arched palate, and pectus excavatum or carinatum.

Brachial artery blood pressure taken in the sitting position
As previously mentioned, elevated blood pressure is typically seen during the PPE. It is important to first make sure that the cuff size is appropriate for the athlete.[14] If the cuff size is appropriate, and the blood pressure is still elevated, the athlete should sit and rest for 5 to 10 minutes; the blood pressure measurement should then be repeated. It is also important to inquire regarding the use of caffeine, nicotine, or other stimulants, as these may account for elevations in blood pressure.[15]

Finally, the presence of arrhythmias should be further evaluated before proceeding with clearance for participation in sports. Primary electrical diseases such as long QT syndrome, Wolff-Parkinson-White syndrome, catecholaminergic polymorphic ventricular tachycardia, Brugada syndrome, and short QT syndrome are some of the causes of sudden cardiac death in athletes.[4] Athletes with a fast heart rate, especially one that comes on suddenly and that resolves with vagal maneuvers, may indicate supraventricular tachycardia, as opposed to sinus tachycardia, which begins and ends gradually. The use of substances such as caffeine, alcohol, tobacco, medications, or illicit drugs should be questioned to rule them out as possible causes of palpitations in athletes who have them. Unless a clear etiology of palpitations is found after a basic work-up, and additional assessment for malignant arrhythmia with Holter or event monitoring is completed, activity should be limited and a cardiology consultation considered.[16]

Musculoskeletal

A general musculoskeletal physical examination should include range of motion, strength, and symmetry. It has been found that history alone is 92% sensitive in detecting significant musculoskeletal abnormalities,[17] but even then, a more detailed examination should be obtained on specific areas with a history of prior injury, swelling, or instability. It has also been suggested that a sport-specific or a joint-specific examination could be done if there are enough time and resources available.[18] For example, a history of labral tear of the shoulder may not be as high-yield for a cyclist, but may place a pitcher at higher of developing problems. Thus, it is important to keep in mind a prior history of injury while trying to correlate it with the intended sport.

Eyes and Visual Acuity

Visual acuity should be evaluated during the PPE with a standard Snellen chart. If the athlete uses eyeglasses or contact lenses, it is important to perform the evaluation while he or she is wearing them.[7] If an athlete is identified to have abnormal visual acuity, he or she should be evaluated by a specialist if the impairment may place him or her at risk for injury. For example, a patient with myopia may be at risk for injury if he or she desires to practice boxing. Anisocoria should be documented, as it may help avoid confusion during the evaluation of an athlete if he or she sustains brain injury.[7]

Lungs

Examination of the lungs may reveal wheezes or rubs, and these should lead to further evaluation. Most examinations may be normal, although this does not exclude asthma or exercised-induced bronchospasm. If there is a concern for such, further evaluation, and perhaps pulmonary function testing, should be pursued.[4]

Abdomen

The abdomen should be examined while the athlete is lying supine. Any abnormal findings such as masses, tenderness, rigidity, or organomegaly should be further investigated prior to clearance.[4]

Male Genitalia

This is performed with the athlete in standing position. Examination should include evaluation of the size and shape of both testicles and the inguinal canal. Any abnormities such as masses or tenderness should be further evaluated, possibly with ultrasonography.[4]

Skin

A thorough evaluation should be performed with the focus on identifying viral, bacterial, or fungal infections, rashes, signs of trauma, and marks of illicit drug use.[19]

Neurologic

Detailed examination should be performed in an athlete with a history of head injuries or neuropraxias. For someone with a history of concussion, examination should be normal and will help as a baseline for comparison if future injury occurs. In athletes with history of neuropraxias, upper extremity and neck range of motion, sensation, strength, reflexes, and Spurling test should be performed.[4] Any concerns or positive findings should be evaluated further.

CLEARANCE

Once the history and examination parts are completed, the decision for clearance may have 4 potential outcomes[4]:

1. Cleared for all activities without restriction
2. Cleared with recommendations for further evaluation or treatment
3. Not cleared, or status to be reconsidered after further evaluation, treatment, or rehabilitation
4. Not cleared for certain types of sports or for any sports

Table 1
Classification of sports according to contact

Contact	Limited-Contact	Noncontact
Basketball	Adventure racing	Badminton
Boxing	Baseball	Bodybuilding
Cheerleading	Bicycling	Bowling
Diving	Canoeing or kayaking (white water)	Canoeing or kayaking (flat water)
Extreme sports	Fencing	Crew or rowing
Field hockey	Field events	Curling
Football, tackle	High jump	Dance
Gymnastics	Pole vault	Field events
Ice hockey	Floor hockey	Discus
Lacrosse	Football, flag or touch	Javelin
Martial arts	Handball	Shot-put
Rodeo	Horseback riding	Golf
Rugby	Martial arts	Orienteering
Skiing, downhill	Racquetball	Power lifting
Ski jumping	Ice skating	Race walking
Snowboarding	In-line skating	Riflery
Soccer	Roller skating	Rope jumping
Team handball	Skiing	Running
Ultimate Frisbee	Cross-country	Sailing
Water polo	Water	Scuba diving
Wrestling	Skateboarding	Swimming
	Softball	Table tennis
	Squash	Tennis
	Volleyball	Track
	Weight lifting	
	Windsurfing or surfing	

Data from Rice SG, American Academy of Pediatrics Council on Sports Medicine and Fitness. Medical conditions affecting sports participation. Pediatrics 2008;121(4):841–8.

In determining the clearance status of a particular athlete, one must consider the athlete's risk for harm to himself or herself or to others,[4] factoring in the type of sport he or she is playing, and the amount of contact or impact the athlete is likely to receive (**Table 1**). If there is concern regarding clearance, the decision should be made based on guidelines, such as the recommendations by the AAP Committee of Sports Medicine and Fitness, or the 36th Bethesda Conference Guidelines on Cardiovascular Abnormalities.[4]

Health care providers should be an athlete's advocate, first and foremost. Communication with parents (if the athlete is a minor), coaching staff, trainer, and other personnel involved is important. Release of information should be first granted by the athlete or parents. A clear explanation of the concerns, next steps, and potential clearance upon completion of further evaluation, treatment, or rehabilitation should be given. Participation in sports is an important part of growth and development. The role of health care professionals should be to ensure the safe participation of athletes, notwithstanding the pressures surrounding sports, such as scholarships and the potential for a professional career.

REFERENCES

1. Ogden CL, Carroll MD, Curtin LR, et al. Prevalence of high body mass index in US children and adolescents, 2007-2008. JAMA 2010;303(3):242–9.
2. National Federation of State High School Associations. High school athletics participation survey. 2012. Available at: http://www.nfhs.org/content.aspx?id=3282. Accessed February 13, 2013.
3. Intensive training and sports specialization in young athletes. American Academy of Pediatrics. Committee on Sports Medicine and Fitness. Pediatrics 2000;106(1):154–7.
4. American Academy of Family Physicians (AAFP), American Academy of Pediatrics (AAP), American College of Sports Medicine (ACSM), American Medical Society for Sports Medicine (AMSSM), American Orthopaedic Society for Sports Medicine (AOMMS), American Osteopathic Academy of Sports Medicine (AOASM). The preparticipation physical evaluation. 4th edition. American Academy of Pediatrics; 2010. p. 1–155.
5. Team Physician consensus statement. Med Sci Sports Exerc 2000;32(4):877–8.
6. Metzl JD. Preparticipation examination of the adolescent athlete: Part 1. Pediatr Rev 2001;22(6):199–204.
7. Myers A, Sickles T. Preparticipation sports examination. Prim Care Clin Office Pract 1998;25(1):226–37.
8. Peterson MC, Holbrook JH, Von Hales D, et al. Contributions of the history, physical examination, and laboratory investigation in making medical diagnoses. West J Med 1992;156(2):163–5.
9. Maron BJ. Sudden death in young athletes. N Engl J Med 2003;349(11):1064–75.
10. Wilber RL, Rundell KW, Szmedra L, et al. Incidence of exercise-induced bronchospasm in Olympic winter sports athletes. Med Sci Sports Exerc 2000;32(4):732–7.
11. Rifat S, Ruffin MT IV, Gorenflow DW. Disqualifying criteria in a preparticipation sports evaluation. J Fam Pract 1995;41(1):42–50.
12. Beckvid Henriksson G, Schnell C, Linden Hirschberg A. Women endurance runners with menstrual dysfunction have prolonged interruption of training due to injury. Gynecol Obstet Invest 2000;49(1):41–6.
13. Lively MW. Preparticipation physical examinations: a collegiate experience. Clin J Sport Med 1999;9(1):3–8.

14. Pickering T, Hall JE, Appel LJ, et al. Recommendations for blood pressure measurement in humans and experimental animals: part 1: blood pressure measurement in humans: a statement for professionals from the Subcommittee of Professional and Public Education of the American Heart Association Council on High School Blood Pressure Research. Circulation 2005;111(5):697–716.

15. Maron BJ, Thompson PD, Ackerman MJ, et al. Recommendations and considerations related to preparticipation screening for cardiovascular abnormalities in competitive athletes: 2007 update: a scientific statement from the American Heart Association Council on Nutrition, Physical Activity, and Metabolism: endorsed by the American College of Cardiology Foundation. Circulation 2007;115(12): 1643–55.

16. Giese EA, O'Connor FG, Depenbrock PJ, et al. The athletic preparticipation evaluation: cardiovascular assessment. Am Fam Physician 2007;75:1008–14.

17. Gomez JE, Landry GL, Bernhard DT. Critical evaluation of the 2-minute orthopedic screening examination. Am J Sports Med 2001;29(3):304–10.

18. Garrick J. Pre-participation orthopedic screening examination. Clin J Sport Med 2004;14(3):123–6.

19. Bender TW III. Cutaneous manifestations of disease in athletes. Skinmed 2003; 2(1):34–40.

A Guide to Exercise Prescription

Jason Crookham, DO, CAQSM

KEYWORDS

- Physical activity • Physical inactivity • Cardiorespiratory fitness
- Metabolic equivalents

KEY POINTS

- Exercise is a foundational component of good health. The American College of Sports Medicine and "Exercise is Medicine" recommend treating exercise as a vital sign, and assessing and prescribing physical activity at every medical visit.
- Meeting the recommended physical activity goals results in a significant reduction in all-cause mortality.
- Physicians can improve health by prescribing exercise.

Strength-of-Recommendation Taxonomy: Key recommendations for practice	
Clinical Recommendation	Evidence Rating[Refs.]
Getting 150 min of moderate-intensity exercise reduces all-cause mortality	B[1,2,3]
Physicians can improve health by prescribing exercise	C[4,5,6,7,8,9]
Prescribe exercise with FITT (Frequency, Intensity, Type, and Time) to improve compliance	C[3,10]
Recommend a plan that the patient is at least 70% confident he can accomplish to improve adherence	C[11,12]

THE PROBLEM OF LOW CARDIORESPIRATORY FITNESS, SEDENTARY TIME, AND PHYSICAL INACTIVITY

Exercise counseling by primary care physicians has been shown to increase participation in physical activity by patients.[4,5,11,13,14] Furthermore, when surveyed, patients state that they would like their physician to prescribe exercise, and report that they would be more interested in exercise if advised by their physician.[4]

The author has nothing to disclose.
Fortius Sport and Health, 3713 Kensington Avenue, Burnaby, British of Columbia, V5B 0A7, Canada
E-mail address: jason.crookham@fortiussport.com

Physical inactivity, low cardiorespiratory fitness (CRF), and prolonged sedentary time are growing public health problems. In one study, the attributable mortality risk of low cardiorespiratory fitness was greater than the risks incurred from smoking, diabetes, and obesity combined.[1] To highlight the epidemic of inactivity, exercise advocate and sports medicine physician, Karim Khan, coined the term "Smokadiabesity".

According to the World Health Organization, physical inactivity constitutes the fourth leading cause of death globally.[15] When measured directly rather than by surveys, physical inactivity is the leading cause of death in the United States.[15] Low CRF also infers significant mortality risk. Although mortality risk factors such as diabetes and obesity track together, Blair[1] has shown that people can be fit and fat. **Fig. 1** illustrates that it is the least fit people in the population who have the highest risk of mortality.[1]

More than half of adults and 80% of adolescents do not meet the Centers for Disease Control and Prevention (CDC) and American College of Sports Medicine Physical Activity Guidelines.[2] Most adolescents and adults in the United States also spend over 8 hours of sedentary time daily.[2] Sedentary time alone is an independent risk factor for mortality, regardless of the level of fitness or physical activity.[16]

SHORT-TERM AND LONG-TERM BENEFITS OF EXERCISE

The benefits of exercise have been well documented by many research studies.[1,4,5,15,16,17] The US Federal Physical Activity Guidelines,[2] American College of Sports Medicine (ACSM),[3] American Heart Association (AHA),[18] and American Diabetes Association (ADA) all recommend 150 minutes per week of moderate-intensity exercise to achieve health benefits. Exercising more than 150 minutes per week will continue to reduce health risks, but the benefits are not as great (**Fig. 2**).

When counseling patients about exercise, it may be helpful to promote the immediate benefits of exercise as well as long-term benefits. Immediate benefits of physical activity are improved cognitive ability, reduced anxiety, and positive sense of well-being.[19] Exercise in school improves concentration and academic outcomes.[20] In one study, improved SAT scores were observed to correlate strongly with time spent doing physical activity.[15]

Long-term benefits of exercise are numerous. Exercise lowers stroke risk by 27%,[6] reduces the incidence of diabetes by approximately 50%,[21] can lower the incidence of

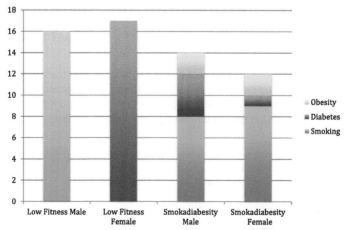

Fig. 1. Attributable risk of all-cause mortality. (*Data from* Blair SN. Physical inactivity: the biggest public health problem of the 21st century. Br J Sports Med 2009;43(1):1–2.)

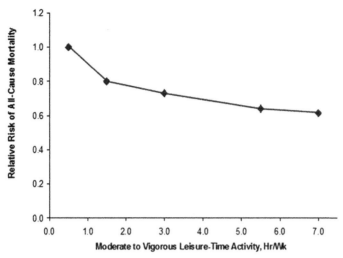

Fig. 2. "Median" shape of the exercise dose-response curve. (*From* US Department of Health and Human Services. Physical activity guidelines for Americans. Available at: http://www.health.gov/paguidelines/Report/G1_allcause.aspx#figureg12. Accessed March 16, 2013.)

colon cancer by more than 60%,[22] and reduce the risk of developing Alzheimer dementia by 40%.[23] Exercise can also reduce mortality and risk of recurrent breast cancer by approximately 50%.[24] Care providers should inform patients of the serious risk of low CRF and physical inactivity. Comparing the risk of low CRF with smokadiabesity may be easy to remember, and motivating.[1]

SUMMARY OF PUBLISHED GUIDELINES ON EXERCISE

The Cochrane Collaboration, the United States Preventative Services Task Force (USPSTF), the ACSM, and the AHA have published recommendations on exercise prescription and physical activity.

Cochrane Database Recommendations on Physical Activity

Cochrane reviews have established that professional advice and continued support encourages people to increase physical activity in the short and medium term.[25] Interventions aimed to increase exercise combined with diet are able to decrease the incidence of type 2 diabetes in people with impaired glucose tolerance and metabolic syndrome.[26] A later Cochrane meta-analysis showed that exercise significantly improves glycemic control in people with type 2 diabetes even without weight loss.[27] Along with improving diabetes outcomes, Cochrane reviews found evidence that exercise-based cardiac rehabilitation is effective in reducing cardiovascular mortality and hospital admissions in men and women who have had myocardial infarction and revascularization.[28] Furthermore, when compared with either waiting or placebo, exercise improved the symptoms of depression in a Cochrane review of 28 randomized trials.[29] As treatment for depression, exercise also had a similar strength of effect when compared head-to-head with cognitive therapy.[7] As suspected by many educators and coaches, exercise improved self-esteem in the short term. This finding suggests that exercise may be an important intervention to improve children's self-esteem and reduce behavioral problems in school.[8] A review of 43 randomized controlled trials investigating exercise in postmenopausal women showed that exercise will improve bone mineral density and reduce the risk of fractures. Women who engaged in a combination of exercises had 3.2% less bone loss and fewer fractures.[30] Cochrane reviews also elucidated the positive health effects of exercise among cancer survivors,[9] and adults living with human immunodeficiency virus/AIDS.[31] A review on weight reduction after childbirth[32] and exercise interventions to help people quit smoking[33] also revealed positive effects. However, both reviews recommended further study. Finally, low back pain (LBP) is a common disorder that tends to recur. Cochrane reviews found moderate evidence that posttreatment exercise programs can prevent recurrences of LBP up to 24 months from the first episode of pain (**Box 1**).[34]

The United States Preventative Services Task Force Recommendations on Physical Activity

The USPSTF provides evidence-based recommendations about clinical preventative services. Many clinicians and health insurance plans use USPSTF guidelines to inform clinical decisions and guide services offered. The USPSTF makes recommendations about physical activity under the topics of "Fall Prevention,"[35] "Healthful Diet and Physical Activity to Prevent Cardiovascular Disease and Obesity in Adults and Children,"[36] and "Screening for and Managing Obesity in Adults."[36] As of the time of writing, the USPSTF is working on a draft research plan on behavioral counseling to promote a healthy diet and physical activity for the prevention of cardiovascular disease in persons with known risk factors.[36] The goal of the research is to systematically review the following questions. Do primary care–relevant behavioral counseling interventions for physical activity in adults with improved cardiovascular disease (CVD) risk factors (1) improve cardiovascular disease health outcomes (eg, prevent morbidity

---

Box 1
Summary of Cochrane Collaboration recommendations on exercise

Professional advice encourages people to increase physical activity in the short and long term[25,35]

Exercise along with diet interventions is able to decrease the incidence of T2D in people with IFG and metabolic syndrome[26]

Exercise improves glycemic control even without weight loss in T2D[27]

Exercise reduces cardiovascular mortality and hospital admission in people with CHD[28]

Exercise improves symptoms of depression[7,29]

Exercise reduces behavioral problems and improves self-esteem in children[8]

Exercise improves bone density and decreases risk of fracture in women[30]

Exercise reduces low back pain[34]

Exercise improves weight loss in women after childbirth[32]

Exercise improves smoking cessation[33]

Exercise is safe and improves health for people with HIV/AIDS[31]

Exercise improves quality of life in cancer survivors[9]

Abbreviations: CHD, coronary heart disease; HIV, human immunodeficiency virus; IFG, impaired fasting glucose; T2D, type 2 diabetes.

and mortality), (2) improve intermediate outcomes associated with CVD (eg, lipid profile, glucose tolerance, weight, body mass index), and (3) change associated health behaviors? And (4) what are the adverse effects of care-relevant behavioral counseling? The exercise inclusion condition will be physical activity that must involve aerobic activities involving large muscle groups, such as cycling, walking, swimming, and resistance training designed to improve strength (**Table 1**).

Table 1
Synopsis of United States Preventative Services Task Force (USPSTF) recommendations related to exercise

Topic	Recommended Intervention	Grade of Evidence
Prevention of falls in community-dwelling adults age 65 or older	Exercise or physical therapy and vitamin D supplementation to prevent falls in community-dwelling adults aged 65 y or older who are at increased risk for falls	B
Behavioral counseling to promote a healthful diet and physical activity for cardiovascular disease prevention in adults[a]	Medium- or high-intensity behavioral interventions to promote a healthful diet and physical activity may be provided to individual patients in primary care settings or in other sectors of the health care system after referral from a primary care clinician. In addition, clinicians may offer healthful diet and physical activity interventions by referring the patient to community-based organizations. Strong linkages between the primary care setting and community-based resources may improve the delivery of these services[a]	C
Screen for obesity. Patients with a body mass index (BMI) of 30 kg/m^2 or higher should be offered or referred to intensive, multicomponent behavioral interventions	Intensive, multicomponent behavioral interventions for obese adults include the following components: Behavioral management activities, such as setting weight-loss goals Improving diet or nutrition and increasing physical activity Addressing barriers to change Self-monitoring Strategizing how to maintain lifestyle changes	B
Screening for obesity in children and adolescents	Screen children 6–18 y and older for obesity and offer intensive behavioral intervention. Effective comprehensive weight-management programs incorporated counseling and other interventions that targeted diet and physical activity	B
Screening for osteoporosis in women age 65 or older, younger women with equal fracture risk	Adequate calcium, vitamin D, and weight-bearing exercise. Consider pharmacologic intervention	B

[a] The AHA has criticized the June 2012 USPSTF recommendation on "Behavioral Counseling to Promote a Healthful Diet and Physical Activity for Cardiovascular Disease Prevention in Adults." The USPSTF statement does not make it clear that it only applies to a small portion of the adult population with no risk factors for cardiovascular disease, and may discourage primary care clinicians from providing behavioral counseling on diet and exercise.[37]

American College of Sports Medicine Recommendations on Physical Activity

The ACSM is the largest sports medicine and exercise science organization in the world. In July 2011, the ACSM published updated recommendations addressing aerobic, resistance, flexibility, and neuromotor exercise.[3] The purpose of the updated guidelines were to provide evidence-based recommendations to health professionals for developing exercise prescriptions and to clarify sometimes conflicting recommendations from professional and governmental organizations such as the surgeon general, AHA, and CDC. The most recent guidelines were made in conjunction with the AHA and the US Department of Health and Human Services 2008 Physical Activity Guidelines for Americans.[38]

In 2007, the ACSM created the Exercise is Medicine Task Force, with the vision of making physical activity a standard part of the disease prevention and treatment paradigm in the United States, and to promote exercise as a "vital sign" to be assessed and recommended at every patient visit.[39]

As an authority on exercise prescription, the ACSM makes a comprehensive recommendation on this topic. For apparently healthy adults, the level of physical activity should be assessed at every clinical visit as a vital sign. A comprehensive program of cardiorespiratory, resistance, flexibility, and neuromotor exercise should be recommended. Irrespective of exercise habits, reducing total time spent in sedentary pursuits and interspersing short bursts of physical activity should be a goal of all adults. Specific recommendations are as follows.

Cardiorespiratory exercise of moderate intensity for 150 minutes per week. Thirty minutes per day for at least 5 days of brisk walking, running, biking, swimming, racquet sports, or team sports such as soccer are acceptable. Another shorter but more vigorous intensity option of 75 minutes per week requires at least 20-minute bouts on 3 days per week.[40,41] Patients should be educated that "some is good, more is better," but even one-half of recommended volume may improve fitness in sedentary individuals.[42,43]

Resistance exercises such as squats, push-ups, or pull-ups to strengthen major muscle groups on 2 to 3 days per week should be recommended. Muscular endurance will improve with 2 to 4 sets of 15 to 20 repetitions. Eight to 12 repetitions improve strength and power. Wait at least 48 to 72 hours between resistance training sessions.[44]

Flexibility exercises on 2 to 3 days per week to improve range of motion. Stretches should be held for 10 to 30 seconds and repeated 2 to 4 times to accumulate 60 seconds per stretch. Flexibility exercise should be performed after warming the muscle or light aerobic exercise. Static, dynamic, ballistic, and proprioceptive neuromuscular facilitation are all effective. A stretching routine can usually be completed in 10 minutes.[45,46]

Neuromotor exercise training on 2 to 3 days per week or more for 20 to 30 minutes. Exercises involving balance, agility, and coordination help to reduce the risk of falls. Examples include activities such as tai chi and yoga (**Table 2**).[47,48]

Table 2 Synopsis of ACSM recommendations related to exercise	
Cardiorespiratory exercise	Moderate-intensity option of 30 min at least 5 d/wk
Resistance exercise	2–3 d/wk of major muscle group strength exercises
Flexibility exercise	2–3 d/wk to improve range of motion
Neuromotor exercise training	2–3 d/wk or more for 20–30 min

PRACTICAL APPROACH TO PRESCRIBING EXERCISE

To successfully prescribe exercise, the clinician should ask about exercise, assess readiness, consider risks and need for exercise stress testing or other screening, choose an appropriate exercise prescription, and plan for reevaluation at follow-up (**Fig. 3**).

Using the "Stages of Change" Model to Assess Readiness for Exercise Prescription

Assessing readiness for exercise prescription is essential. One approach is to use the "Stages of Change" model to improve success. Overly optimistic expectations of inexperienced exercisers may lead to disappointment and attrition. Interventions to ensure realistic expectations might increase success and prevent potential negative effects of failure.[12] The Stages of Changes model includes precontemplation, contemplation, preparation, action, and maintenance, and has improved exercise adherence in some studies.[49] Patients in the precontemplation stage are not ready to start an exercise program, and should receive information about the health benefits of exercise and the risks of a sedentary lifestyle. Patients in the contemplation and preparation stages should receive an exercise prescription appropriate to their level of readiness. Those who are already exercising and meeting the recommendation of 150 minutes of moderate-intensity physical activity will benefit from continued encouragement (**Table 3**).

Using the PAR-Q to Stratify Risk Before Exercise Prescription

Once it has been established that the patient is willing to start an exercise program, the Physical Activity Readiness Questionnaire form (PAR-Q) can then be used to guide who will need formal risk stratification before exercise prescription.

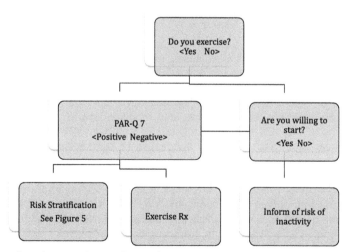

Fig. 3. Flow chart for assessing readiness of exercise prescription. (*Adapted from* The Guidelines of the American College of Sports Medicine and the Canadian Society for Exercise Physiology; and Garber CE, Blissmer B, Deschenes MR, et al. Quantity and quality of exercise for developing and maintaining cardiorespiratory, musculoskeletal, and neuromotor fitness in apparently healthy adults: guidance for prescribing exercise. Med Sci Sports Exerc 2011;43(7):1334–59; and *From* Physical Activity Readiness Questionnaire (PAR-Q) Form 2002. Available at: http://www.csep.ca/cmfiles/publications/parq/par-q.pdf. Accessed May 8, 2013; with permission from the Canadian Society for Exercise Physiology.)

Table 3 Recommended action at each stage of change		
Stage of Change	**Action of Provider**	
Precontemplation (patient not ready to exercise)	Encourage patient to consider exercising; tell patient about health benefits of exercise	
	Independent exerciser	**If supervision necessary**
Contemplation (if patient interested in or thinking about exercise)	Write prescription; refer to nonclinical fitness professional	Refer to clinical exercise professional
Preparation (if patient exercising less that recommended amount)	Write prescription; refer to nonclinical fitness professional	Refer to clinical exercise professional
Action and maintenance (if patient is exercising recommended amount)	Encourage continued exercise	Encourage continued exercise

Created by James O. Prochaska, PhD. Reprinted with permission from Exercise is Medicine® and the American College of Sports Medicine.

Those who answer "No" to all 7 PAR-Q questions likely have a low risk of health complications and can generally begin a vigorous exercise program without supervision at any intensity.[50]

When the patient answers "Yes" to any PAR-Q questions, the clinician needs to stratify risk level, determine the need for preparticipation exercise testing, and determine the need for professional or clinical supervision during exercise (**Fig. 4**).

Deciding Who Needs Further Testing or Who Should be Limited to Nonvigorous Physical Activity

The primary areas of focus when assessing exercise risk are cardiovascular, pulmonary, and metabolic. According to the ACSM guidelines for exercise testing and prescription,[44] patients with cardiovascular, pulmonary, or metabolic disease fall into the "High Risk" category. High-risk patients should be referred to exercise stress testing, have clinical supervision, and modifications, precautions, and contraindications to exercise should be considered.[51] Those without formal diagnosis, but with major signs and symptoms suggestive of cardiovascular, pulmonary, or metabolic disease should also be considered at high risk and be referred for further testing.

For patients without known cardiovascular, pulmonary, or metabolic disease, clinicians need to ask about risk factors concerning coronary heart disease (CHD) to further determine the degree of risk. Risk factors include age, family history, current cigarette smoking, sedentary lifestyle, obesity, hypertension, hyperlipidemia, and prediabetes. Those with 2 or more CHD risk factors are at moderate risk and may safely perform unsupervised moderate-intensity exercise, defined as 65% to 75% of maximum heart rate or 3 to 6 metabolic equivalents (METS). A practical gauge of moderate-intensity exercise is the "Talk but Not Sing Test".[52] This test guides the exerciser to intensity whereby he or she is able to carry on a conversation but would feel breathless if trying to sing. Another guide is perceived exertion of 3 to 4 on a 10-point scale. Patients with 1 CHD risk factor may be considered low risk and do not require further testing before exercise at any intensity (**Box 2, Fig. 5**).

Physical Activity Readiness
Questionnaire - PAR-Q
(revised 2002)

PAR-Q & YOU

(A Questionnaire for People Aged 15 to 69)

Regular physical activity is fun and healthy, and increasingly more people are starting to become more active every day. Being more active is very safe for most people. However, some people should check with their doctor before they start becoming much more physically active.

If you are planning to become much more physically active than you are now, start by answering the seven questions in the box below. If you are between the ages of 15 and 69, the PAR-Q will tell you if you should check with your doctor before you start. If you are over 69 years of age, and you are not used to being very active, check with your doctor.

Common sense is your best guide when you answer these questions. Please read the questions carefully and answer each one honestly: check YES or NO.

YES	NO	
☐	☐	1. **Has your doctor ever said that you have a heart condition _and_ that you should only do physical activity recommended by a doctor?**
☐	☐	2. **Do you feel pain in your chest when you do physical activity?**
☐	☐	3. **In the past month, have you had chest pain when you were not doing physical activity?**
☐	☐	4. **Do you lose your balance because of dizziness or do you ever lose consciousness?**
☐	☐	5. **Do you have a bone or joint problem (for example, back, knee or hip) that could be made worse by a change in your physical activity?**
☐	☐	6. **Is your doctor currently prescribing drugs (for example, water pills) for your blood pressure or heart condition?**
☐	☐	7. **Do you know of _any other reason_ why you should not do physical activity?**

If you answered

YES to one or more questions

Talk with your doctor by phone or in person BEFORE you start becoming much more physically active or BEFORE you have a fitness appraisal. Tell your doctor about the PAR-Q and which questions you answered YES.

- You may be able to do any activity you want — as long as you start slowly and build up gradually. Or, you may need to restrict your activities to those which are safe for you. Talk with your doctor about the kinds of activities you wish to participate in and follow his/her advice.
- Find out which community programs are safe and helpful for you.

NO to all questions

If you answered NO honestly to <u>all</u> PAR-Q questions, you can be reasonably sure that you can:
- start becoming much more physically active – begin slowly and build up gradually. This is the safest and easiest way to go.
- take part in a fitness appraisal – this is an excellent way to determine your basic fitness so that you can plan the best way for you to live actively. It is also highly recommended that you have your blood pressure evaluated. If your reading is over 144/94, talk with your doctor before you start becoming much more physically active.

DELAY BECOMING MUCH MORE ACTIVE:
- if you are not feeling well because of a temporary illness such as a cold or a fever – wait until you feel better; or
- if you are or may be pregnant – talk to your doctor before you start becoming more active.

PLEASE NOTE: If your health changes so that you then answer YES to any of the above questions, tell your fitness or health professional. Ask whether you should change your physical activity plan.

Informed Use of the PAR-Q: The Canadian Society for Exercise Physiology, Health Canada, and their agents assume no liability for persons who undertake physical activity, and if in doubt after completing this questionnaire, consult your doctor prior to physical activity.

No changes permitted. You are encouraged to photocopy the PAR-Q but only if you use the entire form.

NOTE: If the PAR-Q is being given to a person before he or she participates in a physical activity program or a fitness appraisal, this section may be used for legal or administrative purposes.

"I have read, understood and completed this questionnaire. Any questions I had were answered to my full satisfaction."

NAME _____

SIGNATURE _____   DATE _____

SIGNATURE OF PARENT _____   WITNESS _____
or GUARDIAN (for participants under the age of majority)

Note: This physical activity clearance is valid for a maximum of 12 months from the date it is completed and becomes invalid if your condition changes so that you would answer YES to any of the seven questions.

CSEP | SCPE   © Canadian Society for Exercise Physiology www.csep.ca/forms

Fig. 4. PAR-Q 7. (Source: Physical Activity Readiness Questionnaire (PAR–Q) © 2002. Used with permission from the Canadian Society for Exercise Physiology, www.csep.ca.)

Role of Exercise Stress Test

Patients who are stratified in the moderate-risk or high-risk categories may benefit from further testing before beginning an exercise program. Exercise stress testing, along with other cardiovascular tests, can add important information about safe intensity of activity.

Box 2
Medical history, signs and symptoms, and risk factors of risk stratification

High Risk: Cardiovascular, Metabolic, or Pulmonary Disease

Cardiovascular disease

- Coronary artery disease
- Peripheral artery disease
- Heart failure
- Heart valve disease
- Congenital heart disease
- Pacemaker/internal defibrillator

Metabolic disease

- Diabetes mellitus (type 1 or 2)
- Renal, liver or thyroid disease

Pulmonary disease

- Chronic obstructive lung disease
- Asthma
- Interstitial lung disease
- Cystic fibrosis

High Risk: Major Signs and Symptoms of Cardiovascular, Metabolic, or Pulmonary Disease

- Typical chest pain
- Dyspnea on exertion or rest
- Dizziness of syncope
- Orthopnea
- Ankle edema
- Palpitations/unexplained tachycardia
- Intermittent claudication
- Known heart murmur

Moderate Risk: Two Cardiovascular, Metabolic, or Pulmonary Risk Factors

- Female older than 55 years; if with history of hysterectomy or is postmenopausal
- Male older than 45 years
- Blood pressure (BP) higher than 140/90 mm Hg
- On BP medication
- Total cholesterol higher than 200 mg/dL
- First-degree relative with coronary heart disease (<55-year-old male or <65-year-old female)
- Body mass index higher than 30 kg/m^2
- Prediabetes

Data from Jonas S, Edward M. ACSM's Exercise is Medicine: A clinician's guide to exercise prescription. Philadelphia: Kerry O'Rourke; 2009. p. 31–45, 198.

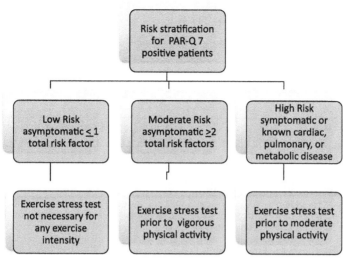

Fig. 5. ACSM risk stratification of patients. (*Data from* Jonas S, Edward M. ACSM's Exercise is Medicine: A clinician's guide to exercise prescription. Philadelphia: Kerry O'Rourke; 2009. p. 31–45, 198.)

Although there is no perfect test for screening the asymptomatic population for coronary artery disease (CAD), exercise testing is one of the most cost-effective methods, and its use is prudent in patients with significant risk factors.[53] However, the exercise stress test has further application beyond screening, including: evaluation of chest pain with possible diagnosis of CAD; screening patients with risk of CAD; determination of prognosis in patients with known CAD; assessment of treatment for CAD; and determination of exercise capacity and safety for an exercise prescription.[54]

When the goal of exercise stress testing is to exclude CAD, it is most valuable in patients with an intermediate (10%–90%) pretest likelihood of CAD.[55]

Three steps can determine pretest probability.[56]

Step 1. Ask 3 questions.
  Is chest pain substernal?
  Is chest pain brought on by exertion?
  Is chest pain relieved within 10 minutes by rest or nitroglycerin?
Step 2. Classify the chest pain.
  1/3 = Nonanginal chest pain
  2/3 = Atypical anginal chest pain
  3/3 = Typical anginal chest pain
Step 3. Refer to the ACC/AHA guidelines for exercise testing **Table 4**.

When the pretest probability of CAD is in the intermediate range (10%–90%), a negative study provides justification for no further testing but continued close observation (see **Table 4**). On the other hand, the likelihood of a false positive is low enough that an abnormal exercise test should be followed by additional studies, including invasive studies. Exercise stress testing in those with low pretest probability is more likely to produce false positives, especially in women[57]; this can lead to unnecessary patient anxiety and further dangers of unnecessary testing. In the high-risk group, a negative exercise stress test is not sensitive enough to exclude significant CAD.

Table 4
Pretest probability of coronary artery disease by age, gender, and symptoms

Age (y)	Gender	Typical Angina Pectoris	Atypical Angina Pectoris	Nonanginal Chest Pain	Asymptomatic
30–39	Men	Intermediate	Intermediate	Low	Very low
	Women	Intermediate	Very low	Very low	Very low
40–49	Men	High	Intermediate	Intermediate	Low
	Women	Intermediate	Low	Very low	Very low
50–59	Men	High	Intermediate	Intermediate	Low
	Women	Intermediate	Intermediate	Low	Very low
60–69	Men	High	Intermediate	Intermediate	Low
	Women	High	Intermediate	Intermediate	Low

High indicates >90%; intermediate, 10%–90%; low, <10%; very low, <5%.

No data exist for patients <30 or >69 years, although it can be extrapolated that the prevalence of coronary artery disease increases with age. In a few cases, patients with ages at the extremes of the decades listed may have probabilities slightly outside the high or low range.

Data from Gibbins RJ, Balady GJ, Beasley JW, et al. ACC/AHA guidelines for exercise testing: executive summary: a report of the American College of Cardiology/American Heart Association Task Force on Practice Guidelines (Committee on Exercise Testing). Circulation 1997;96:345–54.

Although exercise stress testing may provide information to guide exercise prescription for high-risk patients, it is important to remember that testing is not necessary before high-intensity exercise in the low-risk patient or moderate-intensity exercise in the moderate-risk patient.[10]

Another use for exercise stress testing is to determine exercise capacity and objectively evaluate the patient's responses to exercise, including observations of heart rate, blood pressure, perceived exertion, electrocardiogram, and maximal oxygen uptake if applicable.

Choosing the Appropriate Exercise Prescription

When choosing an exercise prescription, the goal is to work to meet the ACSM guidelines of 150 minutes of moderate-intensity exercise per week and to create a plan that the patient can complete regularly. Using the "FITT Principle" can help clinicians remember the components of an exercise prescription. An exercise prescription will include frequency, intensity, time (or duration), and type (FITT).[10] Frequency refers to the number of times the exercise is performed during the week.[3] Intensity is the level of vigor the exercise is performed. Besides the "talk not sing test," another common measure of moderate-intensity physical activity is target heart rate. Calculate the maximum heart rate by the equation: 220 − (Age in years). Moderate physical activity leads to a heart rate of 64% to 75% of maximal heart rate.

Time or duration of physical activity refers to the length of time each bout of activity is continuously performed. Bouts of at least 10 minutes may be added together during a day.[43]

Patients are much more likely to be adherent with exercise if they agree to a plan that they are confident they can complete. Ask the patient to consider a 10-point scale in which 1 is "not confident at all" and 10 is "100% sure it can be done." When the confidence score is 7 or greater, the likelihood of compliance is improved.[58] It is the "regular" that is the difficult part of regular exercise.

Finally, the type of physical activity is important. Exercise should involve large muscle groups in a rhythmic fashion. Walking is the most common form of exercise. Fortunately, many physical activities will meet the requirements, and are outlined in **Table 5**.

Table 5
Examples of types of physical activity (associated intensity in METs)

Light, <3 METs	Moderate, 3–6 METs	Vigorous, >6 METs
Walking		
Walking slowly on flat surface	Walking at a brisk pace 3–4 mph (able talk but not sing)	Very brisk walking 4.5 mph, hiking uphill, jogging 5 mph
Household and Occupational		
Standing performing light work with hands	Cleaning, sweeping, carpentry, mowing lawn	Shoveling, carrying heavy loads
Leisure Time and Sports		
Billiards, darts, fishing, or playing most musical instruments	Basketball, bicycling 10–12 mph, ballroom dancing, swimming leisurely, doubles tennis	Basketball, bicycling >12 mph, cross-country skiing, soccer, moderate-pace swimming, singles tennis

Adapted from Haskell WL, Lee IM, Pate RR, et al. Physical activity and public health: updated recommendation for adults from the American College of Sports Medicine and the American Heart Association. Med Sci Sports Exerc 2007;39(8):1423–34.

Using a Pedometer

Pedometers are another effective way to promote physical activity.[59] A goal of 10,000 steps is recommended (a mile is approximately 2000 steps), but fewer steps may still meet exercise guidelines for aerobic activity.[60] Pedometers are limited in that the "quality" of steps cannot be determined. The baseline number of steps by is determined by wearing the pedometer for a week. If the goal of 10,000 is not met, activity may be increased by 1000 steps per day every 2 weeks. Pedometers can motivate patients to look for opportunities to be more active during the day, such as taking stairs instead of the elevator, parking farther from the work place, and walking on work breaks (**Table 6**).[1]

SPECIAL POPULATIONS
Exercise in Children

As with adults, the prevalence of physical activity in children has declined.[61] The prevalence of obesity in all childhood age groups has nearly tripled, and risk factors for CVD are more prevalent in obese children than in children of normal weight.[62] In

Table 6
"Steps per day" physical activity index for adults

No. of Steps	Activity Level
0–5000	Sedentary
5000–7499	Low active
7500–9999	Somewhat active
10,000–12,500	Active
12,500 or more	Highly active

Adapted from Tudor-Locke C, Lutes L. Why do pedometers work?: a reflection upon the factors related to successfully increasing physical activity. Sports Med 2009;39(12):981–93.

fact, children born today may have a shorter life expectancy than their parents.[63] Regular exercise in children decreases the risk of developing obesity and hypertension, heart disease, and diabetes. Early intervention is important because 80% of children who are overweight at 10 to 15 years old are obese at the age of 25.[64] Furthermore, exercise has specific benefits for children. The benefits of increased bone density can be improved with exercise, and reduce the risk of fracture in adulthood and osteoporosis later in life. Regular exercise also improves self-esteem and school performance, enhances energy levels, and decreases the risk of depression.[8,19,29] Pediatric psychiatrists use exercise prescription for the treatment of symptoms associated with mood disorder.[65] Because children have immature thermoregulatory systems, children and adolescents should exercise in a thermoneutral environment and be properly hydrated. The ACSM position statement on exercise in heat and fluid replacement can be referenced for further information.

The CDC make recommendations for children and adolescents age 6 to 17 years in the Physical Activity Guidelines for Americans. Youth can benefit from moderate and vigorous-intensity physical activity for periods that add up to 60 minutes or more daily. Activities should include aerobic activity, muscle-strengthening activity, and bone-strengthening activity.

Aerobic activity in children may include short bursts that may not technically meet the criteria for aerobic activity in adults. Just as importantly, children should perform age-appropriate activities that are enjoyable and will be continued over time.

Muscle-strengthening exercises require muscles to be overloaded and do more than is required in daily activity. In children, this can be accomplished by unstructured play such as climbing on playground equipment and lifting their own body weight. Older children may perform structured strengthening exercise with weights or resistance bands.

Bone-strengthening activity is of particular importance in children because peak bone mass is achieved at the end of adolescence.[66] Bone-strengthening activities require weight bearing, and can be either aerobic or strengthening (**Box 3**).

Exercise and Obesity

Exercise presents particular challenges to the obese patient. Exercises for weight loss have shown minimal effect in comparison with diet. Patients may be encouraged to know that exercise has a protective effect against obesity-related complications regardless of the weight loss achieved.[67] Individuals who are morbidly obese should

---

Box 3
Physical activity guidelines for children and adolescents

Accumulate 60 minutes or more of physical activity daily.

Most of these 60 or more minutes a day should be spent in either moderate- or vigorous-intensity aerobic physical activity.

Muscle-strengthening physical activity should be included on at least 3 days of the week.

Bone-strengthening physical activity should be included on at least 3 days of the week.

Young people should be encouraged to participate in physical activities that are appropriate for their age, enjoyable, and offer variety.

Adapted from Haskell WL, Lee IM, Pate RR, et al. Physical activity and public health: updated recommendation for adults from the American College of Sports Medicine and the American Heart Association. Med Sci Sports Exerc 2007;39(8):1423–34.

be cautious of orthopedic injury when beginning an exercise program.[68] Obese patients may reduce injury risk by starting with non–weight-bearing exercise such as swimming, water aerobics, cycling, or floor exercises.[69] Childhood obesity and physical activity has been shown to increase rates of minor injuries, such as slipped capital femoral epiphysis and tibia varum.[70] Fortunately, obesity does not appear to be associated with severe injury and should not be a deterrent from meeting exercise guidelines.[71] Compared with dieting, exercise has little impact on weight loss in the first 6 months of a program. However, adequate physical activity is crucial in maintaining weight loss. Exercise may not get the weight off, but it will keep it off (**Box 4**).[72,73]

Exercise in the Elderly

Elderly patients will benefit from regular exercise following the same recommendation of 150 minutes per week of aerobic activity, and strengthening exercise at least 3 days a week. Age ($\geq$45 years in men and $\geq$55 in women) is identified as a cardiovascular risk factor by the ACSM and should be considered during risk stratification before exercise prescription. Age alone is not a contraindication for exercise. In elderly people, exercise training is both safe and beneficial in improving flexibility, strength, and quality of life. Programs that focus on strength and balance can reduce falls.[74] Weight-bearing activity along with vitamin D supplementation helps to maintain bone density in the elderly.[75] Because many elderly are sedentary, even a small amount of physical

---

Box 4
Benefits of exercise in overweight and obese individuals

Cardiovascular

1. Improved cardiovascular performance

2. Decreased myocardial oxygen demand

3. Slowing of atherosclerosis

4. Reduced blood pressure

5. Increased peripheral blood flow

Metabolic

1. Improved lipid profile

2. Decreased risk of type 2 diabetes

3. Reduction in truncal obesity

4. Increased basal metabolic rate

Psychological

1. Improved self-image

2. Decreased anxiety

3. Improvement of symptoms in patients with depression

Reduction in the risk of cancer (reproductive, colon)

Reduction in the risk of osteoporosis and osteoarthritis

Symptomatic and functional improvement in patients with chronic obstructive pulmonary disease

Data from Okay D, Jackson PV, Marcinkiewicz M, et al. Exercise in obesity. Prim Care 2009;36:379–93.

activity such as walking 10 minutes per day can have significant benefit regarding morbidity and mortality.[76] Mounting evidence also supports the use of physical activity for the prevention of dementia and treatment of Alzheimer-related symptoms in the elderly.[77,78]

Exercise in Patients with Osteoarthritis

Osteoarthritis is a common problem encountered in primary care, and is a major source of disability in the United States. In the period 2007 to 2009, 50% of adults 65 years or older reported an arthritis diagnosis, and 1 in 5 of all adults report having a doctor diagnose them with arthritis.[79] Exercise, even running, does not cause osteoarthritis.[80,81] Obesity, joint injury, genetics, nutritional factors, and muscle weakness are the most significant causes of osteoarthritis.[82] Exercise strengthens muscle around joints and stretching reduces stiffness. Beyond physiologic improvements, exercise also decreases pain, and improves function and coping mechanisms.[80] Exercise prescription for patients with osteoarthritis may need to be modified. Minimal weight-bearing exercise such as swimming or cycling can be used for aerobic activity. Resistance training is particularly beneficial for treating pain and improving function in hip and knee osteoarthritis.[83] Patents with arthritis should be counseled that it is normal to experience some discomfort around the joint for a few hours after exercise and that this does not indicate that they are injuring the joint. Patients may also benefit from timing exercise with their period of least severe pain during the day, and after taking pain medication if necessary. If pain continues longer than a few hours, the duration and intensity of the next exercise should be reduced.[10]

SUMMARY

Exercise is a fundamental component of good health. The ACSM and Exercise is Medicine recommend treating exercise as a vital sign, and assessing and prescribing physical activity at every medical visit. Achieving the recommended goals of physical activity results in significant reduction in all-cause mortality. Physicians can improve health by prescribing exercise.

REFERENCES

1. Blair SN. Physical inactivity: the biggest public health problem of the 21st century. Br J Sports Med 2009;43:1–2.
2. Healthy People 2020. Available at: http://www.healthypeople.gov/2020/topicsobjectives2020/objectiveslist.aspx?topicId=33. Accessed March 27, 2013.
3. Garber CE, Blissmer B, Deschenes MR, et al. Quantity and quality of exercise for developing and maintaining cardiorespiratory, musculoskeletal, and neuromotor fitness in apparently healthy adults: guidance for prescribing exercise. Med Sci Sports Exerc 2011;43(7):1334–59.
4. Petrella RJ, Lattanzio CN. Does counseling help patients get active? Systematic review of the literature. Can Fam Physician 2002;48:72–80.
5. Petrella RJ, Koval JJ, Cunningham DA, et al. Can primary care doctors prescribe exercise to improve fitness? The Step Test Exercise Prescription (STEPS) project. Am J Prev Med 2003;24(4):316–22.
6. HU FB, Stampfer MJ, Colditz GA, et al. Physical activity and risk of stroke in women. JAMA 2000;283(22):2961–7.
7. Mead GE, Morley W, Campbell P, et al. Exercise for depression. Cochrane Database Syst Rev 2008;(4):CD004366.

8. Ekeland E, Heian F, Hagen KB, et al. Exercise to improve self-esteem in children and young people. Cochrane Database Syst Rev 2004;(1):CD003683.
9. Mishra SI, Scherer RW, Geigle PM, et al. Exercise interventions on health-related quality of life for cancer survivors. Cochrane Database Syst Rev 2012;(8):CD007566.
10. Jonas S, Edward M. ACSM's exercise is medicine: a clinician's guide to exercise prescription. Philadelphia: Kerry O'Rourke; 2009. p. 31–45, 198.
11. Weidinger KA, Lovegreen SL, Elliott MB, et al. How to make exercise counseling more effective: lessons from rural America. J Fam Pract 2008;57(6):394–402.
12. Jones F, Harris P, Waller H, et al. Adherence to an exercise prescription scheme: the role of expectations, self-efficacy, stage of change and psychological well-being. Br J Health Psychol 2005;10(3):359–78.
13. McDermott AY, Mernitz H. Exercise in older patients: prescribing guidelines. Am Fam Physician 2006;74(3):437–44.
14. Patrick K, Pratt M, Sallis RE. The healthcare sectors role in US national physical activity plan. J Phys Act Health 2009;6(Suppl 2):S211–9.
15. ACSM Exercise is medicine fact sheet. Available at: http://exerciseismedicine. org/documents/EIMFactSheet2012_all.pdf. Accessed April 1, 2013.
16. Owen N, Bauman A, Brown W. Too much sitting: a novel and important predictor of chronic disease risk? Br J Sports Med 2009;43(2):81–3.
17. Kohl HW 3rd, Craig CL, Lambert EV, et al. The pandemic of physical inactivity: global action for public health. Lancet 2012;380(9838):294–305.
18. Balady GJ, Williams MA, Ades PA, et al. Core components of cardiac rehabilitation/secondary prevention programs: 2007 update: a scientific statement from the American Heart Association Exercise, Cardiac Rehabilitation, and Prevention Committee, the Council on Clinical Cardiology; the Councils on Cardiovascular Nursing, Epidemiology and Prevention, and Nutrition, Physical Activity, and Metabolism; and the American Association of Cardiovascular and Pulmonary Rehabilitation. Circulation 2007;115(20):2675–82.
19. Calfas KJ, Taylor WC. Review articles: effects of physical activity on psychological variables in adolescents. Pediatr Exerc Sci 1994;4:406–23.
20. Sallis JF, McKenzie TL, Kolody B, et al. Effects of health-related physical education on academic achievement: project SPARK. Res Q Exerc Sport 1999;70: 127–34.
21. Wei M, Gibbons LW, Mitchell TL, et al. The association between cardiorespiratory fitness and impaired fasting glucose and type 2 diabetes in men. Ann Intern Med 1999;131(5):394.
22. Slattery ML, Potter JD. Physical activity and colon cancer: confounding or interaction? Med Sci Sports Exerc 2002;34(6):913–9.
23. Larsen EB, Wang L, Bowen JD, et al. Exercise is associated with the reduced risk for incident dementia among persons 65 years of age and older. Ann Intern Med 2006;114:73–81.
24. Holmes MD, Chen WY, Feskanich D, et al. Physical activity and survival after breast cancer diagnosis. JAMA 2005;293:2479.
25. Hillsdon M, Foster C, Thorogood M. Interventions for promoting physical activity. Cochrane Database Syst Rev 2005;(1):CD003180.
26. Orozco LJ, Buchleitner AM, Gimenez-Perez G, et al. Exercise or exercise and diet for preventing type 2 diabetes mellitus. Cochrane Database Syst Rev 2008;(3):CD003054.
27. Thomas D, Elliott EJ, Naughton GA. Exercise for type 2 diabetes mellitus. Cochrane Database Syst Rev 2006;(3):CD002968.

28. Heran BS, Chen JM, Ebrahim S. Exercise-based cardiac rehabilitation for coronary heart disease. Cochrane Database Syst Rev 2011;(7):CD001800.

29. Rimer J, Dwan K, Lawlor DA, et al. Exercise for depression. Cochrane Database Syst Rev 2012;(7):CD004366.

30. Howe TE, Shea B, Dawson LJ, et al. Exercise of preventing and treating osteoporosis in post menopausal women. Cochrane Database Syst Rev 2011;(7):CD000333.

31. O'Brien K, Nixon S, Glazier R, et al. Progressive resistive exercise interventions for adults living with HIV/AIDS. Cochrane Database Syst Rev 2004;(4): CD004248.

32. Amorim A, Linne YM, Lourenco PM. Diet or exercise or both for weight reduction in women after childbirth. Cochrane Database Syst Rev 2012;(3):CD005627.

33. Ussher MH, Taylor A, Faulkner G. Exercise interventions for smoking cessation. Cochrane Database Syst Rev 2012;(1):CD002295.

34. Choi BK, Verbeek JH, Tam WW, et al. Exercise for the prevention of recurrences of episodes of low-back pain. Cochrane Database Syst Rev 2010;(1): CD006555.

35. Moyer VA, U.S. Preventive Services Task Force. Prevention of falls in community-dwelling older adults: U.S. Preventive Services Task Force Recommendation Statement. Ann Intern Med 2012;157:197–204.

36. U.S. Preventive Services Task Force. Behavioral counseling interventions to promote a healthful diet and physical activity for cardiovascular disease prevention in adults: U.S. Preventive Services Task Force Recommendation Statement. AHRQ Publication No. 11-05149-EF-2. 2012. Available at: http://www.guideline.gov/content.aspx?id=37711. Accessed March 18, 2013.

37. American Heart Association. Available at: http://www.heart.org/idc/groups/heart-public/@wcm/@adv/documents/downloadable/ucm_437052.pdf. Accessed April 1, 2013.

38. US Department of Health and Human Services. 2008 physical activity guidelines for Americans [Internet]. Washington, DC: ODPHP Publication; 2008. p. 61 Cited 2010 October 10. Available at: http://www.health.gov/paguidelines/pdf/paguide.pdf. Accessed May 30, 2013.

39. Exercise is Medicine Task Force, "about exercise is medicine." Available at: http://exerciseismedicine.org/about.htm. Accessed May 30, 2013.

40. Lee IM, Rexrode KM, Cook NR, et al. Physical activity and coronary heart disease in women: is "no pain, no gain" passé? JAMA 2001;285(11):1447–54.

41. Manson JE, Greenland P, LaCroix AZ, et al. Walking compared with vigorous exercise for the prevention of cardiovascular events in women. N Engl J Med 2002;347:716–25.

42. Church TS, Earnest CP, Skinner JS, et al. Effects of different doses of physical activity on cardiorespiratory fitness among sedentary, overweight or obese postmenopausal women with elevated blood pressure: a randomized controlled trial. JAMA 2007;297(19):2081–91.

43. Haskell WL, Lee IM, Pate RR, et al. Physical activity and public health: updated recommendation for adults from the American College of Sports Medicine and the American Heart Association. Med Sci Sports Exerc 2007;39(8):1423–34.

44. American College of Sports Medicine. Position stand: progression models in resistance training for healthy adults. Med Sci Sports Exerc 2009;41(3):687–708.

45. American Geriatrics Society Panel on Exercise and Osteoarthritis. Exercise prescription for older adults with osteoarthritis pain: consensus practice recommendations. A supplement to the AGS Clinical Practice Guidelines on the management of chronic pain in older adults. J Am Geriatr Soc 2001;49(6):808–23.

46. Decoster LC, Cleland J, Altieri C, et al. The effects of hamstring stretching on range of motion: a systematic literature review. J Orthop Sports Phys Ther 2005;35(6):377–87.

47. Bird M, Hill KD, Ball M, et al. The long-term benefits of a multi-component exercise intervention to balance and mobility in healthy older adults. Arch Gerontol Geriatr 2011;52(2):211–6.

48. Hewett TE, Myer GD, Ford KR. Reducing knee and anterior cruciate ligament injuries among female athletes: a systematic review of neuromuscular training interventions. J Knee Surg 2005;18(1):82–8.

49. Petrella RJ, Lattanzio CN, Shapiro S, et al. Improving aerobic fitness in older adults: effects of a physician-based exercise counseling and prescription program. Can Fam Physician 2010;56(5):e191–200.

50. Arraix GA, Wigle DT, Mao Y. Risk assessment of physical activity and physical fitness in the Canada health survey follow up study. J Clin Epidemiol 1992;45(4):419–28.

51. Exercise is medicine clinicians guides. Available at: http://exerciseismedicine.org/documents/HCPActionGuide_LR.pdf. Accessed March 18, 2013.

52. Foster C, Porcari JP, Anderson J, et al. The talk test as a marker of exercise training intensity. J Cardiopulm Rehabil Prev 2008;28(1):24–30.

53. Fowler GC, Evans CH, Altman MA. Exercise testing. Prim Care 1997;24(2):375–406.

54. Froelicher VF, Quaglietti S. Handbook of exercise testing. Boston: Little, Brown; 1996.

55. Diamond GA. A clinically relevant classification of chest discomfort. J Am Coll Cardiol 1983;1:574–5.

56. Gibbins RJ, Balady GJ, Beasley JW, et al. ACC/AHA guidelines for exercise testing: executive summary: a report of the American College of Cardiology/American Heart Association Task Force on Practice Guidelines (Committee on Exercise Testing). Circulation 1997;96:345–54.

57. Breen DP. Stress tests: how to make a calculated choice. J Fam Pract 2007;56(4):287–93.

58. Moyers TB, Martin JK, Houck JM, et al. From in-session behaviors to drinking outcomes: a causal chain for motivational interviewing. J Consult Clin Psychol 2009;77(6):1113–24.

59. Tudor-Locke C, Lutes L. Why do pedometers work?: a reflection upon the factors related to successfully increasing physical activity. Sports Med 2009;39(12):981–93.

60. Tudor-Locke C, Bassett DR Jr, Rutherford WJ, et al. BMI-referenced cut points for pedometer-determined steps per day in adults. J Phys Act Health 2008;5(Suppl 1):S126–39.

61. Pizarro AN, Ribeiro JC, Marques EA, et al. Is walking to school associated with improved metabolic health? Int J Behav Nutr Phys Act 2013;10:12.

62. CDC Website NHANES Data. Available at: http://www.cdc.gov/nchs/data/hestat/overweight/overweight_child_under02.htm. Accessed March 18, 2013.

63. Olshansky SJ, Passaro DJ, Hershow RC, et al. A Potential decline in life expectance in the United States in the 21st century. N Engl J Med 2005;352(11):1138–45.

64. Whitaker RC, Wright JA, Pepe MS, et al. Predicting obesity in young adulthood from childhood and parental obesity. N Engl J Med 1997;337:869–73.

65. Trivedi MH, Greer TL, Church TS. Exercise as an augmentation treatment for nonremitted major depressive disorder: a randomized, parallel dose comparison. J Clin Psychiatry 2011;72(5):677–84.

66. Teegarden D, Proulx WR, Martin BR, et al. Peak bone mass in young women. J Bone Miner Res 1995;10(5):711–5.
67. Lee S, Kuk JL, Davidson LE, et al. Exercise without weight loss is an effective strategy for obesity reduction in obese individuals with and without Type 2 diabetes. J Appl Physiol 2005;99(3):1220–5.
68. Georgiadis AG, Mohammad FH, Mizerik KT, et al. Changing presentation of knee dislocation and vascular injury from high-energy trauma to low-energy falls in the morbidly obese. J Vasc Surg 2013;57(5):1196–203.
69. Cooper C, Inskip H, Croft P, et al. Individual risk factors for hip osteoarthritis: obesity, hip injury and physical activity. Am J Epidemiol 1998;147(6):516–22.
70. Carrel AL, Bernhardt DT. Exercise prescription for the prevention of obesity in adolescents. Curr Sports Med Rep 2004;3:330–6.
71. Bazelmans C, Coppieters Y, Godin I, et al. Is obesity associated with injuries among young people? Eur J Epidemiol 2004;19(11):1037–42.
72. Wing RR. Behavioral weight control. In: Wadden TA, Stunkard AJ, editors. Handbook of obesity treatment. New York: The Guilford Press; 2002. p. 301–16.
73. Okay DM, Jackson PV, Marcinkiewicz M, et al. Exercise in obesity. Prim Care 2009;36:379–93.
74. Province MA, Hadley EC, Hornbrook MC, et al. The effects of exercise on falls in elderly patients. A preplanned meta-analysis of the FICSIT Trials. Frailty and Injuries: cooperative studies of intervention techniques. JAMA 1995;273(17):1341–7.
75. U.S. Preventative Services Task Force. Behavioral Counseling to Promote a Healthy Diet and Physical Activity for cardiovascular disease prevention in persons with known risk factors: Draft research plan. AHRQ Publication No. 13-05179-EF-5. Available at: http://www.uspreventiveservicestaskforce.org/uspstf11/physactivity/physart.htm. Accessed March 30, 2013.
76. Evans WJ. Exercise training guidelines for the elderly. Med Sci Sports Exerc 1999;31(1):12–7.
77. Vidoni ED, Van Sciver A, Johnson DK, et al. A community-based approach to trials of aerobic exercise in aging and Alzheimer's disease. Contemp Clin Trials 2012;33(6):1105–16.
78. Delfina LF, Willis BL, Radford NB, et al. The association between midlife cardiorespiratory fitness levels and later-life dementia: a cohort study. Ann Intern Med 2013;158(3):162–8.
79. CDC arthritis fact sheet. Available at: http://www.cdc.gov/arthritis/data_statistics/arthritis_related_stats.htm. Accessed April 3, 2013.
80. Hurley MV, Mitchell HL, Walsh N. In osteoarthritis, the psychosocial benefits of exercise are as important as physiological improvements. Exerc Sport Sci Rev 2003;31(3):138–43.
81. Shrier I. Muscle dysfunction versus wear and tear as a cause of exercise related osteoarthritis: an epidemiological update. Br J Sports Med 2004;38:526–35.
82. Felson DT, Lawrence RC, Dieppe PA, et al. Osteoarthritis: new insights. Part 1: the disease and its risk factors. Ann Intern Med 2000;133(8):635–46.
83. Golightly YM, Allen KD, Caine DJ. A comprehensive review of the effectiveness of different exercise programs for patients with osteoarthritis. Phys Sportsmed 2012;40(4):52–65.

Diagnosis and Treatment of Osteoarthritis

Rafaelani L. Taruc-Uy, MD[a],*, Scott A. Lynch, MD[b]

KEYWORDS

- Osteoarthritis • Joint pain • Joint swelling • Joint inflammation • Osteophytes
- Joint deformity

KEY POINTS

- Treatment options for osteoarthritis are generally based on symptom severity and duration, with the goals of symptom alleviation and improvement in functional status.
- Nonpharmacologic options include physical activity through land-based or aquatic exercises, acupuncture, transcutaneous electrical nerve stimulation, splints, and braces.
- Pharmacologic options are instituted in a stepwise approach, and include topical capsaicin, acetaminophen, nonsteroidal anti-inflammatories, cyclooxygenase-2 inhibitors, and intra-articular steroid injections.
- A surgical approach to osteoarthritis is reserved for chronic cases when pharmacologic and nonpharmacologic treatment options have already failed. Options include fusion and joint lavage, arthroscopy, and arthroplasty.

BACKGROUND

Osteoarthritis (OA) refers to a heterogeneous group of conditions that lead to joint symptoms and signs associated with loss of integrity of the articular cartilage, in combination with changes in underlying bone and joint margins.[1] OA affects more than 40 million individuals in the United States alone, and is the leading cause of disability nationwide.[2] It is the most common articular disease worldwide, although frequencies vary by country.[3] The high prevalence of OA makes it one of the principal reasons for office visits in the primary care setting. OA causes with both direct and indirect economic costs to society. Clinician visits, medications, and surgical interventions comprise the direct costs, while comorbidities and time lost from work because of the effects of disability make up the indirect costs.[4] This situation is more evident among the elderly, who may lose their independence and may later need assistance with their daily living activities, thus adding to the economic burden.[5,6]

[a] Family Medicine Program, Department of Family Medicine, Mount Sinai Hospital Chicago, 15th Street at California Avenue, Chicago, IL 60608, USA; [b] Bone and Joint Institute, Penn State Hershey, Penn State College of Medicine, 30 Hope Drive, Building B, Suite 2400, Hershey, PA 17033-0850, USA
* Corresponding author.
E-mail address: ela.taruc@gmail.com

Prim Care Clin Office Pract 40 (2013) 821–836
http://dx.doi.org/10.1016/j.pop.2013.08.003
0095-4543/13/$ – see front matter Published by Elsevier Inc.

primarycare.theclinics.com

OA can be subdivided into primary and secondary forms, with the primary, or idiopathic, form occurring in previously intact joints without any inciting agent.[4] Aging plays an integral part in this form of OA, as the wear and tear on the joints cause damage to the cartilage, leading to an abnormal repair mechanism. Certain diseases including primary generalized OA, erosive OA, and chondromalacia patellae are categorized as subsets of primary OA. The secondary form of OA is caused by an underlying predisposing factor, such as trauma (**Box 1**).

Box 2 lists some of the risk factors that may predispose persons to develop OA. In general, any breach in the integrity of the chondrocyte matrix has the potential to cause OA.[2] Among these, obesity and joint injury are 2 of the strongest modifiable risk factors.[7] Hip OA has an important correlation with weight, genetic factors, sex, previous traumas, occupational factors, and age, whereas knee OA has a significant correlation with weight, lifestyle, and physical activity.[8]

OA develops by the combination of biochemical, cellular, and mechanical processes.[2] It is thought to start from the breakdown, by proteolysis, of the cartilage matrix. The weak matrix is prone to fibrillation and erosion, and results in the release of proteoglycans and collagen fragments into the synovial fluid. This process induces an inflammatory response in the synovium, which causes further cartilage degradation. As the cartilage becomes weak it begins to thin out, causing the joint space to narrow.[4] Damage to the cartilage also causes new bony outgrowths, or spurs, to form around the joints, which are evident on radiographs. The exact mechanism of pain generation in OA is not well understood, but is possibly related to an interplay of several mechanisms enumerated in **Box 3**.

DIAGNOSIS

The diagnosis of OA is primarily based on thorough history and physical examination findings, with or without radiographic evidence.[9] Although some patients may be asymptomatic initially, the most common symptom is pain. Primary OA is usually symmetric and tends to initially affect the weight-bearing joints: the knees, hips, and spine. However, it is not uncommon for the joints of the hands and wrists to also become symptomatic. The pain is usually described as intense, deep, and "achy," worsened by movement or extensive use and relieved by rest and simple analgesics. Later on, as joints become more worn, the pain becomes more noticeable and unresponsive to medications. The pain causes reduction in range of motion and a decrease in

---

Box 1
Secondary causes of osteoarthritis

- Mechanical stress (obesity)
- Repeated trauma or surgery to the joint structures
- Infection
- Congenital abnormalities (abnormal joints at birth)
- Endocrine and metabolic disorders (diabetes, calcium deposition disorders)
- Other articular diseases (gout and pseudogout, rheumatoid arthritis)

Data from Lozada C. Osteoarthritis in Medscape reference. 2012. Available at: http://emedicine. medscape.com/article/330487-overview; and Hinton R, Moody RL, Davis AW, et al. Osteoarthritis: diagnosis and therapeutic considerations. Am Fam Physician 2002;65(5):841–9.

Box 2
Risk factors for osteoarthritis

- Age older than 50 years
- Obesity
- Trauma/injury to joints
- Genetics (significant family history)
- Reduced levels of sex hormones
- Muscle weakness
- Repetitive use (ie, jobs requiring heavy labor and bending)
- Infection
- Crystal deposition
- Acromegaly
- Previous inflammatory arthritis (eg, burnt-out rheumatoid arthritis)
- Heritable metabolic causes (eg, alkaptonuria, hemochromatosis, and Wilson disease)
- Hemoglobinopathies (eg, sickle cell disease and thalassemia)
- Neuropathic disorders leading to a Charcot joint (eg, syringomyelia, tabes dorsalis, and diabetes)
- Underlying morphologic risk factors (eg, congenital hip dislocation and slipped femoral capital epiphysis)
- Disorders of bone (eg, Paget disease and avascular necrosis)
- Previous surgical procedures (eg, meniscectomy)

Data from Lozada C. Osteoarthritis in Medscape reference. 2012. Available at: http://emedicine.medscape.com/article/330487-overview.

Box 3
Osteoarthritic pain mechanisms

- Osteophytic periosteal elevation
- Vascular congestion of subchondral bone, leading to increased intraosseous pressure
- Synovitis with activation of synovial membrane nociceptors
- Fatigue in muscles that cross the joint
- Overall joint contracture
- Joint effusion and stretching of the joint capsule
- Torn menisci
- Inflammation of periarticular bursae
- Periarticular muscle spasm
- Psychological factors
- Crepitus (a rough or "crunchy" sensation)
- Central pain sensitization

Data from Lozada C. Osteoarthritis in Medscape reference. 2012. Available at: http://emedicine.medscape.com/article/330487-overview.

functional capacity. Some patients feel stiffness that develops during rest, with morning joint stiffness for less than 30 minutes (morning stiffness longer than 30 minutes is more commonly associated with rheumatoid arthritis). Some may also report crepitus (a grating or cracking sensation) over the joint, which may or may not be associated with pain. Those with affected weight-bearing joints may exhibit an antalgic gait. Disease progression is characteristically slow, over several years or decades, causing the patient to become less active and more susceptible to morbidities associated with decreased physical activity, such as weight gain.[4]

Physical examination findings, when present, are mostly found on the affected joints. Most common are a reduced range of motion, crepitus, and intra-articular joint swelling, also called an effusion.[2] Sometimes malalignment and bone enlargement can be seen as well. Inflammatory changes, erythema, or warmth over the area are uncommon. These features are more likely to be seen in gouty or crystal arthropathies or in inflammatory arthritis, such as rheumatoid arthritis.[4] In late stages muscle atrophy around a severely affected joint can be seen. In OA of the hand, the distal interphalangeal (DIP), proximal interphalangeal (PIP), and trapeziometacarpal (base of the thumb) joints are affected. Heberden nodes and Bouchard nodes (**Fig. 1**), which are palpable osteophytic growths over the DIP and PIP joints, respectively, are more appreciable in women. In OA of the spine, associated changes are typically seen in the lumbar region, specifically the L3 through L5 levels. Facet arthritic changes cause foraminal narrowing, which may cause compression of the nerve roots. The later complication of lumbar spine OA is acquired spondylolisthesis.[4]

Inflammatory markers such as the erythrocyte sedimentation rate (ESR), C-reactive protein level, immunologic tests, and uric acid levels are typically within their reference range and usually do not need to be ordered, unless other conditions are being ruled out. No specific laboratory abnormalities are associated with OA.[2] Ancillary testing may be warranted if response to treatment is not as expected or the diagnosis remains uncertain. Synovial fluid is characteristically viscous and clear. Analysis usually shows a white blood cell (WBC) count of less than 2000/μL with mononuclear predominance,

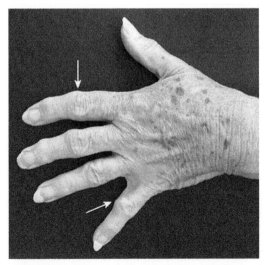

Fig. 1. Heberden nodes and Bouchard nodes (*arrows*). (*From* Waldman S. Physical diagnosis of pain: an atlas of signs and symptoms. 2nd edition. Philadelphia: Saunders; 2010; with permission.)

negative Gram stains and cultures, as well as the absence of crystals when the fluid is viewed under a polarized microscope. Ongoing research on the use of monoclonal antibodies, synovial fluid markers, and urinary pyridinium cross-links (ie, breakdown products of cartilage) as osteoarthritic indicators are under way. Discovery of a marker for early OA will aid in the diagnosis, monitoring, and targeted treatment of OA in the future.[4]

Plain radiography can help confirm the diagnosis, is readily available, and is cost-effective.[2] Typical findings are joint-space narrowing or loss, subchondral bony sclerosis, osteophyte formation, and cyst formation. **Figs. 2–4** illustrate these radiographic findings. Computed tomography (CT) or magnetic resonance imaging (MRI) is rarely used, unless other abnormalities are being ruled out. CT may be used to assist in the diagnosis of patellofemoral malalignment of the patellofemoral joint. Findings on MRI include chondral thinning, subchondral osseous changes, and osteophytes. In addition, direct visualization of the articular cartilage and other joint tissues (eg, meniscus, tendon, muscle, or effusion) is possible with MRI. Ultrasonography is currently being investigated as a tool for monitoring cartilage degeneration and for assistance with joint injections for treatment. Bone scans can help to differentiate OA from osteomyelitis and bone metastases, although these are not typically used in routine diagnosis.

DIAGNOSIS: KEY POINTS

- OA refers to a heterogeneous group of conditions that lead to joint symptoms and signs associated with loss of integrity of the articular cartilage.
- The diagnosis of OA is primarily based on thorough history and physical examination findings, with or without radiographic evidence.

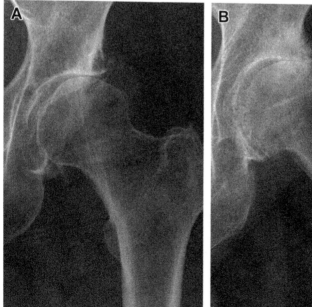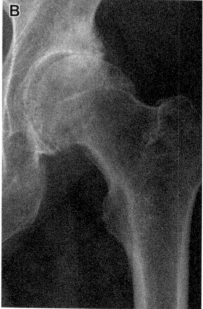

Fig. 2. Radiographs of hip osteoarthritis. (*From* Altman RD, Gold GE. Atlas of individual radiographic features in osteoarthritis, revised. Osteoarthritis Cartilage 2007;15(1):A1–A56; with permission.)

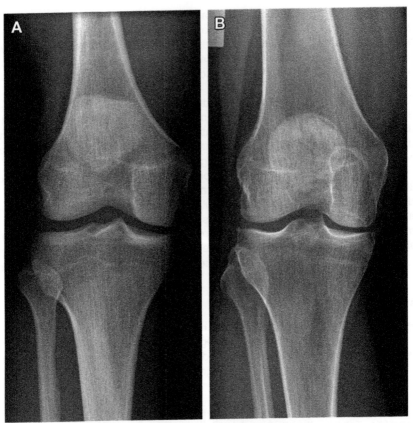

Fig. 3. Radiographs of knee osteoarthritis. (*From* Altman RD, Gold GE. Atlas of individual radiographic features in osteoarthritis, revised. Osteoarthritis Cartilage 2007;15(1):A1–A56; with permission.)

- The most common symptom is pain, described as intense, deep, and "achy," worsened by movement or extensive use and relieved by rest and simple analgesics.
- Most commonly affected are the weight-bearing joints: knees, hips, spine.
- Physical examination findings may include crepitus, effusion, decreased range of motion, and Heberden and Bouchard nodes in the hands.
- Typical radiographic findings include joint-space narrowing, subchondral sclerosis, osteophytic growths, and cysts.

THE AMERICAN COLLEGE OF RHEUMATOLOGY CRITERIA FOR THE CLASSIFICATION AND REPORTING OF OSTEOARTHRITIS OF THE HAND, KNEE, AND HIP

Hand OA

Patients are classified as having OA of the hand if they meet the criteria shown in **Box 4**. Sensitivity for hand OA if all of these criteria are fulfilled is 92%, and specificity is 98%. If at least 3 of these 4 criteria are met, sensitivity increases to 94% while specificity drops to 87%. Radiography was of less value than clinical examination in the classification of symptomatic OA of the hands. The 10 selected joints are the second and third DIP joints, second and third PIP joints, and the trapeziometacarpal joints of both hands.[10]

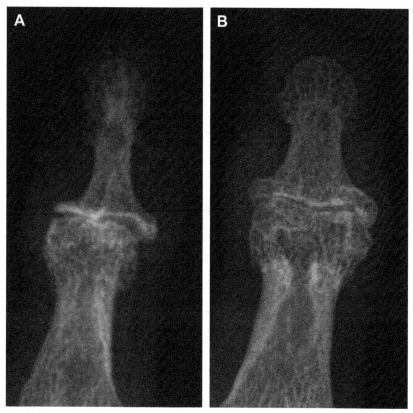

Fig. 4. Radiographs of hand osteoarthritis. (*From* Altman RD, Gold GE. Atlas of individual radiographic features in osteoarthritis, revised. Osteoarthritis Cartilage 2007;15(1):A1–A56; with permission.)

Knee OA

A patient who has knee pain and at least 3 of 6 of the following is classified as having knee OA: age older than 50 years, stiffness of less than 30 minutes, crepitus, bony tenderness, bony enlargement, and no palpable warmth. Diagnosis based on these

---

Box 4
Criteria for classification of idiopathic osteoarthritis of the hand

History

    Hand pain, aching, or stiffness

Physical examination findings

    Hard tissue enlargement involving at least 2 of 10 selected joints

    Swelling of fewer than 3 metacarpophalangeal joints

    Hard tissue enlargement of at least 2 distal interphalangeal joints

Data from Altman R, Alarcon G, Appelrouth D, et al. The American College of Rheumatology criteria for the classification and reporting of osteoarthritis of the hand. Arthritis Rheum 1990;33(11):1601–10.

criteria was found to have a sensitivity of 95% and specificity of 69%. If laboratory findings are considered, an ESR of less than 40 mm/h and synovial fluid analysis are characteristic of OA (clear, viscous, WBC count <2000/mm^3); sensitivity with laboratory tests decreases to 92% but specificity increases to 75%. If radiographic findings of osteophytes are considered, the diagnosis is made with 91% sensitivity and 86% specificity (**Table 1**).[1]

Hip OA

Table 2 describes how hip OA may be diagnosed through clinical findings alone, and with radiographic findings.[11]

TREATMENT

Treatment options for OA are generally classified as pharmacologic, nonpharmacologic, surgical, and complementary and/or alternative.[9] Typically, patients receive a combination of these treatment options to achieve optimal results.[12] Treatment initiation is based on symptom severity and duration, with the goals of symptom alleviation and improvement in functional status.[4] Individualization of treatment options is important.

Nonpharmacologic Modalities

Physical activity has been widely proved to decrease pain and improve function in patients with OA.[13,14] The American College of Rheumatology (ACR) recommends both land-based and aquatic-based programs, depending on patients' comfort level and preferences.

Assistive devices such as walking canes, braces, and appropriate footwear may provide significant improvement in a patient's ability to perform activities of daily living (ADLs). Joint-protection and energy-conservation techniques must also be taught to

---

Table 1
Criteria for classification of idiopathic osteoarthritis of the knee

Clinical	Clinical and Laboratory	Clinical and Radiographic
Knee pain	Knee pain	Knee pain
+	+	+
At least 3 of 6:	At least 5 of 9:	At least 1 of 3:
Age >50 y	Age >50 y	Age >50 y
Stiffness <30 min	Stiffness <30 min	Stiffness <30 min
Crepitus	Crepitus	Crepitus
Bony tenderness	Bony tenderness	+
Bony enlargement	Bony enlargement	Osteophytes
No palpable warmth	No palpable warmth	
	ESR <40 mm/h	
	RF <1:40	
	SF signs of OA: clear viscous, or WBC <2000/mm^3	
95% sensitive	92% sensitive	91% sensitive
69% specific	75% specific	86% specific

Abbreviations: ESR, erythrocyte sedimentation rate; OA, osteoarthritis; RF, rheumatoid factor; SF, synovial fluid; WBC, white blood cell count.

Data from Altman R, Asch E, Bloch D, et al. Development of criteria for the classification and reporting of osteoarthritis: classification of osteoarthritis of the knee. Arthritis Rheum 1986;29(8):1039–49.

Table 2	
Criteria for classification of idiopathic osteoarthritis of the hip	
Clinical	Clinical and Radiographic
1. Hip internal rotation ≥15°, pain present on internal rotation of the hip, morning stiffness of the hip for <60 min, and age >50 y, or 2. Hip internal rotation <15° and ESR ≤45 mm/h; if no ESR obtained, hip flexion ≤115° substituted	Pain + At least 2 of the following criteria: Osteophytes (femoral or acetabular) Joint space narrowing (superior, axial, and/or medial), and ESR <20 mm/h
86% sensitive 75% specific	89% sensitive 91% specific

Data from Altman R, Alarcon G, Appelrouth D, et al. The American College of Rheumatology criteria for the classification and reporting of osteoarthritis of the hip. Arthritis Rheum 1991;34(5):505–14.

prevent further injury. For involvement of the trapeziometacarpal joint, the ACR recommends applying a splint.

Tai Chi is a form of Chinese martial arts consisting of slow, calculated movements, practiced for its health benefits and defense training. A pilot cluster-randomized trial among elderly patients with knee OA concluded that practicing Tai Chi can be efficacious in reducing pain and stiffness.[15]

Physical and occupational therapy are beneficial especially for deconditioned patients and postoperative patients who need to be retrained.

A pulsed electromagnetic field stimulation device and transcutaneous electrical nerve stimulation (TENS) are other possible treatment options for pain relief, both of which are thought to work by decreasing the pressure pain threshold.[16]

Acupuncture is another option for the treatment of chronic pain and physical dysfunction associated with OA.[4] Although data are limited, some studies have shown some benefit to acupuncture, especially when combined with pharmacologic treatment options,[17] although this therapy remains controversial.

Glucosamine sulfate (an amino-monosaccharide), glycosaminoglycans, and proteoglycans are substrates of hyaluronic acid, a major component of joint fluid.[2]

Glucosamine, chondroitin, and the 2 in combination have been the most extensively studied. Some improvement in pain and functional indices and a decrease in the loss of joint-space width have been demonstrated in some, but not all, studies,[18] and this therapy remains controversial.

Balneotherapy, also known as spa therapy or mineral baths, is also used to treat OA, although scientific evidence is weak because of methodological flaws in the studies that have shown efficacy.[19] However, in a randomized, controlled, single-blind study, improvement of pain and function, as well as the quality of life in patients with hand OA, have been demonstrated with balneotherapy combined with magnetotherapy.[20] However, this also remains controversial.

ACR RECOMMENDATIONS FOR NONPHARMACOLOGIC TREATMENT MODALITIES FOR OSTEOARTHRITIS

Nonpharmacologic modalities such as modification of ADLs, joint-protection techniques, assistive devices, and thermal agents are conditionally recommended by the ACR for OA of the hand. In addition, patients with OA involving the trapeziometacarpal joint have been found to benefit from hand splints.[13]

For patients with OA of the knee, it is strongly recommended that they participate in cardiovascular (aerobic) and/or resistance land-based exercise, or aquatic exercise, depending on individual patient preference and safety. It is also strongly recommended for symptomatic, overweight patients to lose weight. Other treatment options include self-management programs, manual therapy in combination with supervised exercises, psychosocial interventions, medially directed patellar taping for patellofemoral OA, medially wedged insoles for those who have lateral compartment OA, laterally wedged subtalar strapped insoles for those who have medial compartment OA, thermal agents, walking aids as needed, and other exercise programs, such as Tai Chi. Traditional Chinese acupuncture and TENS are recommended only when the patient with knee OA has chronic moderate to severe pain and is a candidate for total knee arthroplasty, but either is unwilling to undergo the procedure, has comorbid medical conditions, is taking concomitant medications that lead to relative or absolute contraindications to surgery, or the surgeon is not comfortable recommending the procedure.

For the initial management of hip OA, as for knee OA, it is strongly recommended that patients participate in cardiovascular (aerobic) and/or resistance land-based exercises, or participate in aquatic exercises, depending on individual patient preference and safety. It is also strongly recommended that symptomatic, overweight patients lose weight. Other treatment options include self-management programs, manual therapy in combination with supervised exercises, psychosocial interventions, thermal agents, and walking aids as needed.

Pharmacologic Modalities

Topical capsaicin cream should be considered for adjunctive treatment of focal joint pain.[2] Capsaicin is a component from chili peppers that produces warmth and works by desensitizing neurons by depleting substance P, a pain neurotransmitter. In elderly patients, capsaicin is recommended as first-line treatment of choice for hand OA, although caution is advised because potential serious adverse effects have been observed in clinical trials. Concerns exist that capsaicin-induced nerve desensitization is not fully reversible, and that its autonomic nerve effects may increase the risk of skin ulcers in diabetic patients.[21]

Acetaminophen and nonsteroidal anti-inflammatory drugs (NSAIDs) are the mainstay for the treatment of OA, and cyclooxygenase-2 (COX-2) inhibitors may be used if the former are not well tolerated. The maximum dose of acetaminophen is 4 g/d, and patients must be advised about the potential for overdose and adverse effects, especially when they take over-the-counter medications that have acetaminophen as one of their components. All of these agents have potential gastrointestinal, hepatic, and cardiorenal adverse effects, which increase with dose and duration of treatment. Proton-pump inhibitors (PPIs) should always be considered with an NSAID and with a COX-2 inhibitor in patients at higher gastrointestinal risk.[22]

Intra-articular steroid injections are another treatment option. Corticosteroids work by anti-inflammatory and antinociceptive actions. Corticosteroids have been shown to decrease pain and symptoms associated with OA for up to 3 weeks.[23] However, they must not be administered more than 3 to 4 times per year.[2] Several randomized trials have proven the benefits of intra-articular steroid injections. Although response varies, pain relief and functional improvement can sometimes be obtained for up to 1 year after the injection.[24]

Viscosupplementation, the intra-articular injection of hyaluronic acid or its derivative, is currently approved by the Food and Drug Administration only for patients with knee OA. There is conflicting evidence on its efficacy. Some evidence suggests symptomatic and functional improvement for up to 5 to 13 weeks,[25] whereas others have found minimal or nonexistent effects, Its use in treatment should be individualized because results from trials are not yet generalizable. Its main risk is local adverse reactions from the injection.[26]

Other Agents

Several research studies have focused on other agents with potential for modifying disease progression or treatment of symptoms, but most of these studies still have inconclusive results. S-Adenosylmethionine (SAMe) has been found to have the potential to treat pain and improve functionality, although evidence remains equivocal.[26] Doxycycline is also being investigated for its possible disease-modifying properties and potential to slow cartilage degeneration.[27] Other agents such as strontium ranelate, an agent being used for the treatment of osteoporosis, are being studied for their potential benefit on symptoms of patients with knee OA.[28]

Treatment options using complementary and alternative medicine have gained widespread use among patients because of their ubiquitous presence. In one study topical creams, rubs, and ointments were most commonly used, followed by spiritual methods, alternative providers (such as chiropractors), nutritional supplements, and mind-body therapies.[29] A systematic review has concluded that there is no sufficient evidence to recommend any of the practitioner-based complementary therapies (biofeedback, magnet therapy, chiropractic) for the management of OA, but neither is there sufficient evidence to conclude that they are not effective.[30] In addition, it is important for primary care physicians to discuss with their patients the use of these alternative treatment options, especially when prescribing medications that can cause potential interactions.[30]

ACR RECOMMENDATIONS FOR PHARMACOLOGIC TREATMENT MODALITIES FOR OSTEOARTHRITIS

Pharmacologic modalities recommended for the initial treatment of OA of the hand include either topical or oral NSAIDs, topical capsaicin, or tramadol. Owing to the lack of randomized controlled trials, the ACR has not recommended the use of intra-articular therapies, opioid analgesics, oral methotrexate, or sulfasalazine. Because of a lack of data, no recommendations have been given by the ACR regarding the use of hydroxychloroquine.[13]

For the initial management of knee OA patients may try acetaminophen, oral and topical NSAIDs, tramadol, and intra-articular corticosteroid injections, in a stepwise approach. For patients 75 years and older, topical, instead of oral, NSAIDs are preferred. Because of the lack of randomized controlled trials, the ACR has not recommended chondroitin sulfate, glucosamine, and topical capsaicin for the initial management of knee OA. The ACR has made no recommendations regarding the use of intra-articular hyaluronates, duloxetine, and opioid analgesics. For those with a history of symptomatic or complicated upper gastrointestinal ulcer, use of COX-2 selective inhibitors, or a nonselective NSAID in combination with a PPI, is recommended. In patients with symptomatic knee OA, those unresponsive to previously stated modalities, and those either unwilling to undergo surgery or with contraindications for total arthroplasty, opioid analgesics and duloxetine are possible treatment options. Contraindications to these pharmacologic modalities must be considered, and individual risks and benefits assessed, before initiation.

For the initial management of hip OA, recommendations are similar to those of knee OA, with the exception of the use of topical NSAIDs, intra-articular hyaluronate injections, duloxetine, and opioid analgesics, which are not recommended, as evidence from randomized controlled trial regarding their benefits or safety are insufficient at present. Opioid analgesics are a treatment option in cases of symptomatic hip OA unresponsive to aforementioned modalities when the patients are unwilling or are not candidates for total joint arthroplasty.

Table 3 summarizes the various management recommendations for hand, knee, and hip OA.

Table 3
Nonpharmacologic and pharmacologic recommendations for the initial management of hand, knee, and hip osteoarthritis (OA)

Hand OA	Knee OA	Hip OA
Nonpharmacologic		
Evaluation of ADLs	Aerobic/land-based exercise	Aerobic/land-based exercise
Joint protection techniques	Aquatic exercise	Aquatic exercise
Assistive devices, as needed	Weight loss	Weight loss
Thermal modalities	Self-management programs	Self-management programs
Splints (for trapeziometacarpal joint OA)	Manual therapy in combination with supervised exercise	Manual therapy in combination with supervised exercise
	Psychosocial interventions	Psychosocial interventions
	Medially directed patellar taping	Thermal agents
	Medially wedged subtalar strapped insoles (for those with lateral-compartment OA)	Walking aids, as needed
	Laterally wedged subtalar strapped insoles (for those with medial-compartment OA)	
	Thermal agents	
	Walking aids, as needed	
	Tai Chi programs	
	Traditional Chinese acupuncture	
	Transcutaneous electrical stimulation	
Pharmacologic		
Topical capsaicin	Acetaminophen	Acetaminophen
Topical NSAIDs, including trolamine salicylate	Oral NSAIDs	Oral NSAIDs
Oral NSAIDs, including COX-2 selective inhibitors	Topical NSAIDs	Tramadol
Tramadol	Tramadol	Intra-articular corticosteroid injections
For persons aged ≥75 y, topical rather than oral NSAIDs	Intra-articular corticosteroid injections	

Abbreviations: ADLs, activities of daily living; COX-2, cyclooxygenase-2; NSAIDs, nonsteroidal anti-inflammatory drugs.
Data from Hochberg M, Altman R, April KT, et al. American College of Rheumatology 2012: recommendations for the use of nonpharmacologic and pharmacologic therapies in osteoarthritis of the hand, hip, and knee. Arthritis Care Res 2012;64(4):465–74.

Surgical Approach

If conservative treatment fails, surgical approaches to the treatment of OA can be considered. The most common indications for surgery are intractable pain and worsening disability.[9] Mechanical symptoms may also lead to surgical intervention. Surgical approaches to OA include fusion and joint lavage, osteotomy, arthroscopy, and arthroplasty.

Fusion and Joint Lavage

Fusion, or the union of bones on either side of the affected joint, is a procedure done to relieve pain, usually when knee-replacement procedures fail or as an initial procedure for ankle or foot arthritis. However, this procedure puts more stress on the surrounding joints.[4] Joint lavage, although suggested in observational studies to give promising results, has failed to demonstrate pain relief or improvement of function in patients with knee OA.[31]

High tibial osteotomy is a procedure aimed at shifting the weight from the weakened cartilage on the medial aspect of the knee to the healthy lateral aspect of the knee, used primarily for younger patients with significant malalignment of the lower extremity, usually genu varum or bowleg deformity, and isolated medial compartment OA. It is thought to improve physical activity by decreasing pain, and often delays total knee replacement until about 10 years later.[32] However, total knee replacement is more difficult following this procedure.

Arthroscopy is a minimally invasive procedure used for removal of meniscal tears and debridement of loose articular cartilage. Randomized trials of arthroscopic debridement for OA of the knee have consistently failed to show an advantage over maximal medical therapy combined with physical therapy.[9] However, in some prospective consecutive series, most patients with knee OA associated with unstable cartilage or meniscal injuries have reported good to excellent symptomatic results at short-term and mid-term follow-ups after arthroscopy.[33] Therefore, arthroscopy is not recommended for nonspecific "cleaning of the knee" in OA, owing to its varying success rates.[4]

Arthroplasty is the surgical replacement of joint surface with a metal and plastic prosthesis, and is the treatment of choice for severe symptomatic OA. A variety of prosthetic devices are available, although studies are lacking regarding the advantage of one against the other.[9] Arthroplasty is performed if all other modalities are ineffective, if osteotomy is not appropriate, or if a patient cannot perform ADLs despite maximal use of the other treatment options already mentioned. This procedure alleviates pain and may improve function. Excellent patient outcomes following total joint replacement of the hip, knee, and shoulder have been reported.[9] Possible complications include infection and thrombophlebitis, with or without pulmonary embolism.[34] The use of perioperative antibiotics has decreased the incidence of postoperative infection, while early ambulation and administration of heparin or warfarin as prophylactic treatment for thrombosis are currently being observed. In the absence of complications, a minimum of 10 to 15 years of viability is expected after the procedure.[4]

REFERENCES

1. Altman R, Asch E, Bloch D, et al. Development of criteria for the classification and reporting of osteoarthritis: classification of osteoarthritis of the knee. Arthritis Rheum 1986;29(8):1039–49. Available at: http://www.rheumatology.org/practice/clinical/classification/oaknee.pdf#toolbar=1.

2. Hinton R, Moody RL, Davis AW, et al. Osteoarthritis: diagnosis and therapeutic considerations. Am Fam Physician 2002;65(5):841–9. Available at: http://www. aafp.org/afp/2002/0301/p841.html#afp20020301p841-b4.

3. Centers for Disease Control and Prevention. Prevalence of doctor-diagnosed arthritis and possible arthritis—30 states, 2002. MMWR Morb Mortal Wkly Rep 2004;53:383–5. Available at: http://www.ncbi.nlm.nih.gov/pubmed/15470523.

4. Lozada C. Osteoarthritis in Medscape reference. 2012. Available at: http:// emedicine.medscape.com/article/330487-overview.

5. Bitton R. The economic burden of osteoarthritis. Am J Manag Care 2009;15(Suppl 8): S230–5. Available at: http://www.ncbi.nlm.nih.gov/pubmed/19817509.

6. Murphy L, Cisternas M, Yelin E, et al. Update: direct and indirect costs of arthritis and other rheumatic conditions—United States, 1997. MMWR Morb Mortal Wkly Rep 2004;53(18):388–9. Available at: http://www.cdc.gov/mmwr/PDF/wk/mm5318.pdf.

7. Suri P, Morgenroth DC, Hunter DJ. Epidemiology of osteoarthritis and associated comorbidities. PM R 2012;4(Suppl 5):S10–9. Available at: http://www.ncbi.nlm. nih.gov/pubmed/22632687.

8. De Filippis L, Gulli S, Caliri A, et al. Epidemiology and risk factors in osteoarthritis: literature review data from "OASIS" study. Reumatismo 2004;56(3):169–84 [in Italian]. Available at: http://www.ncbi.nlm.nih.gov/pubmed/15470523.

9. Sinusas K. Osteoarthritis: diagnosis and treatment. Am Fam Physician 2012; 85(1):49–56. Available at: http://www.aafp.org/afp/2012/0101/p49.html.

10. Altman R, Alarcon G, Appelrouth D, et al. The American College of Rheumatology criteria for the classification and reporting of osteoarthritis of the hand. Arthritis Rheum 1990;33(11):1601–10. Available at: http://www.rheumatology.org/practice/ clinical/classification/oa-hand/1990_classification_%20oa_hand.pdf#toolbar=1.

11. Altman R, Alarcon G, Appelrouth D, et al. The American College of Rheumatology criteria for the classification and reporting of osteoarthritis of the hip. Arthritis Rheum 1991;34(5):505–14. Available at: http://www.rheumatology.org/practice/ clinical/classification/oa-hip/1991_classification_oa_hip.pdf#toolbar=1.

12. Zhang W, Moskowitz RW, Nuki G, et al. OARSI recommendations for the management of hip and knee osteoarthritis, Part II: OARSI evidence-based, expert consensus guidelines. Osteoarthritis Cartilage 2008;16(2):137–62. Available at: http://www.ncbi.nlm.nih.gov/pubmed/18279766.

13. Lund H, Weile U, Christensen R, et al. A randomized controlled trial of aquatic and land-based exercise in patients with knee osteoarthritis. J Rehabil Med 2008;40(2): 137–44. Available at: http://www.ncbi.nlm.nih.gov/pubmed/18509579.

14. Vignon E, Valat JP, Rossignol M, et al. Osteoarthritis of the knee and hip and activity: a systematic international review and synthesis (OASIS). Joint Bone Spine 2006;73(4):442–55. Available at: http://www.ncbi.nlm.nih.gov/pubmed/ 16777458.

15. Tsai PF, Chang JY, Beck C, et al. A pilot cluster-randomized trial of a 20-week Tai Chi program in elders with cognitive impairment and osteoarthritic knee: effects on pain and other health outcomes. J Pain Symptom Manage 2012;45(4):660–9. http://dx.doi.org/10.1016/j.jpainsymman.2012.04.009   pii:S0885–3924(12) 00375-2. Available at: http://www.ncbi.nlm.nih.gov/pubmed/23017610.

16. Vance CG, Rakel BA, Blodgett NP, et al. Effects of transcutaneous electrical nerve stimulation on pain, pain sensitivity, and function in people with knee osteoarthritis: a randomized controlled trial. Phys Ther 2012;92(7):898–910. Available at: http://www.ncbi.nlm.nih.gov/pubmed/22466027.

17. Mavrommatis CI, Argyra E, Vadalouka A, et al. Acupuncture as an adjunctive therapy to pharmacological treatment in patients with chronic pain due to osteoarthritis

of the knee: a 3-armed, randomized, placebo-controlled trial. Pain 2012;153(8): 1720–6. Available at: http://www.ncbi.nlm.nih.gov/pubmed/22727499.

18. Ragle RL, Sawitzke AD. Nutraceuticals in the management of osteoarthritis: a critical review. Drugs Aging 2012;29(9):717–31. Available at: http://www.ncbi.nlm. nih.gov/pubmed/23018608.

19. Verhagen AP, Bierma-Zeinstra SM, Boers M, et al. Balneotherapy for osteoarthritis. Cochrane Database Syst Rev 2007;(4): CD006864. Available at: http:// www.ncbi.nlm.nih.gov/pubmed/17943920.

20. Horváth K, Kulisch Á, Németh A, et al. Evaluation of the effect of balneotherapy in patients with osteoarthritis of the hands: a randomized controlled single-blind follow-up study. Clin Rehabil 2012;26(5):431–41. Available at: http://www.ncbi. nlm.nih.gov/pubmed/22144722.

21. Altman RD, Barthel HR. Topical therapies for osteoarthritis. Drugs 2011;71(10): 1259–79. http://dx.doi.org/10.2165/11592550-000000000-00000. Available at: http://www.ncbi.nlm.nih.gov/pubmed/21770475.

22. Adebajo A. Non-steroidal anti-inflammatory drugs for the treatment of pain and immobility-associated osteoarthritis. BMC Fam Pract 2012;13(23). Available at: http://www.medscape.com/viewarticle/764209.

23. Hameed F, Ihm J. Injectable medications for osteoarthritis. PM R 2012;4(Suppl 5): S75–81. Available at: http://www.ncbi.nlm.nih.gov/pubmed/22632706.

24. Cheng OT, Souzdalnitski D, Vrooman B, et al. Evidence-based knee injections for the management of arthritis. Pain Med 2012;13(6):740–53. http://dx.doi.org/10. 1111/j.1526-4637.2012.01394.x. Available at: http://www.ncbi.nlm.nih.gov/ pubmed/22621287.

25. Kelly J. Viscosupplementation for knee OA: little gain, big risks. Ann Intern Med 2012. Published online. Available at: http://www.medscape.com/viewarticle/765492.

26. Rutjes AW, Nüesch E, Reichenbach S, et al. S-Adenosylmethionine for osteoarthritis of the knee or hip. Cochrane Database Syst Rev 2009;(4): CD007321. Available at: http://www.ncbi.nlm.nih.gov/pubmed/19821403.

27. Nüesch E, Rutjes AW, Trelle S, et al. Doxycycline for osteoarthritis of the knee or hip. Cochrane Database Syst Rev 2009;(4): CD007323. Available at: http://www. ncbi.nlm.nih.gov/pubmed/19821404.

28. Reginster JY, Badurski J, Bellamy N, et al. Efficacy and safety of strontium ranelate in the treatment of knee osteoarthritis: results of a double-blind, randomised placebo-controlled trial. Ann Rheum Dis 2013;72(2):179–86. Available at: http:// www.ncbi.nlm.nih.gov/pubmed/23117245.

29. Callahan LF, Wiley Exley EK, Mielenz TJ, et al. Use of complementary and alternative medicine among patients with arthritis. Prev Chronic Dis 2009;6(2):A44. Available at: http://www.cdc.gov/pcd/issues/2009/apr/pdf/08_0070.pdf.

30. Macfarlane GJ, Paudyal P, Doherty M, et al. A systematic review of evidence for the effectiveness of practitioner-based complementary and alternative therapies in the management of rheumatic diseases: osteoarthritis. Rheumatology (Oxford) 2012;51(12):2224–33. Available at: http://www.ncbi.nlm.nih.gov/ pubmed/22923762.

31. Reichenbach S, Rutjes AW, Nüesch E, et al. Joint lavage for osteoarthritis of the knee. Cochrane Database Syst Rev 2010;(5): CD007320. Available at: http:// www.ncbi.nlm.nih.gov/pubmed/20464751.

32. Niinimäki TT, Eskelinen A, Mann BS, et al. Survivorship of high tibial osteotomy in the treatment of osteoarthritis of the knee: Finnish registry-based study of 3195 knees. J Bone Joint Surg Br 2012;94(11):1517–21. http://dx.doi.org/10.1302/0301-620X. 94B11.29601. Available at: http://www.ncbi.nlm.nih.gov/pubmed/23109632.

33. Figueroa D, Calvo R, Villalón IE, et al. Clinical outcomes after arthroscopic treatment of knee osteoarthritis. Knee 2012. [Epub ahead of print]. Available at: http://www.ncbi.nlm.nih.gov/pubmed/23103346.

34. Ravi B, Escott B, Shah PS, et al. A systematic review and meta-analysis comparing complications following total joint arthroplasty for rheumatoid arthritis versus for osteoarthritis. Arthritis Rheum 2012;64(12):3839–49. http://dx.doi.org/10.1002/art.37690. Available at: http://www.ncbi.nlm.nih.gov/pubmed/23192790.

Evaluation and Treatment of Cervical Radiculopathy

Cayce A. Onks, DO, MS, ATC[a,b,]*, Gregory Billy, MD[c]

KEYWORDS

- Cervical radiculopathy • Evaluation • Treatment

KEY POINTS

- The treatment options for cervical radiculopathy continue to evolve as it becomes better defined and gaps in the literature are identified. A thorough history and physical examination is usually adequate to make the diagnosis.
- When the diagnosis is in question, or when invasive treatment is anticipated, imaging should be performed.
- Cervical spine magnetic resonance imaging is the study of choice unless there is a contraindication; computed tomography, or in some cases, computed tomography myelography, are alternatives.
- Conservative therapies including multiple pharmacologic agents, immobilization, physical therapy, manipulation, traction, and transcutaneous electrical nerve stimulation have all been used in the treatment of cervical radiculopathy with variable success.
- Cervical steroid injections have been shown to be beneficial.
- Surgical treatment is indicated in myelopathy or recalcitrant cases.
- Most cases of cervical radiculopathy respond well to initial conservative measures using a multimodal approach.

INTRODUCTION: NATURE OF THE PROBLEM

Cervical radiculopathy was first described clinically in 1817 by Parkinson.[1] In 2010, the North American Spine Society (NASS), a multidisciplinary collaboration, developed the "Diagnosis and Treatment of Cervical Radiculopathy from Degenerative Disorders" evidenced-based guidelines, which is the first known consensus statement on this topic. Their working definition was as follows: "A pain in a radicular pattern in one

No disclosures for either author.
[a] Department of Family and Community Medicine, Penn State Milton S. Hershey Medical Center, Hershey, PA, USA; [b] Department of Orthopaedics and Rehabilitation, Penn State Milton S. Hershey Medical Center, Hershey, PA, USA; [c] Department of Orthopaedics and Rehabilitation, Penn State Orthopaedics, 1850 East Park Avenue, Suite 112, State College, PA 16803, USA
* Corresponding author. Penn State Hershey Medical Group, Mail Code HP21, 3025 Market Street, Camp Hill, PA 17011.
E-mail address: conks@hmc.psu.edu

or both upper extremities related to compression and/or irritation of one or more cervical roots. Frequent signs and symptoms include varying degrees of sensory, motor and reflex changes as well as dysesthesias and paresthesias related to nerve root(s) without evidence of spinal cord dysfunction (myelopathy)."[2]

Studies and subsequent estimates have shown that up to 75% of patients diagnosed with cervical radiculopathy have their symptoms secondary to foraminal encroachment/degenerative changes,[1] which serve as the focus for the NASS guidelines, and may assist in clinical decisions for these patients. A herniated nucleus pulposus is believed to account for the other 20% to 25% of cases.[1]

Cause of Cervical Radiculopathy	Percentage
Foraminal encroachment	70–75
Herniated nucleus pulposus	20–25

The natural history of cervical radiculopathy has been difficult to define as there are limited data available. The available data does not report on the results of untreated patients, which limits the conclusions about its natural history. Cervical radiculopathy from degenerative disorders is believed to be self-limiting and spontaneous resolution occurs over variable lengths of time with or without specific treatment.[2]

The incidence of cervical radiculopathy has been reported to be 107.3 per 100,000 for men and 63.5 per 100,000 for women.[1] Typically, a peak incidence is seen in the sixth decade.

PATIENT HISTORY

The initial history should focus on the chief complaint. These patients often describe pain, weakness, numbness, or paresthesias. In greater than 70% of patients with cervical radiculopathy or stenosis, the complaint is pain.[3] It can be beneficial to obtain patient-perceived pain using a visual analog scale. This can serve as an objective measure of pain as a baseline, as well as in response to treatment.[4]

The history of present illness should attempt to determine the onset as either acute or insidious, which can assist in making the diagnosis. Cervical radicular pain is typically perceived in the upper limb, which should not be confused with pain perceived in the neck. The mechanism, investigation, and treatment are different for these 2 distinct entities.[5] The patient often describes myotomal and/or dermatomal distributions. The description of pain may be described in a range from dull to severe burning pain. This pain should be differentiated from other causes of radicular pain through the history. Other conditions that should be considered in the differential are listed in **Box 1**:

In many patients, there is a history of similar symptoms. It is useful to find out about previous diagnostic tests and their results. It is also helpful to know what treatments have or are currently being used, and their level of effectiveness.

A history of myelopathic features should never be overlooked. Any patient who presents with a history concerning for myelopathy should be questioned about specific symptoms that would suggest the underlying process. **Table 1** lists some of the symptoms described in myelopathy.

Box 1
Differential diagnosis for cervical radiculopathy

Cervical structure referred pain

Pancoast tumor

Heart/aortic disease

Thoracic outlet syndrome

Acute brachial neuritis (Parsonage-Turner)

Rotator cuff disease

Peripheral entrapment neuropathies

Torticollis

Meningitis

Acromioclavicular joint pathology

Adhesive capsulitis

Sympathetically driven syndrome

Bicipital disease

Herpes zoster

Neoplasm

Glenohumeral arthritis

Cervical trigger points/spasm

Posture-related syndromes

Multisystem vasculitidies

Table 1
Red flag signs and symptoms of myelopathy

Symptoms	Examination Findings
Loss of coordination	Hyperreflexia
Sensory disturbance multiple levels	Weakness
Stiffness of the upper and lower limbs	Lhermitte sign (electric shock moving down the spine initiated by flexion of the neck from a supine position)
Acute change in bowel or bladder function	
Frequent falling	Upper motor neuron (UMN) signs
	Clonus, ankle (involuntary rhythmic muscular contractions and relaxations elicited by moving the foot from plantarflexion to terminal dorsiflexion)
	Hoffmann sign (flexion of the index fingers with flexion and adduction of the thumb when the examiner flexes then releases the terminal phalanx of the long finger in a flipping motion)
	Upgoing toe as described by Babinski (first digit extension in response to a stroke over the lateral foot moving distally from the calcaneus to the metatarsal bases and then medially to the first base)

Data from Polston D. Cervical radiculopathy. Neurol Clin 2007;25:373–85; and Carette S, Phil M, Fehlings M. Cervical radiculopathy. N Engl J Med 2005;353:392–9.

Social history may reveal helpful data such as cigarette smoking, axial load bearing, high-risk occupations, and previous lumbar radiculopathy that have been implicated as strong indicators of cervical degeneration.[6]

Providers need to be especially discerning when a patient presents complaining of neck or back pain, as this is a common complaint of drug seekers trying to obtain narcotic medications.[7] The NASS has made the recommendation that emotional and cognitive factors should be considered when addressing treatment of cervical radiculopathy from degenerative disorders.[2]

PHYSICAL EXAMINATION

A thorough physical examination should always be completed. Observation of the patient may reveal a rigid posture. Findings of kyphosis, scoliosis, and loss of normal lordosis of the cervical spine should be considered. General asymmetries throughout the biomechanical chain should be identified. Palpation is important for detecting cervical bony tenderness, especially if there is a history of trauma. Documenting ranges of motion is also helpful, especially when monitoring success of therapeutic interventions.

The critical aspect of the physical examination is the neurologic examination. The most common physical findings include numbness or sensory changes, weakness, and abnormal deep tendon reflexes.[2] Sensory changes are best evaluated with testing of sharp stimulus sensation, and may be perceived in a dermatomal pattern with pain following a myotomal distribution.[1] **Table 2** presents these patterns for each nerve root.

There are several provocative tests that can assist in making the diagnosis of cervical radiculopathy. Efforts to confirm the validity and reliability of these maneuvers have been difficult because of methodological differences and inability to perform meta-analysis. Most reviews on this topic do recommend their use and the NASS has recommended that they be considered in evaluation of patients with clinical signs and symptoms consistent with the diagnosis of cervical radiculopathy.[2] Common provocative maneuvers are as follows:

Table 2
Nerve root patterns

Root	Level	Pain Distribution	Abnormalities		
			Motor	Sensory	Reflex
C4	C3-C4	Lower neck, trapezius	Usually none	Cape distribution (upper shoulders)	N/A
C5	C4-C5	Neck, shoulder, lateral arm	Deltoid, supraspinatus, infraspinatus	Lateral arm	Biceps
C6	C5-C6	Neck, radial arm, thumb	Biceps, brachioradialis, wrist extension	Lateral forearm and thumb	Brachioradialis
C7	C6-C7	Neck, lateral forearm, middle finger	Triceps, wrist flexion, finger extension	Dorsal mid-forearm and third digit	Triceps
C8	C7-C8	Neck, medial forearm, ulnar digits	Finger flexion	Fourth, fifth digits and medial hand, forearm	N/A
T1	C8-T1	Ulnar forearm	Intrinsics	Proximal ulnar forearm	N/A

Data from Refs.[3,8,9]

- Spurling test. The patient is in a seated position while the examiner passively moves the head into extension and then rotates the head to the affected side. It can be performed with or without an axial load once in position. A positive test reproduces radicular pain into the affected extremity. It has been shown to be 93% specific and 30% sensitive.[10] A systematic review showed low to moderate sensitivity and high specificity.[11]
- Shoulder abduction test (relief sign). The shoulder of the affected side is abducted above the patient's head. A positive test relieves the pain. It has been shown to have low to moderate sensitivity and moderate to high specificity.[11]
- Traction/neck distraction (axial manual distraction test). The patient lies in a supine position while the examiner cups the occiput and supports the angle of the mandible. Gentle traction is then applied. A positive finding is relief from pain. It is believed to have low to moderate sensitivity and high specificity.[2,11]
- Valsalva maneuver. An attempt to exhale against a closed airway leading to an increase in intrathoracic and intrathecal pressure. A positive sign is an increase in pain from impingement secondary to the increased pressure. This has been shown to have low to moderate sensitivity and high specificity.[11]
- Upper limb tension test (same concept as straight leg raising of the lower extremity). The patient lies supine on the table. The shoulder is passively depressed and brought into abduction. The forearm is then supinated with the wrist brought into extension. Then, the shoulder should be externally rotated and the elbow extended. Contralateral, then ipsilateral, side bending of the cervical spine is subsequently performed. A positive test results in pain. The test has been shown to be the most sensitive of all provocative maneuvers. There are mixed findings for specificity.[11,12]

It is extremely important to be able to identify the warning signs or red flag symptoms. These correspond to signs and symptoms of myelopathy. Myelopathy typically refers to any pathologic change to the spinal cord itself and is often seen more commonly in the elderly.[13] These changes are often progressive and are not reversible without surgical decompression. These signs and symptoms are listed in **Table 1**. Including the physical examination maneuvers in the evaluation of patients presenting with cervical radiculopathy can be reassuring and may help to distinguish those who have high pain levels and are symptomatic from those who may need additional workup.

Completing a thorough history and physical examination is often all that is needed to make a diagnosis of cervical radiculopathy, which is a clinical diagnosis. Initial treatment strategies can be implemented in most cases without further data collection.

> Magnetic resonance imaging (MRI) is the study of choice. Computed tomography (CT) may be used as an alternative in patients who have a contraindication for MRI.

IMAGING AND ADDITIONAL TESTING

Imaging of the cervical spine is often indicated, especially in cases where conservative therapy is failing. These examinations should be ordered and interpreted with caution. It has been reported that 100% of men and 96% of women ages 70 years show radiographic evidence of cervical spondylosis.[14,15] It has been reported that 36.6% of former National Football League athletes aged 30 to 49 years have arthritis of the cervical spine compared with 16.9% of the general population.[16,17] Cervical plain films have been shown to have low sensitivity and specificity in terms of identifying the presence or absence of nerve root lesions.[8,18] It has been shown that asymptomatic lumbar disk herniation occurs with increasing incidence with age.[19] MRI findings of asymptomatic disk bulge or protrusion have been found in up to 20% of patients aged 45 to 54 years and frank cord compression from this protrusion in 8%.[18]

Many investigators advocate obtaining cervical radiographs as an initial step in the evaluation of cervical radiculopathy.[3,6,8,18,20] However, there is no recommendation in the recent NASS clinical guidelines regarding plain films in the evaluation of patients with clinical symptoms of cervical radiculopathy.[2] Historically, plain films have been used to identify obvious fractures, disk space narrowing, osteophyte formation, instability, tumors, spondylolysis, or spondylolisthesis. There is still benefit from using plain films from a cost and availability standpoint, but because of their poor sensitivity and specificity, they may give a clinician a false sense of reassurance.

NASS clinical guidelines recommend that for confirmation of correlative compressive lesions (disk herniations and spondylosis) in the cervical spine of patients for whom conservative therapy has failed and are candidates for interventional or surgical treatment, MRI is the study of choice. It is also recommended that CT be used as an alternative in patients who have a contraindication for MRI.[2]

When the diagnosis is still in question after MRI because of clinical findings that are not confirmed by that imaging modality, it is recommended that CT myelography be used, especially if there is a question of foraminal compression.[2]

Electromyography (EMG) has also been used to clarify the diagnosis of cervical radiculopathy in confusing clinical scenarios.[3,6,8,9,13,20,21] It has been shown to be the most useful in demonstrating positive sharp wave potentials and fibrillation potentials that can be present in the corresponding myotome within 3 weeks.[6,9] EMG testing can be of particular value in trying to determine the culprit level when imaging shows multilevel findings. Studies have shown better clinical outcomes when EMG showed denervation preoperatively. Another study showed that MRI was more accurate and more sensitive than EMG.[22,23]

PHARMACOLOGIC TREATMENT

The visual analog scale has been validated as a means to measure pain objectively both at the initial examination and subsequent visits to measure the success of treatment.[2] Many other measures such as the modified Prolo, patient-specific functional scale, health status questionnaire, sickness impact profile, modified million index, McGill pain scores, and the modified Oswestry disability index can be used to access outcome measures.[2]

Several medications have been used in the treatment of cervical radiculopathy. Common medications used include steroids, antiinflammatories, antidepressants, muscle relaxers, neuropathic medications, Chinese herbal medicine, and opioids. Few good studies have been published regarding their use in cervical radiculopathy. The NASS guidelines goes as far as to say that no studies adequately address the role of pharmacologic treatment in the management of cervical radiculopathy from degenerative disease. There have been multiple Cochrane reviews on the use of these medications with back, neck, and neuropathic pain, which may be somewhat helpful in the treatment of cervical radiculopathy. **Table 3** lists a summary of the Cochrane reviews.

Prednisone has been considered an option for first-line therapy for radicular pain by most experts. The basis of its use come from studies that have shown that perineural inflammatory mediators are present at the site of herniated disks, and that their

Table 3 Cochrane reviews on pain medications		
Medication Class	**Review Context**	**Results**
Antidepressants	Neuropathic pain	TCAs (nortriptyline/amytriptyline) and venlafaxine (SNRI) have NNT around 3
Chinese herbal medicine	Chronic neck pain in degenerative disease	Low-quality evidence that Qishe reduces pain over placebo. Extractum nucis vomicae and Jingfukang reduced pain better than diclofenac
NSAIDs	Low back pain	Effective for short-term symptomatic relief in patients with acute and chronic pain without sciatica. COX-2 with lower side effects, but with possible cardiac side effects
Opioids	Neuropathic pain	Intermediate term (median = 28 d) significant efficacy over placebo. Risks because of addiction potential
Tramadol	Neuropathic pain	Significant reduction. NNT 3.8

Abbreviations: COX-2, cyclooxygenase-2; NNT, number needed to treat; NSAID, nonsteroidal antiinflammatory drug; SNRI, serotonin norepinephrine reuptake inhibitor; TCA, tricyclic antidepressant.
Data from Refs.[24–28]

presence may be the underlying cause of radicular pain.[29,30] A recent meta-analysis looked at the efficacy and tolerance of systemic steroids in sciatica and found that steroid efficacy was not greater than placebo. It was also noted that there was an adverse event rate of 13.3% with steroids and the number needed to harm was 20.[31] This does not address cervical radiculopathy specifically, and highlights the need for more research to answer the question about whether there is true benefit from oral systemic steroid use in cervical radiculopathy.

Gabapentin and pregabalin have also been studied and used in patients with radiculopathy. One study in particular looked at the use of pregabalin with cervical or lumbar radiculopathy in the primary care setting. They found that using it as monotherapy or as add-on therapy, patients had significant reduction of pain and disability compared with the group without it.[32] Other studies have also concluded that gabapentin provides significant decrease in pain and disability for either acute or chronic lumbar radiculopathy.[33,34]

The International Association for the Study of Pain released their evidence-based guidelines for pharmacologic management of neuropathic pain and listed tricyclic antidepressants, serotonin norepinephrine reuptake inhibitors, gabapentin, pregabalin, and topical lidocaine as first-line choices for neuropathic pain.[35] Opioid analgesics and tramadol were recommended as good second-line options, and in selected cases, first-line therapies. Examples of this would be acute neuropathic pain, neuropathic cancer pain, acute exacerbations, and during titration of other first-line choices.[35]

Muscle relaxants can also be used treat related neck pain caused by increased tension at muscle insertion sites in the setting of cervical radiculopathy.[36] There are no studies to address their use in this setting, but our experience is that they can be a helpful adjunct to therapy.

NONPHARMACOLOGIC TREATMENT

Several nonpharmacologic conservative measures have been used in the treatment of cervical radiculopathy, typically in addition to other therapies. Immobilization was recently looked at with a randomized controlled trial using a cervical collar started during the day of injury and continued for the first 3 weeks of symptoms. A significantly lower neck index disability score compared with controls, as well as a substantial reduction in arm and neck pain, were noted.[37] Our clinical experience also suggests that use of the collar at night improves sleep and reduces pain the following morning on awakening.

A review looking at exercise for neck pain found that there was low-quality evidence that supported neck strengthening in cervical radiculopathy for pain relief in the short term.[38] Traction is another modality that is commonly used in the treatment of cervical radiculopathy and its efficacy or effectiveness for neck pain with or without radiculopathy has not been proved.[39] Manipulation has been used and it has been concluded that, for neck pain, it can provide immediate or short-term change in pain and function.[40] Good randomized controlled studies are difficult to conduct and, in some circumstances, impossible. This is 1 of the limitations to providing definitive data regarding these modalities.

Transcutaneous electrical nerve stimulation (TENS) has also had mixed reviews. Studies have been inconsistent and conclusions regarding its use in acute pain have not been reached.[41] High-frequency TENS was shown to be more effective against uterine muscle spasm and in turn led to more effective reduction of pain than placebo for patients suffering from primary dysmenorrhea.[42] Future randomized studies should be performed looking at the use of TENS in muscle spasm reduction, which may in turn relieve the pain with cervical radiculopathy through a mechanism similar to that achieved with muscle relaxers. There is an ongoing Cochrane review in progress looking at the use of TENS for neuropathic pain.

INTERVENTIONAL TREATMENT

Translaminar and transforaminal epidural injections of corticosteroids under fluoroscopic guidance have shown favorable results.[9] A best evidence synthesis of more than 1200 studies found that there was short-term symptomatic improvement of radicular symptoms.[43] The NASS guidelines suggest that the use of transforaminal epidural steroid injections may be considered, but that they do not make recommendations regarding the safety and efficacy of translaminar steroid injections.[2] There are risks with any procedure, but in the cervical spine, some of the complications can be devastating; brainstem or spinal cord sequelae should be considered. Complication rates have varied between 0% and 16.8%.[44] There have been no definitive evidence-based recommendations on when these injections should be administered in the course of the disease process, how many a patient should receive, which corticosteroid, and how much to administer.

It has been suggested that surgery should be considered in patients unresponsive to conservative management for more than 6 weeks, neurologic deficits persisting for greater than 6 weeks, neurologic decline after the onset of signs or symptoms at any point, myelopathy, or instability.[45] Surgical intervention has been recommended for rapid relief of symptoms.[2,43] A Cochrane review cited 2 eligible small trials that did not provide reliable evidence because that were believed to have significant risk of bias. The conclusion was that there was low-quality evidence that surgery may provide pain and subjective improvement in the short term, but no difference in the long term for radiculopathy and mild myelopathy.[46] However, the NASS guidelines suggest that there may be benefit with a single-level repair, with favorable outcomes greater than 4 years in degenerative cervical radiculopathy.[2] As with cervical injections, the risks of surgery should be considered when discussing these treatment options with patients.

EVALUATION OF OUTCOME AND LONG-TERM RECOMMENDATIONS

Initial strategies in the treatment of cervical radiculopathy are typically conservative. Because little is known regarding the natural history and specific treatment outcomes, initial treatments are focused on decreasing radicular pain. Some smaller studies have shown up to 92% success with nonsurgical treatment.[47] Most have advocated for initial conservative therapy.[3,6,8,9,13,20,21] Long-term goals focus on returning to normal motion, flexibility, strength, neurologic function, and prevention of recurrences. The desired goal is to return the patient to their predisease function.

There seems to be a role for cervical steroid injections. Surgery has more defined indications for when it should be considered.

Although no studies have addressed a multimodal approach to the treatment of cervical radiculopathy, this is usually a practical approach that takes into account the patient's history, examination, and personal preferences.

SUMMARY

Treatment option for cervical radiculopathy continue to evolve as it becomes better defined and gaps in the literature are identified. A thorough history and physical examination are usually adequate to make the diagnosis. When the diagnosis is in question, or when invasive treatment is anticipated, imaging should be performed. Cervical spine MRI is the study of choice unless there is a contraindication. CT, or in some cases, CT myelography, can be used as alternatives. Conservative therapies, including multiple pharmacologic agents, immobilization, physical therapy, manipulation, traction, and TENS, have all been used in the treatment of cervical radiculopathy with variable success. Cervical steroid injections have been shown to be beneficial. Surgical treatment is indicated in myelopathy or recalcitrant cases. Most cases of cervical radiculopathy respond well to initial conservative measures using a multimodal approach.

REFERENCES

1. Radhakrishnan K, Litchy W, O'Fallon M, et al. Epidemiology of cervical radiculopathy: a population-based study from Rochester, Minnesota, 1976 through 1990. Brain 1994;117:325–35.
2. North American Spine Society. Evidence-based clinical guidelines for multidisciplinary spine care. Diagnosis and treatment of cervical radiculopathy from degenerative disease. 2010. Available at: www.spine.org. Accessed July 10, 2013.
3. Eubanks J. Cervical radiculopathy: nonoperative management of neck pain and radicular symptoms. Am Fam Physician 2010;81(1):33–40.
4. Price D, McGrath P, Rafii A, et al. The validation of visual analogue scales as ratio scale measures for chronic and experimental pain. Pain 1983;17:45–56.
5. Bogduk N. The anatomy and pathophysiology of neck pain. Phys Med Rehabil Clin N Am 2003;14:455–72.

6. Roth D, Mukai A, Thomas P, et al. Cervical radiculopathy. Dis Mon 2009;55: 737–56.
7. Don't be scammed by a drug user. The US Department of Justice Drug Enforcement Administration, Office of Diversion Control 1999;1(1). Available at: http://www. deadiversion.usdoj.gov/pubs/brochures/drugabuser.htm#recognize. Accessed February 17, 2013.
8. Polston D. Cervical radiculopathy. Neurol Clin 2007;25:373–85.
9. Carette S, Phil M, Fehlings M. Cervical radiculopathy. N Engl J Med 2005;353: 392–9.
10. Tong H, Haig A, Yamakawa K. The spurling test and cervical radiculopathy. Spine 2002;27:156–9.
11. Rubinstein S, Pool J, van Tulder M, et al. A systematic review of the diagnostic accuracy of provocative tests of the neck for diagnosing cervical radiculopathy. Eur Spine J 2007;16:307–19.
12. Kleinrensink G, Stoeckart R, Mulder P, et al. Upper limb tension tests as tools in the diagnosis of nerve and plexus lesions: anatomical and biomechanical aspects. Clin Biomech 2000;15:9–14.
13. Cohen I, Jouve C. Cervical radiculopathy. In: Frontera W, Silver J, Rizzo T, editors. Essentials of physical medicine and rehabilitation. 2nd edition. Philadelphia: Saunders Elsevier; 2008. p. 17–22.
14. Ruggieri P. Cervical radiculopathy. Neuroimaging Clin N Am 1995;5(3):349–66.
15. Irvine D, Foster J, Newell D, et al. Prevalence of cervical spondylosis in a general practice. Lancet 1965;285(7395):1089–92.
16. Triantafillou K, Laurman W, Kalantar S. Degenerative disease of the cervical spine and its relationship to athletes. Clin Sports Med 2012;31:509–20.
17. Weir D, Jackson J, Sonnega A. University of Michigan Institute for Social Research, National Football League Player Care Foundation study of retired NFL players. Available at: http://www.ns.umich.edu/Releases/2009/Sep09/FinalReport.pdf. Accessed February 12, 2013.
18. Mink J, Gordon R, Deutsch A. The cervical spine: radiologists perspective. Phys Med Rehabil Clin N Am 2003;14:493–548.
19. Jensen M, Brant-Zawadzki M, Obuchowski N, et al. Magnetic resonance imaging of the lumbar spine in people without back pain. N Engl J Med 1994;331(2):69–73.
20. Malanga G. The diagnosis and treatment of cervical radiculopathy. Med Sci Sports Exerc 1997;29(7):236–45.
21. Wainner R, Gill H. Diagnosis and nonoperative management of cervical radiculopathy. J Orthop Sports Phys Ther 2000;30(12):728–44.
22. Alrawi M, Khalil N, Mitchell P, et al. The value of neurophysiological and imaging studies in predicting outcomes in the surgical treatment of cervical radiculopathy. Eur Spine J 2007;16(4):495–500.
23. Ashkan K, Johnston P, Moore A, et al. A comparison of magnetic resonance imaging neurophysiological studies in the assessment of cervical radiculopathy. Br J Neurosurg 2002;16(2):146–8.
24. Saarto T, Wiffen P. Antidepressants for neuropathic pain. Cochrane Database Syst Rev 2007;(4):CD005454. http://dx.doi.org/10.1002/14651858.CD005454.pub2.
25. Cui X, Trinh K, Wang Y. Chinese herbal medicine for chronic neck pain due to cervical degenerative disc disease. Cochrane Database Syst Rev 2010;(1):CD006556. http://dx.doi.org/10.1002/14651858.CD006556.pub2.
26. Roelofs P, Deyo R, Koes B, et al. Non-steroidal anti-inflammatory drugs for low back pain. Cochrane Database Syst Rev 2008;(1):CD000396. http://dx.doi.org/10.1002/14651858.CD000396.pub3.

27. Eisenberg E, McNicol E, Carr D. Opioids for neuropathic pain. Cochrane Database Syst Rev 2006;(3):CD006146. http://dx.doi.org/10.1002/14651858.CD006146.
28. Duehmke R, Hollingshead J, Cornblath D. Tramadol for neuropathic pain. Cochrane Database Syst Rev 2006;(3):CD003726. http://dx.doi.org/10.1002/14651858.CD003726.pub3.
29. Kang J, Georgescu H, McIntyre-Larkin L, et al. Herniated lumbar intervertebral discs spontaneously produce matrix metalloproteinases, nitric oxide, interleukin-6, and prostaglandin E_2. Spine 1996;21(3):271–7.
30. Saal J. The role of inflammation in lumbar pain. Spine 1995;20(16):1821–7.
31. Roncoroni C, Baillet A, Durand M, et al. Efficacy and tolerance of systemic steroids in sciatica: a systematic review and meta analysis. Rheumatology 2011;50(9):1603–11.
32. Saldana M, Navarro A, Perez C, et al. Patient reported outcomes in subjects with painful lumbar or cervical radiculopathy treated with pregabalin: evidence from medical practice in primary care settings. Rheumatol Int 2010;30:1005–15.
33. Yildirim K, Deniz O, Gureser G, et al. Gabapentin monotherapy in patients with chronic radiculopathy: the efficacy and impact on quality of life. J Back Musculoskeletal Rehabil 2009;22:17–20.
34. Kasimcan O, Kaptan H. Efficacy of gabapentin for radiculopathy caused by lumbar spinal stenosis and lumbar disc hernia. Neurol Med Chir (Tokyo) 2010; 50:1070–3.
35. Dworkin R, O'Conner A, Backonja M, et al. Pharmacologic management of neuropathic pain: evidence –based recommendations. Pain 2007;132: 237–51.
36. Levine M, Albert T, Smith M. Cervical radiculopathy: diagnosis and nonoperative management. J Am Acad Orthop Surg 1996;4:305–16.
37. Kuijper B, Tans J, Beelen A, et al. Cervical collar or physiotherapy versus wait and see policy for recent onset cervical radiculopathy: randomized trial. BMJ 2009; 339:b3883.
38. Kay T, Gross A, Goldsmith C, et al. Exercises for mechanical neck disorders. Cochrane Database Syst Rev 2012;(8):CD004250. http://dx.doi.org/10.1002/14651858.CD004250.pub4.
39. Graham N, Gross A, Goldsmith C, et al. Mechanical traction for neck pain with or without radiculopathy. Cochrane Database Syst Rev 2008;(3):CD006408. http://dx.doi.org/10.1002/14651858.CD006408.pub2.
40. Gross A, Miller J, D'Sylva J, et al. Manipulation or mobilisation for neck pain. Cochrane Database Syst Rev 2010;(1):CD004249. http://dx.doi.org/10.1002/14651858.CD004249.pub3.
41. Walsh D, Howe T, Johnson M, et al. Transcutaneous electrical nerve stimulation for acute pain. Cochrane Database Syst Rev 2009;(2):CD006142.
42. Proctor M, Farquhar C, Stones W, et al. Transcutaneous electrical nerve stimulation for primary dysmenorrhea. Cochrane Database Syst Rev 2002;(1):CD002123.
43. Carragee E, Hurwitz E, Cheng I, et al. Treatment of neck pain: injections and surgical interventions: results of the Bone and Joint Decade 2000-2010 Task Force on Neck Pain and Its Associated Disorders. Spine 2008;33(Suppl 4): S153–69.
44. Abbasi A, Malhotra G, Malanga G, et al. Complications of interlaminar cervical epidural steroid injections. Spine 2007;32:2144–51.
45. Albert T, Murrell S. Surgical management of cervical radiculopathy. J Am Acad Orthop Surg 1999;7(6):368–76.

46. Nikolaidis I, Fouyas I, Sandercock P, et al. Surgery for cervical radiculopathy or myelopathy. Cochrane Database Syst Rev 2010;(1):CD001466. http://dx.doi.org/10.1002/14651858.CD001466.pub3.
47. Saal JS, Saal JA, Yurth E. Nonoperative management of herniated cervical intervertebral disc with radiculopathy. Spine 1996;21(16):1877–83.

Choosing the Right Diagnostic Imaging Modality in Musculoskeletal Diagnosis

Andrea L. Aagesen, DO, MS[a],*, Maged Melek, MD, MBCH[b]

KEYWORDS

- Diagnostic imaging • Radiology • Radiographs • Magnetic resonance imaging
- Computed tomography • Arthrogram

KEY POINTS

- Routine radiographs are the first imaging modality of nearly all musculoskeletal disorders.
- Magnetic resonance imaging (MRI) is highly sensitive to fractures and soft tissue injuries.
- Computed tomography is superior to MRI for fracture characterization, particularly involving bones of the hand or the hook of the hamate in the wrist.
- Magnetic resonance arthrogram is recommended for intra-articular disorders such as an injury to the triangular fibrocartilage complex in the wrist, the glenoid labrum in the shoulder, or the acetabular labrum of the hip.

INTRODUCTION

Nature of the Problem

Musculoskeletal injuries and pain are a common presenting complaint among patients in primary care and sport medicine offices. Obtaining a detailed history and physical examination is paramount for establishing an accurate diagnosis. Imaging is an important tool to confirm a diagnosis or rule out a competing diagnosis when the history and physical examination are unable to reliably establish the diagnosis. Selecting the most appropriate imaging test is essential to minimize patient risk, expedite diagnosis and treatment of the patient, and limit health care cost.

Definition

Radiological studies each vary in sensitivity and specificity in identifying abnormalities in different structures. Imaging protocols must take into account the specific clinical

Disclosures: There are no financial disclosures or conflicts of interest for either author.
[a] Department of Physical Medicine and Rehabilitation, University of Michigan Health Systems, 325 East Eisenhower Parkway, Ann Arbor, MI 48108, USA; [b] Department of Family Medicine, Mount Sinai Hospital, 1500th South California Avenue, Chicago, IL 60608, USA
* Corresponding author.
E-mail address: aquandt@med.umich.edu

Prim Care Clin Office Pract 40 (2013) 849–861
http://dx.doi.org/10.1016/j.pop.2013.08.005
0095-4543/13/$ – see front matter © 2013 Elsevier Inc. All rights reserved.

scenario, patient risk and contraindications, and the associated cost of each imaging modality.

Symptom Criteria

Obtaining a careful history and physical examination is necessary to establish the pre-test probability of each competing diagnosis for the musculoskeletal disorder. Accurately choosing the preferred radiological study depends on identifying the affected joint(s) and/or surrounding tissue. In addition, it requires an astute clinician to determine whether the abnormalities identified on the radiological studies are related to the patient's symptoms or whether they are incidental findings unrelated to the patients symptoms.

CLINICAL FINDINGS
History

Imaging algorithms depend on patient age, detailed history, and key physical examination findings to establish the pretest probability for a particular musculoskeletal injury. Key points of the history include the quality and specific location of the pain, onset of pain, related trauma, mechanical symptoms, exacerbating and alleviating factors, pain with weight bearing, instability, and pain while sleeping.

Physical Examination

Physical examination is particularly useful for localizing a patient's pain to a specific joint and the musculoskeletal structure(s) that are involved. Important physical examination findings that support intra-articular disorders include joint swelling (effusion), locking, catching, deformity, and limited or painful range of motion. Instability or laxity suggests ligamentous or capsular injury.[1]

IMAGING
Routine Radiographs

Routine radiographs should almost always be performed as the initial imaging modality for musculoskeletal injuries. Although the densities of calcium, soft tissues, fat, and air can be discerned with radiographs, the resolution of osseous anatomy is superior to that of soft tissues. Radiographs often yield a diagnosis or aid in appropriate selection and interpretation of advanced imaging, particularly with magnetic resonance imaging (MRI). A minimum of 2 radiography projections taken at right angles to each other of the body part of interest are necessary for evaluation. A 3-view radiographic evaluation is recommended for distal extremities in the setting of trauma, because prior studies have shown that up to 6.7% of fractures are only detected on the oblique view and would otherwise have been missed.[2] Certain joints require specific views to depict abnormalities on radiographs (discussed later). In addition, fluoroscopic positioned spot views can be used to avoid bony overlap in certain cases. The sensitivity of routine radiographs varies depending on the mineralization of the bone involved, the specific disorders, and the chronicity of the disorders.[3] The indications, relative cost, and relative radiation exposure of routine radiographs are summarized in **Table 1**.[3]

Computed Tomography

Computed tomography (CT) uses a rotating x-ray source that is reformatted to a cross-sectional image using a computer processor. CT is superior to routine radiographs for evaluating the complex structures of the axial skeleton, the osseous structures of the

Table 1 Summary of routine radiography	
Indications	Bone injury (fracture, degenerative changes)
Cost ($)	50–300[a]
Risks/contraindications	Mild radiation exposure[b]

[a] Cost varies among hospitals and depending on the specific studies performed.
[b] Radiation exposure depends on the specific projections performed.

foot, ankle, pelvis, shoulder, wrist, and hand.[3] CT is superior to radiography in showing subtle cortical bone injury. Specific CT reformatting techniques are often performed for surgical planning, which is beyond the scope of this article but should be considered when selecting between MRI and CT.[3,4] The indications, relative cost, and relative radiation exposure of CT are summarized in **Table 2**.[3,4]

MRI

MRI uses a fixed or superconducting magnet that creates a strong magnetic field. This magnetic field causes the protons of hydrogen nuclei to have a similar alignment, which are then excited by a radiofrequency pulse. The absorbed energy is released as an electromagnetic wave that is detected by a receiving coil, processed, and an image is produced. The field strength of the magnet is directly related to image resolution obtained. The field strength is typically between 1.5 T and 3 T, but may be lower in an open MRI scanner. MRI is optimal to evaluate soft tissue, occult fractures, articular cartilage, masses, marrow abnormalities, synovitis, and infectious processes. MRI is the most sensitive modality for detecting fractures and is recommended if there is clinical suspicion for fracture and radiographs are negative.[4] The indications, relative cost, and contraindications of MRI are summarized in **Table 3**.[4]

Ultrasound

Ultrasound uses high-frequency sound waves directed into musculoskeletal structures. Each tissue comprising the musculoskeletal system varies in density and its ability to transmit and reflect sound waves. The reflected sound waves are converted into an image. Similar to MRI, the image quality depends on the frequency and type of the transducer. In addition, clinical expertise with ultrasound varies and can affect the sensitivity and specificity of ultrasound for evaluation of various injuries. Ultrasound may be used to evaluate masses in soft tissues, vasculature, ligaments, tendons, bone, cartilage,

Table 2 Summary of CT	
Indications	Fracture, cortical bone injury
Cost ($)	100–200[a]
Risks	Moderate radiation exposure[b]
Contraindications	No absolute contraindications. CT of the lumbar spine, abdomen, and pelvis of the pregnant woman should be avoided when possible

[a] Cost varies among hospitals and depends on the specific studies performed.
[b] Helical CT or CT angiogram produces significantly higher radiation exposure.

Table 3 Summary of MRI	
Indications	Soft tissue mass, vascular disease, ligament/tendon injuries, fracture, osteonecrosis, articular disorders, abnormal cartilage, effusion, foreign bodies, guidance for injection
Cost ($)	500–4000[a]
Risks	No radiation exposure to patient
Contraindications[b]	Cardiac pacemaker, cochlear implants, some prosthetic heart valves, bone growth or neurostimulators (TENS), brain aneurysm clips or coils, periorbital metal fragments, some penile prosthesis, older cardiac stents

Abbreviation: TENS, transcutaneous electrical nerve stimulation.
[a] Cost varies widely among hospitals and depends on specific study performed.
[b] Newer implantable devices may be magnetic resonance compatible. Manufacture's recommendations should be consulted on an individual basis.

effusions, and foreign bodies.[3] The indications and relative cost of ultrasound are summarized in **Table 4.**[3]

Bone Scan (Scintigraphy)

Bone scans detect changes in the skeleton's level of bone formation by using an intravenously administered radiopharmaceutical that binds to the hydroxyapatite crystals in the bone matrix proportionately to local blood flow and osteoblastic activity, thus highlighting areas of increased bone turnover and bone perfusion. Therefore, bone scans can detect abnormalities in bone, such as fractures, stress fractures, osteomyelitis, and osteoblastic metastases, before anatomic changes can be detected on radiograph. In addition, bone scans have a higher sensitivity for stress reactions than CT.[5] Although bone scans are highly sensitive for any bone injury that results in bone formation, the specificity is limited. Single-photon emission CT (SPECT) is used in conjunction with planar bone imaging based on the clinical indication or radionuclide uptake pattern to provide a three-dimensional image and improve specificity and sensitivity. Bone scan with SPECT can increase the sensitivity for detecting vertebral bone lesions and distinguish between aggressive and nonaggressive lesions.[5] In addition to osseous disorders, a 3-phase bone scan can detect abnormal sympathetic activity in an extremity, which is often associated with complex regional pain syndrome. A characteristic finding on the planar 3-phase bone scan is diffuse generalized increased uptake of bone agent throughout all the bones of 1 extremity in all 3 phases, which is caused by increased generalized blood flow.[5] The indications, relative cost, and radiation exposure of bone scans are summarized in **Table 5.**[5]

Table 4 Summary of musculoskeletal ultrasound	
Indications	Soft tissue mass, vascular disease, ligament/tendon injuries, bone (fracture, osteoporosis), articular disorders, cartilage, effusion, foreign bodies, guidance for injection
Cost ($)	100–300[a]
Risks/contraindications	None

[a] Cost varies among hospitals and depends on the specific study performed.

Table 5
Summary of bone scintigraphy (bone scan)

Indications	Stress fracture, differentiation of osteomyelitis from cellulitis, avascular necrosis or bone infarction, reflex sympathetic dystrophy, peripheral vascular disease, subtle lumbar lesions such as pars defect[a]
Cost ($)	150–650[b]
Risks/contraindications	Minimal radiation exposure to patient, rare allergic reaction to radiopharmaceutical used

[a] Bone scintigraphy with SPECT is recommended to evaluate for pars defect.
[b] Cost varies among hospitals and specific study performed.

DISORDERS
Shoulder Imaging

The complex anatomy of the shoulder joint makes choosing diagnostic imaging tests challenging. The history of trauma, age of the patient, and specific location of pain are among the most important factors for developing a differential diagnosis and selecting the most appropriate imaging studies. In most cases, routine radiographs are an appropriate initial study. Depending on the nature of the trauma and location of pain, specific radiograph views may be necessary for thorough evaluation (**Table 6**). In the

Table 6
Summary of radiographic shoulder views

View	Indication(s)	Specific Structure(s) Evaluated
Standard AP in ER	Trauma	Greater tuberosity of humerus
Standard AP in IR	Trauma	Lesser tuberosity of humerus
Grashey (true AP)	Limited ROM Instability	Joint congruity Joint space narrowing Humeral head subluxation
Axillary	Dislocation	Dislocation Anterior/posterior glenoid rim (Bankart fracture)
West point axillary	Dislocation	Anteroinferior glenoid rim (Bankart fracture)
Garth view	Dislocation	Inferior glenoid rim (Bankart fracture) Posterior margin of superolateral humeral head (Hill-Sachs deformity)
Stryker notch	Dislocation	Posterolateral humeral head (Hill-Sachs deformity)
Scapular Y view	Dislocations Trauma	Evaluate supraspinatus outlet Dislocation Scapular fracture Assess for dislocation
Supraspinatus outlet	Impingement Limited ROM	Acromion Humeral head subluxation
Zanca view	Trauma	Acromioclavicular joint
Rockwood view	Impingement	Acromion

Routine shoulder series typically includes AP (in neutral, IR, and/or ER), Grashey, axillary, scapular Y. Routine shoulder series may vary slightly by imaging center or institution.[4]
Abbreviations: AP, anteroposterior; ER, external rotation; IR, internal rotation; ROM, range of motion.
Data from Manaster BJ, Roberts CC, Andrews CL, et al. Diagnostic and surgical imaging anatomy: musculoskeletal. Salt Lake City: Amirsys; 2006.

absence of trauma, deformity, or abnormal range of motion, routine radiographs rarely identify clinically significant abnormalities.[6,7]

Ultrasound and MRI have equivalent sensitivity for rotator cuff disorders and dislocations. Selecting between magnetic resonance (MR) and ultrasound for advanced imaging is based on the specific clinical scenario. Ultrasound is less costly, is better tolerated by patients, and is a dynamic examination that can confirm subluxation of the biceps tendon or subacromial impingement. A labral or osseous injury is better detected with an MR arthrogram and MRI, respectively.[8] Specific MR sequences improve the sensitivity of detecting disorders. For example, the long echo time (TE) sequence and fat-suppressed T2-weighted sequence show increased signal in the rotator cuff tendon in the presence of injury. T1-weighted sequences are similarly used to assess marrow signal related to fracture or bone contusion.[4] CT can be used to characterize fractures and for surgical planning. MR arthrogram is the gold standard for evaluation of the glenoid labrum. CT arthrogram is a good alternative to evaluate labral injury in individuals who cannot undergo MRI.[4] Specific indications for each imaging modality are listed in **Table 7**.[4]

Hand and Wrist Imaging

Imaging of acute and chronic hand and wrist pain should begin with routine radiographs. Radiographs with only 2 projections are inadequate for evaluation in most

Table 7
Summary of indications for common imaging modalities

Imaging Modality	Shoulder Structures/Disorders Detected
Routine radiographs	Dislocations (acromioclavicular and glenohumeral) Fractures (proximal humerus, clavicle, and scapula) Osseous finding associated with rotator cuff disorders Glenohumeral osteoarthritis Acromioclavicular joint arthritis Sternoclavicular joint arthritis
Musculoskeletal ultrasound	Joint effusion Rotator cuff injury (tendinopathy, tear) Biceps tendon injury (dislocation/subluxation, tendinopathy, tear) Muscle atrophy/denervation
MRI	Rotator cuff injury (tendinopathy, tear) Avascular necrosis Biceps tendon injury (tendinopathy/tear) Inflammatory processes Tumors Muscle atrophy/denervation Fracture
CT	Characterize fractures/evaluate bone contours Dislocations Assess for bone tumor Characterize glenoid and humeral head anatomy Soft tissue calcifications
MR arthrography	Labral injury (gold standard for diagnosis) Glenohumeral ligament injuries
CT arthrography	Anterior and posterior labrum Joint capsule

cases. A 3-view radiograph consisting of a posteroanterior, lateral, and oblique view is recommended for wrist and hand trauma, particularly if the joint is involved. Some trauma protocols include a fourth projection that is a posteroanterior view, with the wrist in ulnar deviation. Specialized views may be indicated for certain clinical scenarios. A scaphoid view should be added to the 3-view wrist radiograph to improve sensitivity for a scaphoid fracture. The hook of the hamate is best visualized with the addition of a carpal tunnel view.[9]

Imaging the wrist with high-resolution MR may be indicated when there is clinical concern for a radiographically occult carpal fracture, soft tissue injury, mass, bone marrow abnormalities, synovitis, or an infectious process.[3,4,10] Radiological studies have found that approximately half of symptomatic wrists imaged with MR detected abnormalities that have resulted in a change in working diagnosis, and 46% showed findings that resulted in a change in management.[11] However, when evaluating for a suspected hook of the hamate fracture, CT is recommended if radiographs are negative. Injuries involving the transcarpal ligaments, triangular fibrocartilage complex (TFCC), and/or articular cartilage are best detected with MR arthrography. The sensitivity of MR arthrography is less than that of direct visualization with arthroscopy, so, in cases when the injury is amenable to arthroscopic treatment, advanced imaging may not be indicated.[4,10–12]

In the presence of trauma, tenderness directly over the scaphoid (the anatomic snuffbox) necessitates imaging to evaluate for a scaphoid fracture. Routine radiographs are often insensitive for nondisplaced scaphoid fractures until osteoblastic activity can result in radiographic change, around 10 to 14 days following injury.[10] Initial imaging with routine wrist radiographs should include a scaphoid view. Wrist immobilization and follow-up radiographs are recommended after 2 weeks if clinical concern for fracture remains. If immediate diagnosis is necessary, an MRI may be performed directly after initial radiographs are negative to confirm or exclude a scaphoid fracture. The false-negative rate of scaphoid fracture on follow-up radiograph is as high as 9%.[13] The pooled sensitivity for scaphoid fracture is similar that for MRI (96%), CT (93%) and bone scan (97%), whereas the specificity is inferior for bone scan (89%) compared with MRI (99%) and CT (99%).[14] If clinical suspicion remains high for scaphoid fracture despite negative radiographs, MRI is recommended to confirm or exclude fracture.[15]

Hip and Pelvis Imaging

The complexity of the hip and pelvic anatomy, as well as radicular symptoms potentially originating from spinal disorders, can make diagnosing hip and pelvic pain challenging. Imaging can be useful for establishing the diagnosis. Clinical correlation is important to determine whether the imaging abnormalities detected are related to the patient's pain.

Routine radiographs are the initial imaging study to evaluate nearly all acute and chronic hip and/or pelvic disorders. An anteroposterior (AP) view of the pelvis should include both hips to detect asymmetry. A lateral view detects osseous abnormalities of the femoral head and neck. MRI is highly sensitive and specific for osseous and articular hip injuries, as well as soft tissues injuries of the hip and pelvis, and is the recommended imaging modality in most cases after a radiograph is negative.[4,13,15] Exceptions include evaluation for labral injury, osteoid osteoma, and snapping hip syndrome, which are best detected on MR arthrogram, CT, and ultrasound, respectively.[13,15] Radiographs are insensitive for nondisplaced femoral neck fractures, particularly in an osteoporotic patient. If there is a history of fall, clinical concern for insufficiency fractures, or recent trauma in a patient with hip pain, MRI is recommended before allowing the patient to bear weight on the affected leg.

MR arthrogram involves undergoing an intra-articular hip injection of gadolinium before performing MRI, which improves the sensitivity for labral injury up to 90%.[13] Diagnostic and therapeutic joint injections can be performed at the time of an MR arthrogram to provide clinical information regarding the patient's pain generator. If the detected abnormalities on MR are the source of pain, the patient should experience pain relief following the injection.

Ultrasound is the recommended imaging modality for evaluating snapping hip syndrome, because both static and dynamic imaging can be obtained. CT may be performed to better characterize osseous abnormalities such as osteoid osteoma, and may be used in preoperative planning.[13,14]

Knee Imaging

Radiographs of the knee are commonly performed for evaluation of traumatic and atraumatic knee pain, but are often negative. To decrease the number of unnecessary radiographs, numerous criteria guidelines have been created with the objective of guiding appropriate use of radiographs for acute knee injury. The most widely cited criteria are the Ottawa Knee Rules (**Box 1**).[16–18] Numerous validation studies have found that these guidelines are 100% sensitive for detecting knee fractures and decrease the radiograph rate by 28% to 35%, depending on the specific study.[14,16,17,19] Radiography is not sensitive for meniscal or ligamentous injury. Physical examination is important to establish the pretest probability for internal derangement (disruption of the meniscus, ligaments, and/or osteochondral injury). When clinical suspicion is high for meniscal or ligamentous injury, MRI is the best modality to detect such injuries. Imaging should be performed judiciously, because asymptomatic abnormalities, particularly to the meniscus, are frequently detected on MRI.[20]

Radiographic criteria for detecting osteoarthritis were established in the 1950s and include osteophytes, sclerosis, joint space narrowing, and subchondral cystic bone.[21] Current practice relies more on joint space narrowing, which is more sensitive with a weight-bearing AP view or a weight-bearing AP view with flexion. MRI is a more sensitive modality for early osteoarthritic changes. The usefulness of imaging for detection of osteoarthritis is not clear because the severity of joint degeneration on imaging infrequently correlates with pain.[22]

Foot and Ankle Imaging

In the setting of acute trauma to the foot or ankle, 3-view radiographs should be performed if the patient experiences tenderness over the navicular, base of the fifth metatarsal, medial or lateral malleolus (see **Box 1**), or if the patient does not meet the

---

Box 1
Ottawa Knee Rules for radiography in the setting of acute knee injury

Age greater than or equal to 55 years

Palpable tenderness over head of fibula

Isolated patellar tenderness

Unable to flex knee to 90°

Unable to bear weight immediately and in emergency department (4 steps)

Radiographic examination is recommended for acute knee injuries in patients with 1 or more of these criteria.

inclusion criteria for the Ottawa Rules.[15,23] These rules have been validated for adults and children and have a sensitivity of 99%.[15] However, the exclusion criteria of cases in which the Ottawa Rules should not be applied are extensive and include penetrating trauma, skin wound, polytrauma, neurologic abnormality involving the foot, pregnancy, underlying bone disease, return visit, or presenting with radiographs more than 10 days old.[23] An acute forefoot injury concerning for a Lisfranc injury should always be imaged. Three-view radiographs may be performed as the initial imaging and should include a weight-bearing AP view. Advanced imaging is often necessary even if radiographs are normal when clinical suspicion is high for this injury. MR can detect a ligamentous injury as well as a fracture. If a fracture is identified, CT is often used by orthopedic surgeons to characterize fractures for preoperative planning. Ligamentous injuries to the ankle are common and do not necessitate imaging in most cases.

In the setting of chronic ankle or foot pain, radiographs are typically the appropriate initial study. Routine radiographs of the foot should always include AP and lateral views. Oblique and occasionally specialized views are indicated depending on the clinical presentation. Advanced imaging is often recommended if radiographs are not diagnostic. Selection of MR, CT, bone scan, or ultrasound depends on the specific clinical presentation.

Routine radiographs of the ankle should include AP, lateral, and ankle mortise views. Osteochondral injuries are often not detected on routine radiographs and further imaging with MRI, MR arthrogram, or SPECT/CT may be indicated if clinical suspicion is high.[22] When chronic foot or ankle pain cannot be localized to a particularly structure on examination, MR is usually the recommended modality because it can detect soft tissues as well as osseous abnormalities. Ultrasound is particularly useful for evaluating pain occurring only with particular positions because it allows a dynamic evaluation **Box 2**.[24]

Spine Imaging

Traumatic cervical spine injures

The NEXUS (National Emergency X-Radiography Utilization Study) criteria (midline neck pain or tenderness, neurologic findings, altered mental status, intoxication, and/or distracting injury) have been established and validated to guide selection of patients who require cervical spine imaging for vertebral bone blunt cervical trauma injury with 99% sensitivity and a negative predicted value of 99.8%.[25] Performance of a multidetector-

---

Box 2
Indications for radiography in the setting of acute foot or ankle injury[a]

Navicular tenderness

Tenderness over base of fifth metatarsal

Tenderness over medial or lateral malleolus

Inability to bear weight

Presence of neuropathy affecting feet

Clinical suspicion for Lisfranc injury[b]

[a] Based on Ottawa Rules and exclusion criteria.
[b] MRI is also an appropriate initial imaging study to detect Lisfranc ligamentous injury and should always follow up a normal radiograph if clinical suspicion is high. CT may be required to characterize fractures detected on radiograph or MRI.

row CT (MDCT) has replaced routine cervical radiographs in patients with a suspicion for cervical spine injury because it can be performed more rapidly and has an increased sensitivity. Recent studies have found that radiographs detect only 36% of cervical spine injuries identified on CT in patients who meet one or more of the NEXUS criteria.[26] Thin-slice, reformatted CT imaging is often necessary, even in the presence of a cervical injury detected by radiography, for complete evaluation of the cervical spine for traumatic injuries, including evaluation for subtle injuries, spinal canal compromise, and fragment positioning. When a burst fracture is identified with radiography, a total spine CT should be performed to assess whether fracture fragments compromise the spinal canal and to evaluate for additional injures.[3] Nonosseous structures such as the spinal cord, nerve roots, and soft tissue are not well visualized on CT and often require MRI for thorough evaluation, if clinically indicated. In addition, MRI may identify posterior ligament injuries on the T2-weighted images that were not detected on CT or radiographs.[3] Ligamentous injuries can be detected with flexion/extension radiograph views of the cervical spine, but with a lower sensitivity than MRI. In addition, in the acute setting, there may be significant cervical muscle splinting resulting in a false-negative test. Flexion/extension films should only be obtained after a comprehensive neurologic examination has been completed to exclude any spinal cord or plexus injury.[15]

Traumatic thoracolumbar spine injuries
Although validated criteria have not been established for imaging of the thoracolumbar spine, criteria similar to the NEXUS criteria have been recommended.[15] As with evaluating the cervical spine, MDCT has replaced conventional radiography for evaluation of osseous disorders of the thoracolumbar spine resulting from a trauma because of its superior sensitivity compared with radiographs.[15] In addition, identification of one spinal fracture increases the likelihood of a subsequent spinal fracture and may justify the need for a total spine CT.[3] When a thoracic spine fracture is identified on radiograph, fragment position and spinal canal compromise may require further evaluation with CT.[3,27] MRI is recommended when there is any clinical concern for injury to the spinal cord, nerve roots, and/or soft tissue, which are not well visualized on CT.[3,15]

Spondylolysis and spondylolisthesis
Radiographs are routinely the initial imaging study performed to evaluate a young athlete with low back pain with clinical concern for spondylolysis. Lateral views detect subluxation (spondylolisthesis), which may occur in the presence of a bilateral pars interarticularis defect. AP and oblique views may identify a pars defect (spondylolysis), but with limited sensitivity. Oblique views are slightly more sensitive than AP views but increase the patient's exposure to radiation and are no longer routine in protocols at many institutes. Bone scintigraphy with SPECT is a highly sensitive imaging test for early spondylolysis and is often recommended when radiographs are normal, particularly in elite athletes.[15,28,29] This test shows increased uptake in a pars defect, which is associated with bone healing. This test does not differentiate between a stress reaction or an overt fracture, which results in a high false-positive rate for diagnosing a pars fracture. A pars defect detected on radiographs that is acute is indistinguishable from one that has healed with a fibrous union.[15] Bone scintigraphy with SPECT is important for differentiating these cases and is positive in the former and negative in the latter. A limited CT (reverse gantry axial plane at the area of increased uptake on the bone scintigraphy) is also commonly performed to characterize the extent of fragmentation, neuroforaminal patency, and the extent of healing when the bone scan is positive.[27] When subluxation is identified, flexion and extension radiographs should be performed to assess stability. If there is a clinical concern for radiculopathy,

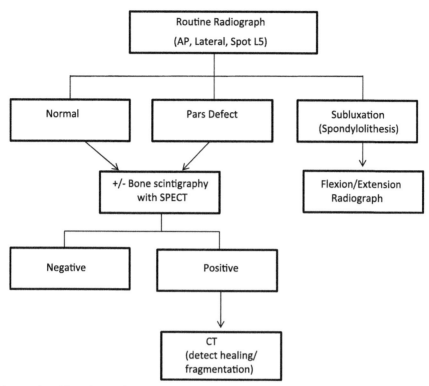

Fig. 1. Algorithms for evaluating spondylolysis in a young athlete. AP, anteroposterior; CT, computed tomography; SPECT, single-photon emission computed tomography.

MRI is recommended to evaluate neural involvement. MRI (particularly T2-weighted fat-saturated images) may also detect edema, reactive marrow changes, and synovitis. Some recent studies suggest that MRI has equivalent sensitivity to CT for detecting a pars fracture (**Fig. 1**).[27,28]

Atraumatic spine disorders

Spinal disorders with insidious onset and/or those without a history of trauma are initially evaluated with routine radiographs. Radiographs detect osseous changes

Table 8		
Radiograph views for evaluating spinal disorders		
Anatomic Region	**Indication**	**Radiography Views**
Cervical spine	Trauma/routine	AP, lateral, AP odontoid, both obliques (including C7–T1 level on both)
	Instability	Flexion/extension
Thoracolumbar spine	Routine	AP, lateral
	Scoliosis	Lateral bending
	Pars defect	AP, lateral, spot L5, both obliques[a]

[a] Oblique views for pars defect is no longer universally performed because of increased radiation dose with modestly increased sensitivity for fracture compared with performing AP and lateral views only.

including osteophyte formation, loss of lordosis, and facet degeneration. Intervertebral disc disorders can be indirectly detected with loss of disc height; however, MRI is usually necessary to evaluate for neuroforaminal stenosis, disc herniation, mass, and/or infection. CT myelography is also used to evaluate for disc herniation, particularly for surgical planning, or when MRI is contraindicated **Table 8**.[3]

SUMMARY

Diagnostic imaging can be a valuable tool when used in conjunction with a thorough history and physical examination for establishing a diagnosis and treatment plan. Radiographs are the initial imaging modality in most cases of musculoskeletal injury or pain. MRI is often the recommended imaging in the setting of a normal radiograph for most injuries. CT is the optimal imaging study for traumatic injury to the hands or the hook of the hamate. Ultrasound can be used to detect myotendinous injuries, ligamentous injuries, fractures, and masses. MR arthrography is recommended for evaluation of specific intra-articular soft tissue structures such as the TFCC in the wrist, glenoid labrum in the shoulder, and the acetabular labrum in the hip. Additional imaging algorithms and the usefulness of imaging studies can be found in the American College of Radiology Appropriateness Criteria.[15]

REFERENCES

1. DeLee JC, Drez D Jr, Miller MD. DeLee & Drez's orthopaedic sports medicine: principles and practice. Philadelphia: Saunders; 2010.
2. De Smet AA, Doherty MP, Norris MA, et al. Are oblique views needed for trauma radiography of the distal extremities? Am J Roentgenol 1999;172:1561–5.
3. Berquist TH. Musculoskeletal imaging companion. Philadelphia: Wolters Kluwer Lippincott Williams & Wilkins; 2007.
4. Manaster BJ, Roberts CC, Andrews CL, et al. Diagnostic and surgical imaging anatomy: musculoskeletal. Salt Lake City (UT): Amirsys; 2006.
5. Brenner AI, Koshy J, Morey J, et al. The bone scan. Semin Nucl Med 2012;42: 11–26.
6. Fraenkel L, Lavalley M, Felson D. The use of radiographs to evaluate shoulder pain in the ED. Am J Emerg Med 1998;16:560–3.
7. Fraenkel L, Shearer P, Mitchell P, et al. Improving the selective use of plain radiographs in the initial evaluation of shoulder pain. J Rheumatol 2000;27:200–4.
8. Teefey S, Rubin D, Middleton W, et al. Detection and quantification of rotator cuff tears. Comparison of ultrasonographic, magnetic resonance imaging, and arthroscopic findings in seventy-one consecutive cases. J Bone Joint Surg Am 2004; 86(4):708–16.
9. Goldfarb CA, Yin Y, Gilula LA, et al. Wrist fractures: what the clinician wants to know. Radiology 2001;219:11–28.
10. Rettig ME, Amadio PC. Wrist arthroscopy. Indications and clinical applications. J Hand Surg Br 1994;19:774–7.
11. Hobby JL, Dixon AK, Bearcroft PW, et al. MR imaging of the wrist: effect on clinical diagnosis and patient care. Radiology 2001;220:589–93.
12. Mack MG, Keim S, Balzer JO, et al. Clinical impact of MRI in acute wrist fractures. Eur Radiol 2003;13:612–7.
13. Jacobson JA, Bedi A, Sekiya JK, et al. Evaluation of the painful athletic hip: imaging options and imaging-guided injections. Am J Roentgenol 2012;199: 516–24.

14. Khoury V, Cardinal E, Bureau N. Musculoskeletal sonography: a dynamic tool for usual and unusual disorders. Am J Roentgenol 2007;188:W63–73.
15. American College of Radiology: appropriateness criteria. Available at: http://www.acr.org/Quality-Safety/Appropriateness-Criteria/Diagnostic/Musculoskeletal-Imaging. Accessed March 27, 2013.
16. Stiell IG, Greenberg GH, Wells GA, et al. Prospective validation of a decision rule for the use of radiography in acute knee injuries. JAMA 1996;275:611–5.
17. Stiell IG, Wells GA, McDowell I, et al. Use of radiography in acute knee injuries: need for clinical decision rules. Acad Emerg Med 1995;2:966–73.
18. Jenny JY, Boeri C, El Armani H, et al. Should plain X-rays be routinely performed after blunt knee trauma? A prospective analysis. J Trauma 2005;58:1179–82.
19. Jackson JL, O'Malley PG, Kroenke K. Evaluation of acute knee pain in primary care. Ann Intern Med 2003;139:575–91.
20. LaPrade RF, Burnett QM 2nd, Veenstra MA, et al. The prevalence of abnormal magnetic resonance imaging findings in asymptomatic knees. With correlation of magnetic resonance imaging to arthroscopic findings in asymptomatic knees. Am J Sports Med 1994;22:739–45.
21. Kellgren JH, Lawrence JS. Radiological assessment of osteoarthritis. Ann Rheum Dis 1957;16:494–501.
22. Claessens AA, Schouten JS, Van den Ouweland FA, et al. Do clinical findings associate with radiographic osteoarthritis of the knee? Ann Rheum Dis 1990; 49:771–4.
23. Bachmann LM, Kolb E, Koller MT, et al. Accuracy of Ottawa ankle rules to exclude fractures of the ankle and midfoot: systematic review. BMJ 2003;326:417.
24. Verhagen RA, Maas M, Dijkgraaf MG, et al. Prospective study on diagnostic strategies in osteochondral lesions of the talus. Is MRI superior to helical CT? J Bone Joint Surg Br 2005;87:41–6.
25. Hoffman JR, Mower WR, Wolfson AB, et al. Validity of a set of clinical criteria to rule out injury to the cervical spine in patients with blunt trauma. National Emergency X-Radiography Utilization Study Group. N Engl J Med 2000;343:94–9.
26. Bailitz J, Starr F, Beecroft J, et al. CT should replace three-view radiographs as the initial screening test in patients at high, moderate, and low risk for blunt cervical spine injury: a prospective comparison. J Trauma 2009;66:1605–9.
27. Wintermark M, Moushine E, Theumann N, et al. Thoracolumbar spine fractures in patients who have sustained severe trauma: depiction with mutidector row CT. Radiology 2003;227:681–9.
28. Sys J, Michielsen J, Bracke P, et al. Nonoperative treatment of active spondylolysis in elite athletes with normal x-ray findings: literature review and results of conservative treatment. Eur Spine J 2001;10:498–504.
29. Masci L, Pike J, Malara F, et al. Use of the one-legged hyperextension test and magnetic resonance imaging in the diagnosis of active spondylolysis. Br J Sports Med 2006;40:940–6.

Evaluation and Treatment of Musculoskeletal Chest Pain

Amba Ayloo, MD*, Teresa Cvengros, MD, CAQSM,
Srimannarayana Marella, MD

KEYWORDS

- Musculoskeletal chest pain • Costochondritis • Stretching exercises
- Pectoralis muscle pain • Fibromyalgia • Myofascial pain • Evaluation • Treatment

KEY POINTS

- Costochondritis is one of the most common causes of musculoskeletal chest pain.
- Stretching exercises have been shown to be effective in relieving the pain in costochondritis.
- Rib fractures, either traumatic or stress fractures, can be a source of chest pain.
- Slipping rib syndrome may occur in children with chronic chest and abdominal pain.
- Muscle strains may cause musculoskeletal chest pain, with intercostal muscle strains being the most common.
- Pectoralis muscle injury needs accurate and early diagnosis for optimal functional recovery in athletes.
- Myofascial pain and fibromyalgia are other causes of musculoskeletal chest pain.
- Herpes zoster should be considered in elderly patients with nonspecific musculoskeletal chest pain.
- It is important to assess all patients with chest pain for non-musculoskeletal causes of pain that could cause increased morbidity or mortality if not identified promptly.

INTRODUCTION

Chest pain is one of the most common reasons for seeking medical attention worldwide. In the United States alone, there are about 7.16 million visits annually to the emergency room with chest pain and most of these patients have noncardiac causes of chest pain.[1] Chest pain accounts for 1% to 3% of office visits to the primary care provider. Of these visits, 21% to 49% of patients are diagnosed with musculoskeletal chest pain, making it the most common cause of chest pain.[2]

Causes of chest pain include cardiovascular, pulmonary, musculoskeletal, gastroenterologic, and psychogenic. Pain can also radiate to the chest from the shoulders,

Funding Sources: None.
Conflict of Interest: None.
Family Medicine Residency Program, Department of Family Medicine, Mount Sinai Hospital, California Avenue at 15th Street, Chicago, IL 60608, USA
* Corresponding author.
E-mail address: ambaayloo@gmail.com

cervical and thoracic spine, lower neck, and structures below the diaphragm (**Fig. 1**).[3]

An important mechanism of chest pain may be referred pain from intrathoracic structures, including the heart, lungs, and esophagus.[3] Pain occurs because free nerve endings that transmit pain from visceral thoracic structures, including the heart, synapse on the same spinal cord dorsal horn interneurons that receive afferent input from the skin, muscles, and joints. The convergence of visceral and somatic pain fibers on the same interneurons causes the referred visceral pain that is perceived in somatic areas remote from involved viscera.[2] Thus, it can sometimes be difficult to delineate the precise cause of chest pain as musculoskeletal or visceral in origin.[2]

It is important to rule out visceral causes of chest pain, including cardiac, esophageal, or pulmonary causes, such as angina, myocardial infarction, malignancies, or pulmonary embolism, before definitively diagnosing musculoskeletal chest pain.[3,4] For example, anginal pain may occur along with underlying costochondritis or subacromial bursitis, which may influence the distribution of anginal pain.[3] In middle-aged and elderly patients with strong, relevant risk factors for cardiac disease, it is recommended to order an electrocardiogram, echocardiogram, and even stress testing as necessary to definitively rule out cardiac causes of chest pain before treating for musculoskeletal chest pain.[3,4]

Musculoskeletal chest pain includes pain related to the anterior chest wall bony and cartilaginous structures, chest wall musculature, and the thoracic spine.[3] In addition, other causes of pain may include skin conditions, neoplasms, and infections of chest

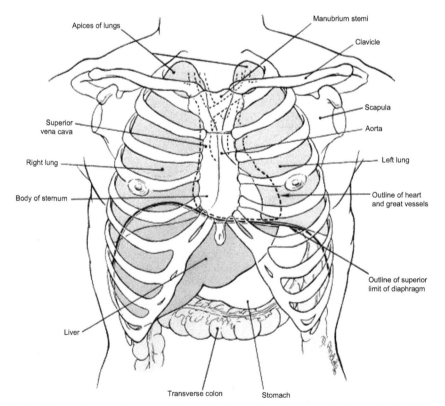

Fig. 1. Diverse origins and causes of chest pain. (*From* Cava JR, Sayger PL. Chest pain in children and adolescents. Pediatr Clin North Am 2004;51(6):1553–68. Philadelphia: Elsevier; with permission.)

wall structures, metabolic causes (vitamin D deficiency),[5] and rheumatologic disorders (**Box 1**).[3,6] The term chest wall syndrome refers to nontraumatic causes of musculoskeletal chest wall pain, which may include diagnoses such as costochondritis, atypical chest pain, and cervicothoracic angina.[7] A good history and physical examination are crucial to accurately diagnosing musculoskeletal chest pain (**Box 2, Table 1**).[3]

MUSCULOSKELETAL CHEST PAIN RELATED TO BONY AND CARTILAGINOUS STRUCTURES OF THE CHEST WALL
Costochondritis and Tietze Syndrome

These are conditions characterized by pain and tenderness in costochondral junctions. The comparative characteristics between the 2 conditions are listed in **Table 2**.[3,4]

The possible mechanism of pain is believed to be mechanical derangement, muscular imbalance, or neurogenic inflammation.[8] The pathogenesis of costochondritis is unclear. Because of its frequent association with other primary causes of chest pain, including anginal pain, it is important, especially in patients with relevant risk factors, to rule out any associated cardiac chest pain.[4]

Box 1
Diverse causes of musculoskeletal chest pain

- **Pain related to bony and cartilaginous structures of the chest wall**

    Costochondritis

    Tietze syndrome

    Rib pain

    - Fractures related to trauma

    - Stress fractures

    Slipping rib syndrome

    Painful xiphoid syndrome

- **Pain related to muscles**

    Muscle strains

    - Pectoralis muscle strains

    - Injuries to internal oblique/external oblique muscles

    - Serratus anterior muscle injury

    Myofascial pain

    Fibromyalgia

    Precordial catch syndrome

    Epidemic myalgia

- **Pain related to thoracic spine**

    Thoracic disc herniation

- **Miscellaneous causes of chest wall pain**

    Skin-related conditions

    - Herpes zoster

    - Neoplasms

    SAPHO syndrome

Table 1		
Key points in history taking		
Pain[3]	Onset	Usually acute or insidious
	Location	Well localized
	Character	Nonsqueezing, reproducible
	Duration	May become chronic
	Precipitating factor	By posture or movement
	Aggravating factor	
	Relieving factor	
History of acute or repeated excessive activity		
Recent or remote trauma[3]		

Data from Fam AG, Smythe HA. Musculoskeletal chest wall pain. Can Med Assoc J 1985;133:379–89.

Box 2
Key points in physical examination

Thorough systematic examination of anterior and posterior chest wall for

Swelling

Erythema

Heat

Tenderness

Neurologic examination to rule out compressions of nerve roots originating in lower cervical or thoracic segments of spinal cord

Sensory disturbances

Muscular strength

Peripheral reflexes of upper and lower extremities

Data from Fam AG, Smythe HA. Musculoskeletal chest wall pain. Can Med Assoc J 1985;133:379–89.

Chest pain involving costochondral joints has also been described in association with vitamin D deficiency.[5] The mechanism involved is believed to be defective bone mineralization caused by lack of vitamin D. This mechanism is shown by findings of rachitic rosary in children with rickets and tenderness of costochondral joints in adult patients with osteomalacia. Low vitamin D should be suspected in people with poor dietary intake of vitamin D or limited exposure to sunlight. Supplementation of vitamin D was associated with improvement of chest pain and overall quality of life. Further studies are needed to definitively associate vitamin D deficiency and costochondritis.[5]

Box 3
Prevalence of costochondritis

Emergency room	30% of chest pain visits were because of costochondritis
Primary care office	20% of chest pain visits were because of musculoskeletal chest pain
	Of these visits, 13% were because of costochondritis

Data from Proulx AM, Zryd TW. Costochondritis: diagnosis and treatment. Am Fam Physician 2009;80(6):617–21.

Table 2
Comparisons between costochondritis and Tietze syndrome

Characteristics	Costochondritis	Tietze Syndrome
Signs of inflammation	Absent	Present
Swelling	Absent	Presence or absence indicate severity of problem
Joints affected	Multiple and unilateral >90% Usually second to fifth costochondral junctions involved (**Fig. 2**)	Usually single and unilateral Usually second and third costochondral junctions involved[3,9,10]
Prevalence[4]	Relatively common (**Box 3**)	Uncommon
Age group affected	All age groups, including adolescents and elderly	Common in younger age group
Nature of pain	Aching, sharp, pressure like	Aching, sharp, stabbing initially, later persists as dull aching
Onset of pain	Repetitive physical activity provokes pain, rarely occurs at rest[11]	New vigorous physical activity such as excessive cough or vomiting, chest impact[9]
Aggravation of pain[9]	Movements of upper body, deep breathing, exertional activities	Movements
Association with other conditions	Seronegative arthropathies, angina pain[12]	No known association
Diagnosis	Crowing rooster maneuver[3] and other physical examination findings	Physical examination, exclude rheumatoid arthritis, pyogenic arthritis[2,3]
Imaging studies	Chest radiograph, computed tomography scan, or nuclear bone scan to rule out infections or neoplasms if clinically suspected[4]	Bone scintigraphy and ultrasonography can be used for screening for other conditions[10,11]
Treatment	Reassurance, pain control, NSAIDs, application of local heat and ice compresses, manual therapy with stretching exercises.[8,13] Corticosteroid or sulfasalazine injections in refractory patients[12]	Reassurance, pain control with NSAIDs,[3,9] and application of local heat. Corticosteroid and lidocaine injections to the cartilage, or intercostal nerve block in refractory patients[3,10]

Abbreviation: NSAIDs, nonsteroidal antiinflammatory drugs.

Evaluation
Physical examination helps in diagnosis. The "crowing rooster" maneuver reproduces the pain of costochondritis (**Fig. 3**).

Treatment
Conservative treatment is generally recommended (see **Table 2**). Stretching exercises have been studied recently in the treatment of costochondritis. In a retrospective open study of patients with a definitive diagnosis of costochondritis who were taking nonsteroidal antiinflammatory drugs (NSAIDs) in the last 2 to 3 months, there was statistically significant improvement in pain in the study group treated with exercises and NSAIDs, compared with the group on NSAIDs only (**Fig. 4**).[8]

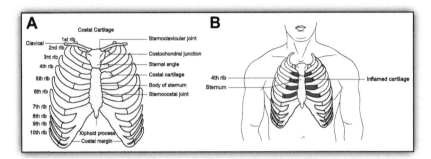

Fig. 2. Rib cage with costal cartilages and inflamed cartilages in costochondritis. (*A*) Labeling of rib cage. (*B*) Inflammation of coastal cartilages.

Rib Pain

Rib pain can be caused by swelling, erosions, and trauma causing fractures (**Figs. 5 and 6**).[3,14]

Evaluation

There is usually a history of initial vague chest pain that increases with inspiration, with movements of the chest and upper limb movements.[3,14] Dull, aching pain is more localized around the scapula, neck, and clavicle and may radiate to the sternum in first rib fractures.[15] Physical examination reveals point tenderness at the site of trauma, with or without local swelling on palpation.[14–16]

It is important to suspect and look for trauma to underlying viscera, including lung contusions, injury to liver, spleen, kidney, or any pneumothorax or hemothorax in multiple rib fractures and also in fractures of the first 4 or last 2 ribs, because these are not commonly seen. Child abuse should always be suspected in any child presenting with rib fractures, especially in infants and toddlers, because routine causes of injury and trauma in children do not cause rib fractures (**Fig. 7**). Imaging studies can help in diagnosing or confirming the fracture (**Box 4**).[15–18]

Treatment

Symptomatic treatment with good pain control for at least 3 weeks is generally recommended for non–sports related injuries.[14] Deep breathing is encouraged to prevent lung

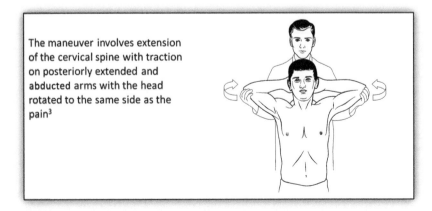

The maneuver involves extension of the cervical spine with traction on posteriorly extended and abducted arms with the head rotated to the same side as the pain[3]

Fig. 3. Crowing rooster maneuver.

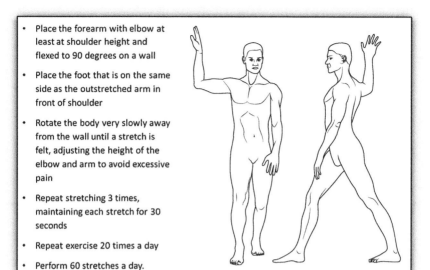

- Place the forearm with elbow at least at shoulder height and flexed to 90 degrees on a wall

- Place the foot that is on the same side as the outstretched arm in front of shoulder

- Rotate the body very slowly away from the wall until a stretch is felt, adjusting the height of the elbow and arm to avoid excessive pain

- Repeat stretching 3 times, maintaining each stretch for 30 seconds

- Repeat exercise 20 times a day

- Perform 60 stretches a day.

Fig. 4. Stretching exercises for costochondritis.

collapse, atelectasis, and lung infections. Splinting, local nerve blocks, and anesthetic injections are not routinely indicated because of poor efficacy and the associated risk of causing pneumothorax.[14] For athletes with first rib fractures, rest is recommended until symptoms resolve, followed by a gradual return to overhead activity, with correction of technique and biomechanical modification. Full recovery may take up to a year.[16,18] Fractures of the fourth to eighth ribs may need pain control and rest, with gradual return to activity at 4 to 6 weeks, then full activity as tolerated at 8 to 10 weeks.[16]

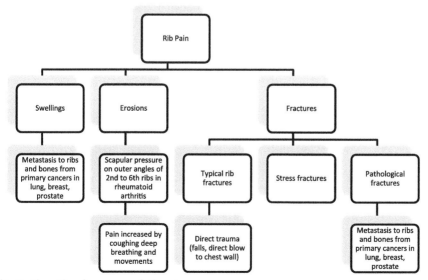

Fig. 5. Algorithm for causes of rib pain.

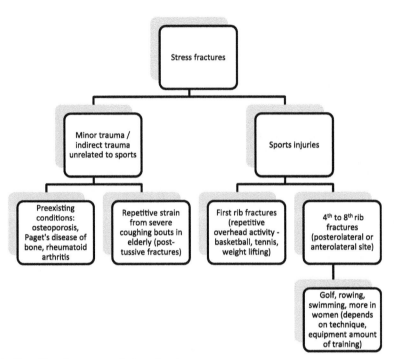

Fig. 6. Algorithm for causes of stress fractures.

Slipping Rib Syndrome

This condition occurs when interchondral fibrous attachments between the lower ribs, usually the 9th and 10th ribs, are inadequate, or rupture and loosen, allowing costal cartilage tips to curl up and override the inner aspect of the rib above, impinging on the intercostal nerve.[20,21] It is a recognized cause of chronic pain syndrome in children with recurrent pain in the lower chest and upper abdomen, but is less common compared with adults because of more flexible chests in children.[21] Repetitive trunk motion in athletes involved in sports such as running can cause slippage of a hypermobile rib under the superior rib, causing nerve impingement and pain.[15,16]

There may be a remote history of trauma.[2] Pain is insidious in onset, severe, sharp, and felt in the abdominal wall or anterior costal cartilage. It may be felt as local somatic

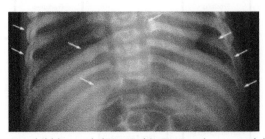

Fig. 7. Rib fractures in a child (*arrows*). (*From* Rubio EI. How do you read these images? Hone your interpretive skills. Rib fractures in a child. 2008. Available at: http://www. pediatricsconsultantlive.com/display/article/1803329/1405067. Accessed March 30, 2013; with permission.)

Box 4
Rib fracture imaging findings

Radiographs show a fracture line in about a half to two-thirds of fractures

In cases with no initial radiographic evidence of fracture, a healing callus may be seen after a few weeks on the radiograph or ultrasonogram

Triple phase bone scan or magnetic resonance imaging (MRI) may be used for early diagnosis.

Data from Refs.[3,15–17,19]

---

pain or as visceral pain, which may mimic biliary colic, peptic ulcer disease, and renal colic.[3,16,21]

Evaluation
Diagnosis is clinical. Examination shows increased tenderness and mobility of the anterior end of the costal cartilage, with an occasional painful click over the tip of affected cartilage. This pain can be reproduced by the hooking maneuver (**Fig. 8**).[2,16,20–23]

Treatment
Reassurance, pain control with analgesics, and avoidance of movements and positions that cause the loose costal cartilage to move upwards suddenly and provoke pain are recommended.[2,16,22] Strapping and local infiltration of lidocaine and corticosteroids for intercostal nerve block may be needed, more commonly in children.[16,20–22] Subperichondrial resection of involved costal cartilages is reserved for refractory cases in children (**Box 5**).

Painful Xiphoid Syndrome

Painful xiphoid syndrome is characterized by pain and tenderness in the region of the xiphoid cartilage. Pain may be low substernal or epigastric, with radiation to the precordium or abdomen.[3,16]

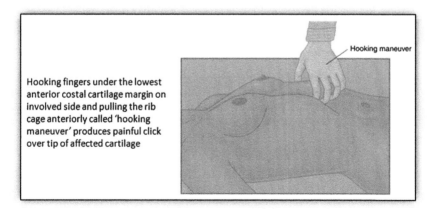

Hooking fingers under the lowest anterior costal cartilage margin on involved side and pulling the rib cage anteriorly called 'hooking maneuver' produces painful click over tip of affected cartilage

Hooking maneuver

Fig. 8. Hooking maneuver for slipping rib syndrome. (*From* Waldman S. Atlas of pain management injection techniques. 3rd edition. Philadelphia: Saunders; 2013. p. 274–6, with permission; and *Data from* Koren W, Shahar A. Xiphodynia masking acute myocardial infarction: a diagnostic cul-de-sac. Am J Emerg Med 1998;16(2):177–8.)

Box 5
Subperichondrial resection

It is important to mark the point of maximum tenderness on the patient while they are awake and supine before going to the operating room

Affected cartilage is excised and perichondrium is preserved

Surgery can be performed as an outpatient procedure

Cryotherapy can help decrease postoperative pain[21]

Data from Fu R, Iqbal CW, Jaroszewski DE, et al. Costal cartilage excision for the treatment of pediatric slipping rib syndrome. J Pediatr Surg 2012;47(10):1825–7.

Evaluation

Painful xiphoid syndrome is a diagnosis of exclusion. Clinical examination by exerting pressure on xiphoid cartilage reduplicates the pain and tenderness. It is important to definitively rule out other serious causes of chest pain, such as myocardial infarction, before reaching this diagnosis.[24]

Treatment

Symptomatic treatment with good pain control is generally recommended. Local injections of corticosteroids or lidocaine are recommended in refractory cases. Surgical excision of xiphoid cartilage is reserved for severe cases.[3]

MUSCULOSKELETAL CHEST PAIN RELATED TO MUSCLES

Muscle strains comprise one of the most common causes of musculoskeletal chest pain. They are usually acute in onset, caused by trauma or overuse.[3] Gradual onset of the muscle pain has also been reported as a result of tension or anxiety in the patient.[2] The commonly involved muscles include the intercostal muscles, pectoralis muscles, internal and external oblique muscles, and serratus anterior muscles.

Intercostal Muscle Strains

Intercostal muscles are the most commonly affected muscles, in almost 50% of patients,[2] followed by the pectoralis muscle group. There may be a history of excessive exertion of untrained muscles with activities like painting a ceiling, chopping wood, or coughing, and in sports with intense upper body activity, such as rowing.[3,16]

Evaluation

Diagnosis is clinical, based on a good history and physical examination. Localized pain or tenderness over the affected muscle groups is seen, which increases with stretching or contracting the involved muscles with activities such as deep inspiration and coughing.[3,16] Muscle tenderness on manual palpation is the most common finding.

Treatment

Reassurance, local application of heat, or use of analgesics for good pain control are recommended, along with avoiding activities that cause recurrence of the pain. Local injections of lidocaine or corticosteroids are reserved for refractory cases.[3,15,16]

Pectoralis Muscle Strains

The pectoralis muscle is one of the most important muscles for various movements of the upper limbs and chest wall (**Fig. 9**).[25] Tears to the pectoralis muscle can be caused

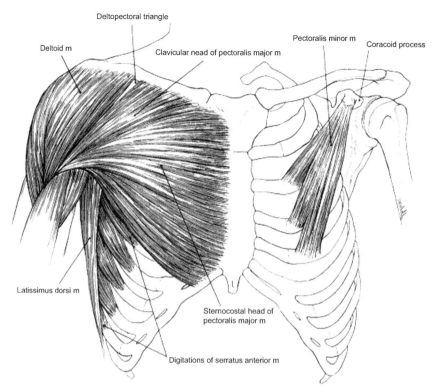

Deltopectoral triangle

Pectoralis minor m   Coracoid process

Deltoid m

Clavicular head of pectoralis major m

Latissimus dorsi m

Sternocostal head of pectoralis major m

Digitations of serratus anterior m

Fig. 9. Pectoralis muscle structure. (*From* Cava JR, Sayger PL. Chest pain in children and adolescents. Pediatr Clin North Am 2004;51(6):1553–68. Philadelphia: Elsevier; with permission.)

by direct blow or indirect trauma.[26–28] The tears can be classified by either cause or location of tear (**Figs. 10** and **11**). Indirect injury occurs when muscle under full tension is subjected to additional stress (eccentric muscle contraction), causing high-grade injuries in athletes in sports such as weight lifting or rugby.[29] Non–sports injury occurs most commonly because of forced abduction with extension or external rotation during a fall or when lifting weights.[25,30]

Evaluation

History and physical examination can help in diagnosis, but imaging is usually advised for correct diagnosis, because clinical assessment can be misled by hematoma or muscle injury.[25] Tears can present as sudden pain in the arm or shoulder accompanied with an audible pop, followed by swelling and ecchymosis. Inspection shows loss of the anterior axillary fold and asymmetry when compared with the other side with palpation of a defect on the side of injury. Loss of arm adduction may be a subtle but important finding in athletes such as weight lifters.[25] Radiographs at initial assessment may show soft tissue swelling with absent pectoralis shadow. Ultrasonography and MRI are modalities of choice and help in making correct decisions about optimal management (**Box 6**).[25]

Treatment

Proper documentation and determination of injury site and mechanism determine the management (**Box 7**).[25,29]

Classification of pectoralis muscle injury (tear)

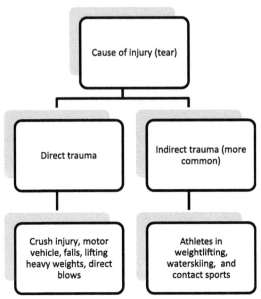

Fig. 10. Algorithm for pectoralis muscle injury based on cause of injury. (*Data from* Hopper MA, Tirman P, Robinson P. Muscle injury of the chest wall and upper extremity. Semin Musculoskelet Radiol 2010;14(2):122–30.)

Injuries to Internal Oblique/External Oblique Muscles

Injuries at the rib and costal cartilage insertion of internal and external oblique muscles are commonly referred to as side strains (**Fig. 12**).[31] They are uncommon, mostly seen

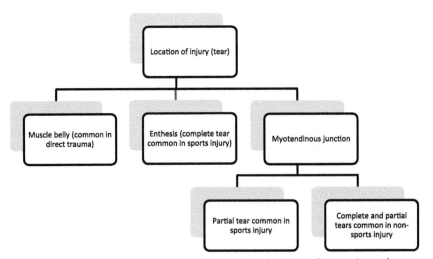

Fig. 11. Algorithm for pectoralis muscle injury based on location of injury. (*Data from* Hopper MA, Tirman P, Robinson P. Muscle injury of the chest wall and upper extremity. Semin Musculoskelet Radiol 2010;14(2):122–30.)

Box 6
Ultrasonography and MRI for diagnosis of pectoralis muscle tears

Ultrasonography is helpful in initial rapid assessment of acute muscle injury and surrounding structures when performed by an experienced clinician[30]

MRI is gold standard for:

   Accurate assessment of site and severity of injury and bony structures

   Identifying patients who benefit most from surgery

Data from Hopper MA, Tirman P, Robinson P. Muscle injury of the chest wall and upper extremity. Semin Musculoskelet Radiol 2010;14(2):122–30.

---

in athletes such as bowlers (cricket), javelin throwers, rowers, swimmers, or ice hockey players. The mechanism of injury is muscle lengthening followed by sudden eccentric contraction.[14,25,31,32] The injury is particularly seen in cricket fast bowlers and is seen in the nonbowling arm.[14]

Evaluation
Physical examination elicits pain and tenderness over the lower 4 costal cartilages, increased by resisted side flexion to the affected side.[31] Diagnosis is clinical, but imaging helps in evaluating the severity of injury and in determining the course of management (**Box 8**, **Figs. 13** and **14**).[25]

   MRI may show hematoma, periosteal stripping, or any stress injury to the underlying rib.[31] It is particularly useful in assessing acute concomitant injury to external oblique muscles. It can help in the follow-up of patients who failed to respond to conservative measures, but can be complicated by respiratory motion artifact.[25,33]

Treatment
Conservative treatment is recommended, with rest, strengthening exercises, and return to activity gradually. A period of 4 to 6 weeks may be needed for complete return to activity, especially in fast bowlers.[14] Reoccurrence of injury is common, especially in the first 2 years of initial injury.[14]

Box 7
Treatment of pectoralis muscle tears

Early surgical intervention[25,29,30]:

   Complete pectoralis major tendon avulsion at humeral attachment

   Helps athletes in early return to sports

      Optimum functional recovery

      Good cosmetic results

Nonsurgical treatment[29]:

   Muscular or musculotendinous tears

   Low-grade partial tears

   Older, sedentary patients for whom loss of strength may not cause significant impairment or debility

Data from Hopper MA, Tirman P, Robinson P. Muscle injury of the chest wall and upper extremity. Semin Musculoskelet Radiol 2010;14(2):122–30.

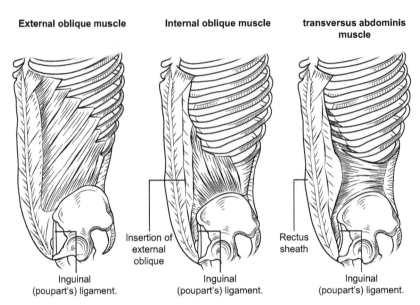

External oblique muscle **Internal oblique muscle** **transversus abdominis muscle**

Insertion of external oblique

Rectus sheath

Inguinal (poupart's) ligament.   Inguinal (poupart's) ligament.   Inguinal (poupart's) ligament.

Fig. 12. Insertion of external and internal oblique muscles.

Serratus Anterior Muscle Injury

Serratus anterior muscle injury is seen in athletes involved in sports such as rowing and weight lifting caused by overuse. Pain is typically located around the medial border of the scapula on the affected side and may radiate to the anterior chest.[15]

Evaluation

Diagnosis is clinical. Physical examination shows reproducible typical pain on resisted scapular protraction.[15]

Treatment

Improvement is seen with rest from activities that increase the pain, but may take several weeks.[15]

Box 8
Ultrasonographic findings in internal oblique muscle injury

Acute injury shows:

 Hematoma

 Fluid between muscle layers

 Loss of normal architecture

 Gap in the insertion of the internal oblique into costal cartilages and ribs (see **Fig. 14**)

Not sensitive to assess chronic injury and small muscle tears[32]

Data from Hopper MA, Tirman P, Robinson P. Muscle injury of the chest wall and upper extremity. Semin Musculoskelet Radiol 2010;14(2):122–30; and Obaid H, Nealon A, Connell D. Sonographic appearance of side strain injury. AJR Am J Roentgenol 2008;191(6):W264–7.

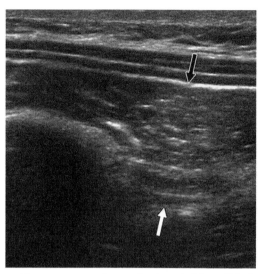

Fig. 13. Ultrasonographic appearance of normal external oblique (*black arrow*) and internal oblique (*white arrow*) muscles. (*From* Obaid H, Nealon A, Connell D. Sonographic appearance of side strain injury. AJR Am J Roentgenol 2008;191(6):265. Available at: http://www.ajronline.org/doi/full/10.2214/AJR.07.3381. Accessed March 12, 2013; with permission.)

Myofascial Pain

As the name implies, myofascial pain is defined as pain originating from muscles or fascia. This type of pain is described as dull and aching, with a stiff feeling. It may be caused by muscle injury or overuse.[34] Myofascial pain may be aggravated by muscle

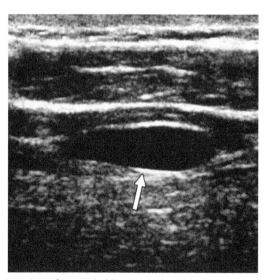

Fig. 14. Gap in the insertion of internal oblique muscle caused by tear (*arrow*). (*From* Obaid H, Nealon A, Connell D. Sonographic appearance of side strain injury. AJR Am J Roentgenol 2008;191(6):265. Available at: http://www.ajronline.org/doi/full/10.2214/AJR.07.3381. Accessed March 12, 2013; with permission.)

use, postural imbalance, cold, anxiety, and psychological stressors.[35] What defines myofascial pain clinically is the identification of a trigger point.[34] A trigger point is "a hyperirritable spot in skeletal muscle that is associated with a hypersensitive palpable nodule in a taut band" of muscle.[36] Additional clinical features of trigger points are listed in **Box 9**.[34,35,37]

Trigger points in the pectoral major and minor muscles, intercostal muscles, anterior serratus muscles, scalenus muscles, and sternalis muscles can be a source of pain referred to the chest wall.[35,38,39] For example, trigger points in the pectoral major or minor muscle may cause ipsilateral chest pain that radiates down the ulnar side of the arm. Sternalis muscle trigger points may cause a deep substernal ache.[35] Myofascial trigger points are common yet often not identified or treated properly, because the initial training of so few medical providers includes adequate education in their identification and treatment.[37]

Evaluation

Carefully examine the chest wall and cervical muscles for active trigger points. The physical examination skills for identifying trigger points are not commonly taught in medical training, and practice is required in order to become competent at this skill. Myofascial pain may not be the sole reason for the pain, but may be a contributing factor in some cases. Therefore, evaluation for other causes of pain is important.[34]

Treatment

It is important to address postural and ergonomic factors and proper stretching and strengthening of muscles when treating myofascial pain. There are several options for local treatment of active trigger points (**Box 10**).[34,37]

Medications that may be helpful include NSAIDs, tricyclic antidepressant drugs, or muscle relaxants, particularly tizanidine (Zanaflex). Consider referral to a provider with experience in treating trigger points and myofascial pain. If myofascial pain is not treated appropriately and underlying predisposing factors are not addressed, it may lead to chronic pain syndromes such as fibromyalgia, through the mechanism of central sensitization.[34]

Fibromyalgia

Fibromyalgia is a distinct complex clinical syndrome that belongs to a group of clinical syndromes characterized by chronic pain, called the central sensitization syndromes.[40–42] The other members of this group include restless leg syndrome, functional gastrointestinal disorders, and chronic fatigue syndrome. Fibromyalgia and other central sensitivity syndromes are characterized by a range of symptoms that include chronic pain, sleep disturbances with decreased rapid eye movement

---

Box 9
Trigger points

Tender ropelike induration in muscle

May produce a twitch response, which is contraction of the muscle, when palpated or needled

May cause restricted range of motion or weakness in the affected muscle

May cause radiation of pain or parasthesias in a myotomal distribution

Firm pressure on a trigger point for at least 5 seconds may elicit referred pain in a myotomal distribution

---

Box 10
Local treatment of trigger points

Ischemic pressure

Injection of trigger point with anesthetic solution such as lidocaine (wet needling)

Injection of trigger point without anesthetic (dry needling)

Stretching the muscle while spraying with vapocoolant

---

sleep, other somatic symptoms, and psychological symptoms.[43] The current hypothesis is that these syndromes represent a spectrum of disorders that result in expression of different symptoms over time, as a result of a complex interplay of various psychological, social, and biological factors, called the biopsychosocial model.[44]

According to various studies that evaluated the prevalence of fibromyalgia in patients with musculoskeletal causes of noncardiac chest pain, prevalence ranges between 2.7% and 30%.[9] Both fibromyalgia and noncardiac chest pain seem to share the same pathogenesis of long-standing pain hypersensitivity, which presents as allodynia and hyperalgesia.[40] The other accompanying somatic and visceral complaints are believed to be caused by hypothalamic-pituitary-adrenal axis abnormalities and autonomic dysfunction.[45] Mechanism of central sensitization with somatic or visceral hypersensitivity manifests as noncardiac chest pain in patients with fibromyalgia.[46]

Fibromyalgia is characterized by chronic widespread pain, unexplained somatic symptoms, which include nonrestorative sleep, dysesthesias, cognitive difficulties, dizziness, syncope, dry mouth, and headaches, and psychological symptoms, such as anxiety or depression.[47] Another characteristic feature of fibromyalgia is the presence of specific points of tenderness at 9 symmetric body sites (**Fig. 15**). It is more common in women, in those 50 years or older, and in those with low educational and household income levels.[48]

Evaluation

History and physical examination are important in diagnosing fibromyalgia. The American College of Rheumatology (ACR) established diagnostic and severity criteria in 1990, which were revised in 2000 (**Box 11**).

Treatment

Various pharmacologic and nonpharmacologic treatments have been shown to be beneficial in fibromyalgia (**Box 12**).

A holistic approach that addresses the various symptoms of fibromyalgia including pain, fatigue, sleep, and mood disorders has been shown to be effective and deliver the most effective results in the long-term.[52]

Precordial Catch Syndrome

Precordial catch syndrome is an uncommon condition characterized by episodes of localized, stabbing, or sharp pain catches in the anterior chest, usually in the left parasternal area or near the cardiac apex in healthy young individuals.[3,53] Pain occurs in a bent-over or slouched position and is increased by deep breathing. It is relieved by shallow respirations and by correcting posture. Local tenderness is absent. The cause is believed to be intercostal muscle spasm caused by postural defects.[3]

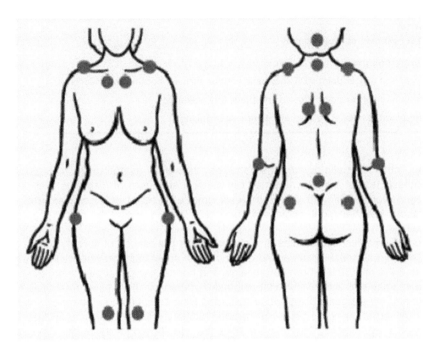

Fig. 15. Tender points in fibromyalgia. (*From* Shipley M. Chronic widespread pain and fibromyalgia syndrome. Medicine 2010;38(4):202–4; with permission.)

Evaluation

Precordial catch syndrome is a diagnosis of exclusion.

Treatment

Reassurance, correcting postural defects, and good pain control are generally recommended.[3,53]

Epidemic Myalgia

Epidemic myalgia is also called devil's grip, caused by acute viral illness with pain in the chest wall and epigastrium.[3] The usual causes are the group B coxsackie viruses, which usually affect intercostal and upper abdominal wall muscles, and rarely the pleura. A prodrome of 1 to 10 days is followed by severe, sharp pain in the lateral chest

---

Box 11
Diagnostic and severity criteria for fibromyalgia

ACR criteria (1990)[49]: presence of chronic widespread pain and tenderness at 11 of 18 body sites

Chronic widespread pain is presence of pain in the upper and lower body, axial skeletal, and left and right sides for at least 3 months, without any history of lesion or trauma to explain the symptoms

ACR revised criteria (2000)[50]: presence of chronic widespread pain and a symptom severity scale (includes fatigue, cognitive disturbances, nonrestorative sleep, and other somatic symptoms)

New criteria offer greater sensitivity for diagnosis of fibromyalgia

---

Box 12
Treatment of fibromyalgia

Pharmacologic treatment: for pain control

- Antidepressants: amitryptiline, cyclobenzaprine, fluoxetine[51]

- Opiates: tramadol

- Central nervous system agents: gabapentin, pregabalin

Nonpharmacologic treatment

- Graded aerobic exercise regimen[52]: helps with pain, avoid overexhaustion

- Sleep evaluation and treatment: helps with nonrestorative sleep and to correct other sleep problems, such as obstructive sleep apnea

- Cognitive behavioral therapy: promotes and reinforces positive behaviors, helps with treatment of pain, fatigue, and other somatic symptoms

Treatment of other coexisting symptoms (psychological, somatic, such as gastrointestinal, etc)

---

wall in adults or the upper abdomen in children. Pain is increased by breathing, coughing, and other thoracic movements and lasts 3 to 7 days, with frequent recurrences.[3]

Evaluation
Diagnosis is usually clinical, with good history and physical examination, with local tenderness of involved muscle groups. Isolation of the virus from the throat or feces or showing increasing titer levels of type-specific neutralizing antibodies can confirm the diagnosis.[3]

Treatment
Symptomatic treatment with good pain control is recommended.[3]

MUSCULOSKELETAL CHEST PAIN RELATED TO THORACIC SPINE
Acute Thoracic Disc Herniation in Athletes

Thoracic disc herniation does not have a typical clinical presentation and most commonly presents as a nonspecific, often acute-onset, midline pain in the thoracic area. It can be unilateral or bilateral. It can be intermittent or constant and may be increased by coughing and straining.[54] Radicular distribution of pain depends on the thoracic spinal segment involved and may be followed by sensory and motor disturbances caused by spinal cord compression. The usual cause is believed to be degeneration, although acute trauma has to be considered in young patients, especially in athletes.[54]

Evaluation
MRI is the imaging of choice and shows thoracic disc herniation.[54]

Treatment
Conservative management is successful in most patients. Selective spinal root or intercostal nerve blockade and epidural steroid injections are used. If there is no improvement in symptoms after 2 to 3 months, or if there is progression of symptoms with new neurologic deficits, operative treatment is recommended, with a success rate of about 80%.[54]

Long-term prognosis is considered to be good, but recurrences of pain and other symptoms are not uncommon. It is important to explain the possibility of recurrent pain to patients, especially young athletes, because it can cause them to prematurely end their sporting careers.[54]

MISCELLANEOUS CAUSES OF MUSCULOSKELETAL CHEST PAIN
Herpes Zoster of the Chest Wall

Herpes zoster is caused by the reactivation of the latent varicella zoster virus, which has been dormant in dorsal root ganglion of the spinal cord since the initial chicken pox infection.[55] About 50% of elderly patients older than 80 years are believed to develop this infection over their lifetime.[55] It presents as a vesicular eruption of the skin, and is dermatomally distributed. The rash is usually unilateral and confined to a single dermatome, but involvement of multiple, bilateral dermatomes is seen. Severe pain is a hallmark of herpes zoster and often precedes, accompanies, and follows resolution of rash (**Box 13**).[56]

Involvement of thoracic dermatomes, especially in elderly patients, can cause diagnostic confusion with cardiac and pulmonary causes of pain, particularly before development of the rash.[62,63] Rash usually involves thoracic dermatomes with grouped vesicles and pustules present on erythematous base. Infection typically resolves completely in 4 weeks. Scarring and depigmentation in the area of the rash may be seen.[6]

Evaluation

Diagnosis during the prodromal phase before appearance of skin lesions is difficult.[6,64] A history of varicella zoster in the past and hyperesthesia and skin tenderness on physical examination that follows a dermatomal distribution are clues to the diagnosis.[6,64] A dermatomally distributed skin rash with grouped vesicles and pustules on an erythematous base is diagnostic (**Fig. 16**). Clinical diagnosis can be confirmed by Tzanck smear (swabs from the base of the vesicles show varicella zoster virus DNA on polymerase chain reaction testing).

Treatment

Pain control and antivirals are mainstays of treatment (**Box 14**).

SAPHO Syndrome

SAPHO syndrome is a chronic disease that is characterized by association of synovitis, acne, pustulosis, hyperostosis, and osteitis.[68] It usually presents with cutaneous manifestations (neutrophilic eruptions, such as palmoplantar pustulosis and hidradenitis suppurativa) and aseptic inflammatory bone lesions with associated findings that include hyperostosis and arthritis of adjacent joints (osteoarthropathy).[69] SAPHO syndrome has a predilection to affect the bony structures of the anterior chest, including

---

Box 13
Characteristics of pain in herpes zoster

Preherpetic neuralgia: prodromal pain that precedes the development of skin eruption (usually by 4 days)[56,57]

- Leads to diagnostic confusion depending on the dermatomes affected
- Fever, malaise, and skin tenderness over affected area may accompany the pain

Postherpetic neuralgia: pain that persists or is recurrent more than 1 month after the onset of initial herpes zoster infection[58]

- More common in elderly women with history of severe prodromal pain and severe skin rash
- Pain is debilitating and resistant to treatment[58,59]

Zoster sine eruption: prodromal pain is not followed by skin eruption

- Leads to diagnostic difficulties[60,61]

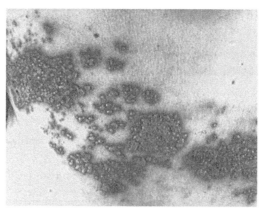

Fig. 16. Dermatomal distribution of herpes zoster skin rash. (*From* Swartz MH. Textbook of physical diagnosis: history of examination. Philadelphia: Saunders; 2009. p. 137–95; with permission.)

the sternum and medial end of clavicle. Anterior chest pain is one of the most common symptoms.[69]

The pathogenesis of SAPHO syndrome is unclear. One of the proposed mechanisms is a possible autoimmune response triggered by a microorganism producing sterile inflammation in the joints and bones.[69–71] *Propionibacterium acnes* is the most commonly cultured microorganism in skin and bone specimens obtained from patients with SAPHO syndrome.[72] Genetic factors and stress are other important factors that are correlated with the syndrome.[69–71]

Evaluation

Although there are no validated criteria, standard diagnostic criteria agreed on by most clinicians and researchers can be used in diagnosis (**Box 15**).[73]

Laboratory findings are nonspecific and include mild leukocytosis, mild anemia, and an increased erythrocyte sedimentation rate. Serum levels of complement C3 and C4 may be increased or normal and serum IgA levels are usually increased.[69]

Treatment

Symptomatic relief with NSAIDs and analgesics are the mainstay of therapy. Corticosteroids, sulfasalazine, and isotretinoin have been used in some cases. Use of tumor necrosis factor inhibitors (such as infliximab and etanercept) and immunomodulators (such as leflunomide and methotrexate) have been proposed in some studies.[69,72,74,75]

Box 14
Treatment of herpes zoster

Start treatment with antiviral agents (acyclovir, valcyclovir) within 72 hours of appearance of skin eruption and continue for 7 days[65]

Postherpetic neuralgia: gabapentin, pregabalin, topical agents (capsaicin cream) and tricyclic antidepressants are commonly recommended[59,66]

Epidural injections of steroid and local anesthetic are used in selective cases[67]

> **Box 15**
> **Standard diagnostic criteria for SAPHO syndrome**
>
> Local bone pain with gradual onset
>
> Multifocal lesions involving long tubular bones and spine
>
> Failure to culture an infectious microorganism
>
> Neutrophilic skin eruptions (palmoplantar pustulosis, nonpalmoplantar pustulosis, psoriasis vulgaris, or severe acne)
>
> Protracted course for several years, with exacerbations and improvement with antiinflammatory drugs
>
> *Data from* Schuster T, Bielek J, Dietz HG, et al. Chronic recurrent multifocal osteomyelitis (CRMO). Eur J Pediatr Surg 1996;6(1):45–51.

SUMMARY

Musculoskeletal chest pain can be a cause of significant morbidity and anxiety for a patient. Better understanding of the various causes of musculoskeletal chest pain can help prevent unnecessary testing and anxiety for patients and ensure timely treatment.

REFERENCES

1. National Hospital Ambulatory Medical Care Survey: 2009 Emergency Dept Summary Tables–Table 10. 2009. Available at: http://www.cdc.gov/nchs/data/ahcd/nhamcs_emergency/2009_ed_web_tables.pdf. Accessed February 20, 2013.
2. Stochkendahl MJ, Christensen HW. Chest pain in focal musculoskeletal disorders. Med Clin North Am 2010;94(2):259–73.
3. Fam AG, Smythe HA. Musculoskeletal chest wall pain. Can Med Assoc J 1985; 133:379–89.
4. Proulx AM, Zryd TW. Costochondritis: diagnosis and treatment. Am Fam Physician 2009;80(6):617–21.
5. Oho RC, Johnson JD. Chest pain and costochondritis associated with vitamin D deficiency: a report of two cases. Case Rep Med 2012;2012:375730.
6. Muir J, Yelland M. Skin and breast disease in the differential diagnosis of chest pain. Med Clin North Am 2010;94(2):319–25.
7. Verdon F, Burnand B, Herzig L, et al. Chest wall syndrome among primary care patients: a cohort study. BMC Fam Pract 2007;8:51.
8. Rovetta G, Sessarego P, Monteforte P. Stretching exercises for costochondritis pain. G Ital Med Lav Ergon 2009;31(2):169–71.
9. Semble EL, Wise CM. Chest pain: a rheumatologist's perspective. South Med J 1988;81(1):64–8.
10. Kamel M, Kotob H. Ultrasonographic assessment of local steroid injection in Tietze's syndrome. Br J Rheumatol 1997;36:547–50.
11. Habib PA, Huang GS, Mendiola JA, et al. Anterior chest pain: musculoskeletal considerations. Emerg Radiol 2004;11:37–45.
12. Freeston J, Karim Z, Lindsay K, et al. Can early diagnosis and management of costochondritis reduce acute chest pain admissions? J Rheumatol 2004;31: 2269–71.

13. Rabey MI. Costochondritis: are the symptoms and signs due to neurogenic inflammation. Two cases that responded to manual therapy directed towards posterior spinal structures. Man Ther 2008;13:82–6.

14. Singer K, Fazey P. Thoracic and chest pain. In: Brukner P, Khan K, editors. Clinical sports medicine. 4th edition. Sydney (Australia): McGraw Medical; 2012. p. 449–62.

15. Karlson KA. Thoracic region pain in athletes. Curr Sports Med Rep 2004;3(1): 53–7.

16. Gregory PL, Biswas AC, Batt ME. Musculoskeletal problems of the chest wall in athletes. Sports Med 2002;32(4):235–50.

17. Sik EC, Batt ME, Heslop LM. Atypical chest pain in athletes. Curr Sports Med Rep 2009;8(2):52–8.

18. Coris EE, Higgins HW. First rib stress fractures in throwing athletes. Am J Sports Med 2005;33(9):1400–4.

19. Dragoni S, Giombini A, Di Cesare A, et al. Stress fractures of the ribs in elite competitive rowers: a report of nine cases. Skeletal Radiol 2007;36(10):951–4.

20. Fu R, Iqbal CW, Jaroszewski DE, et al. Costal cartilage excision for the treatment of pediatric slipping rib syndrome. J Pediatr Surg 2012;47(10):1825–7.

21. Mooney DP, Shorter NA. Slipping rib syndrome in childhood. J Pediatr Surg 1997;32(7):1081–2.

22. Udermann BE, Cavanaugh DG, Gibson MH, et al. Slipping rib syndrome in a collegiate swimmer: a case report. J Athl Train 2005;40(2):120–2.

23. Heinz GJ III, Zavala DC. Slipping rib syndrome: diagnosis using the "hooking manuever". JAMA 1977;237(8):794–5.

24. Koren W, Shahar A. Xiphodynia masking acute myocardial infarction: a diagnostic cul-de-sac. Am J Emerg Med 1998;16(2):177–8.

25. Hopper MA, Tirman P, Robinson P. Muscle injury of the chest wall and upper extremity. Semin Musculoskelet Radiol 2010;14(2):122–30.

26. Kretzler HH Jr, Richardson AB. Rupture of the pectoralis major muscle. Am J Sports Med 1989;17(4):453–8.

27. Wolfe SW, Wickiewicz TL, Cavanaugh JT. Ruptures of the pectoralis major muscle. An anatomic and clinical analysis. Am J Sports Med 1992;20(5):587–93.

28. Bak K, Cameron EA, Henderson IJ. Rupture of the pectoralis major: a meta-analysis of 112 cases. Knee Surg Sports Traumatol Arthrosc 2000;8(2):113–9.

29. Hanna CM, Glenny AB, Stanley SN, et al. Pectoralis major tears: comparison of surgical and conservative treatment. Br J Sports Med 2001;35(3):202–6.

30. Rehman A, Robinson P. Sonographic evaluation of injuries to pectoralis muscles. AJR Am J Roentgenol 2005;184(4):1205–11.

31. Humphries D, Jamison M. Clinical and magnetic resonance imaging features of cricket bowler's side strain. Br J Sports Med 2004;38(5):E21.

32. Obaid H, Nealon A, Connell D. Sonographic appearance of side strain injury. AJR Am J Roentgenol 2008;191(6):W264–7.

33. Connell DA, Jhamb A, James T. Side strain: a tear of internal oblique musculature. AJR Am J Roentgenol 2003;191(6):1511–7.

34. Bennett R. Myofascial pain syndromes and their evaluation. Best Pract Res Clin Rheumatol 2007;21(3):427–45.

35. Alvarez DJ, Rockwell PG. Trigger points: diagnosis and management. Am Fam Physician 2002;65(4):653–60.

36. Simons DG, Travell JG, Simons LS. Glossary. In: Travell & Simons' myofascial pain and dysfunction: the trigger point manual, vol. 1, 2nd edition. Baltimore (MD): Williams & Wilkins; 1999. p. 1–10.

37. Simons DG. Understanding effective treatments of myofascial trigger points. J Bodyw Mov Ther 2002;6(2):81–8.
38. Moseley GL. Pain: why and how does it hurt? In: Brukner P, Khan K, editors. Clinical sports medicine. 4th edition. Sydney (Australia): McGraw-Hill; 2012. p. 41–53.
39. Choi YJ, Choi SU, Shin HW, et al. Chest pain caused by trigger points in the scalenus muscle: a case report. Korean J Anesthesiol 2007;53(5):680–2.
40. Nielsen LA, Henriksson KG. Pathophysiological mechanisms in chronic musculoskeletal pain (fibromyalgia): the role of central and peripheral sensitization and pain disinhibition. Best Pract Res Clin Rheumatol 2007;21(3):465–80.
41. Yunus MB. Role of central sensitization in symptoms beyond muscle pain and the evaluation of a patient with widespread pain. Best Pract Res Clin Rheumatol 2007;21:481–97.
42. Almansa C, Wang B, Achem SR. Noncardiac chest pain and fibromyalgia. Med Clin North Am 2010;94(2):275–89.
43. Moldofsky H. The significance of dysfunctions of the sleeping/waking brain to the pathogenesis and treatment of fibromyalgia syndrome. Rheum Dis Clin North Am 2009;35(2):275–83.
44. Ferrari R. The biopsychosocial model: a tool for rheumatologists. Baillieres Best Pract Res Clin Rheumatol 2000;14:787–95.
45. Crofford LJ, Pillemer SR, Kalogeras KT, et al. Hypothalamic-pituitary-adrenal axis perturbations in patients with fibromyalgia. Arthritis Rheum 1994;37:1583–92.
46. Hollerbach S, Bulat R, May A, et al. Abnormal processing of esophageal stimuli in patients with noncardiac chest pain (NCCP). Neurogastroenterol Motil 2001;12(6):555–65.
47. Clouse R, Carney RM. The psychological profile of non-cardiac chest pain patients. Eur J Gastroenterol Hepatol 1995;7:1160–5.
48. Wolfe F, Ross K, Anderson J, et al. The prevalence and characteristics of fibromyalgia in the general population. Arthritis Rheum 1995;38(1):19–28.
49. Wolfe F, Smythe HA, Yunus MB, et al. The American College of Rheumatology 1990 criteria for the classification of fibromyalgia. Report of the Multicenter Criteria Committee. Arthritis Rheum 1990;33:160–72.
50. Wolfe F, Clauw D, Fitzcharles MA, et al. Clinical diagnostic and severity criteria for fibromyalgia [abstract]. Arthritis Rheum 2009;60(Suppl 10):S210.
51. Hauser W, Bernardy K, Ucelyer N, et al. Treatment of fibromyalgia syndrome with anti-depressants: a meta-analysis. JAMA 2009;301(2):198–209.
52. Goldenberg DL, Burckhardt C, Crofford L. Management of fibromyalgia syndrome. JAMA 2004;292(19):2388–95.
53. Gumbiner CH. Precordial catch syndrome. South Med J 2003;96(1):38–41.
54. Baranto A, Borjesson M, Danielsson B, et al. Acute chest pain in a top soccer player due to thoracic disc herniation. Spine 2009;34(10):E359–62.
55. Johnson RW. Herpes zoster and postherpetic neuralgia: a review of the effects of vaccination. Aging Clin Exp Res 2009;21(3):236–43.
56. Johnson RW. Zoster associated pain: what is known, who is at risk and how can it be managed? Herpes 2007;14(Suppl 2):30–4.
57. Gilden DH, Dueland AN, Cohrs R, et al. Preherpetic neuralgia. Neurology 1991;41:1215–8.
58. Jung BF, Johnson RW, Griffin DR, et al. Risk factors for postherpetic neuralgia in a patient with herpes zoster. Neurology 2004;62(9):1545–51.

59. Zareba G. Pregabalin: a new agent for the treatment of neuropathic pain. Drugs Today (Barc) 2005;41(8):509–16.
60. Barrett AP, Katelaris CH, Morris JG, et al. Zoster sine herpete of the trigeminal nerve. Oral Surg Oral Med Oral Pathol 1993;75(2):173–5.
61. Schuchmann JA, McAllister RK, Armstrong CS, et al. Zoster sine herpete with thoracic motor paralysis temporally associated with thoracic epidural steroid injection. Am J Phys Med Rehabil 2008;87(10):853–8.
62. Goh CL, Khoo L. A retrospective study of the clinical presentation and outcome of herpes zoster in a tertiary dermatology outpatient referral clinic. Int J Dermatol 1997;36(9):667–72.
63. Franken RA, Franken M. Pseudo-myocardial infarction during an episode of herpes zoster. Arq Bras Cardiol 2000;75(6):523–30.
64. Morgan R, King D. Characteristics of patients with shingles admitted to a district general hospital. Postgrad Med J 1998;74(868):101–3.
65. Dworkin RH, Johnson RW, Breuer J, et al. Recommendations for the management of herpes zoster. Clin Infect Dis 2007;44(Suppl 1):S1–26.
66. Saarto T, Wiffen PJ. Antidepressants for neuropathic pain. Cochrane Database Syst Rev 2005;(4):CD005454. http://dx.doi.org/10.1002/14651858.CD005454.pub2.
67. Van Wijck AJ, Opstelten W, Moons KG, et al. The PINE study of epidural steroids and local anaesthetics to prevent postherpetic neuralgia: a randomized controlled trial. Lancet 2006;367(9506):219–24.
68. Chamot AM, Benhamou CL, Kahn MF, et al. Acne-pustulosis-hyperostosis-osteitis syndrome. Result of a national survey. 85 cases. Rev Rhum Mal Osteoartic 1987; 54:187–96.
69. Zigang Z, Ying L, Yuanyuan L, et al. Synovitis, acne, pustulosis, hyperostosis and osteitis (SAPHO) syndrome with review of the relevant published work. J Dermatol 2011;38(2):155–9.
70. Grossman ME, Rudin D, Scher R. SAPHO syndrome: report of three cases and of the literature. Cutis 1999;64:253–8.
71. Earwaker JW, Cotton A. SAPHO: syndrome or concept? Imaging findings. Skeletal Radiol 2003;32:311.
72. Hurtado-Nedelec M, Chollet-Martin S, Nicaise-Roland P, et al. Characterization of the immune response in the synovitis, acne, pustulosis, hyperostosis, osteitis (SAPHO) syndrome. Rheumatology 2008;47:1160–7.
73. Schuster T, Bielek J, Dietz HG, et al. Chronic recurrent multifocal osteomyelitis (CRMO). Eur J Pediatr Surg 1996;6(1):45–51.
74. Gupta AK, Skinner AR. A review of the use of infliximab to manage cutaneous dermatoses. J Cutan Med Surg 2004;8:77–89.
75. Robert I, Matthias L, Costakis G, et al. Mechanism of action for leflunomide in rheumatoid arthritis. Clin Immunol 1999;3:198–208.

The Evaluation and Treatment of Rotator Cuff Pathology

Viviane Bishay, MD[a], Robert A. Gallo, MD[b],*

KEYWORDS

- Rotator cuff • Supraspinatus • Shoulder pain • Shoulder injury • Shoulder weakness

KEY POINTS

- Detailed history including age, onset of symptoms, history of overuse or trauma, duration of symptoms, and previous therapy is very helpful in diagnosis.
- Physical examination should include both affected and unaffected shoulders as well as observation and palpation for atrophy and asymmetry, shoulder range of motion, motor and sensory examination, and special tests.
- Advanced imaging should be reserved for cases that have failed conservative treatment or when a high probability of tear exists.
- Radiographic imaging is more affordable and can spot other sources of shoulder pain, such as calcific tendinitis, glenohumeral arthritis, and proximal humerus fractures.
- Magnetic resonance imaging (MRI), though very costly, has become the method of choice in diagnosing soft-tissue abnormality of the shoulder, given the high sensitivity and specificity in diagnosis.
- Ultrasonography is relatively inexpensive and allows for dynamic assessment of rotator cuff tendons, but accuracy of the results is limited to the skills of the radiologist interpreting these studies.
- Shoulder arthrography is beneficial in cases where traditional imaging methods do not clearly delineate suspected abnormality.
- Contrast-enhanced computed tomography is mostly used to visualize rotator cuff tendons in cases where MRI cannot be used and ultrasonography is not available.

INTRODUCTION/EPIDEMIOLOGY

Shoulder pain is the third most common musculoskeletal complaint at the primary care office.[1] Rotator cuff–related ailments account for the vast majority (65%) of shoulder-related visits. The remainder of presenting complaints pertains to pericapsular soft-tissue pain (11%), acromioclavicular joint pain (10%), and referred pain from

[a] Department of Family Medicine, Mount Sinai Hospital, 1500 South California Avenue, Chicago, IL 60608, USA; [b] Department of Orthopedics, Bone and Joint Institute, Milton S. Hershey Medical Center, Pennsylvania State University College of Medicine, 30 Hope Drive, PO Box 859, Hershey, PA 17033, USA
* Corresponding author.
E-mail address: rgallo@hmc.psu.edu

Prim Care Clin Office Pract 40 (2013) 889–910
http://dx.doi.org/10.1016/j.pop.2013.08.006
0095-4543/13/$ – see front matter © 2013 Elsevier Inc. All rights reserved.

cervical spine pathology (5%).[2] Although there is no evidence that the incidence and type of rotator cuff pathology varies according to race, age and physical activity seem to be influential.[3]

ANATOMY AND PATHOPHYSIOLOGY

The rotator cuff consists of 4 muscles: the supraspinatus, infraspinatus, subscapularis, and teres minor. Individually, these muscles internally rotate (subscapularis), externally rotate (infraspinatus, teres minor), and abduct (supraspinatus) the humeral head. Collectively, these 4 muscles depress the humeral head within the glenoid. In cases of chronic "massive" rotator cuff tears, (ie, tears involving multiple tendons), deltoid overpull causes superior migration of the humeral head and so-called rotator cuff tear arthropathy (**Fig. 1**).

The supraspinatus and subscapularis tendons are prone to impingement by the acromion, coracoacromial ligament, acromioclavicular joint, and/or the coracoid process during the tendons' courses through potentially narrow subacromial and subcoracoid spaces, respectively. Theoretically, impingement can result in inflammatory changes that can progress to tendinosis and secondary degeneration of these tendons. Ultimately this degeneration may contribute to tendon weakness, easy fatigability, and, potentially, a full-thickness rotator cuff tear.

CLINICAL PRESENTATION

Rotator cuff injuries can present acutely, chronically, or acute-on-chronic. Acute onset of pain often occurs as the sequela of a traumatic event, such as falling onto the shoulder or lifting a heavy object. Although they can affect any individual, acute injuries typically occur in younger populations,[4] and can be associated with a dramatic increase in pain and rapid decline in function. Chronic injuries tend to afflict older adults[4] or those subjected to repetitive overhead activities, such as overhead athletes and laborers. These patients experience a more subtle, gradual decrease in strength. Some with

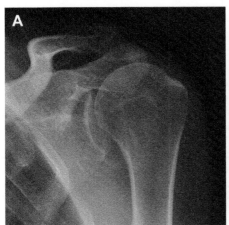
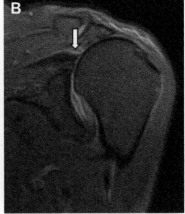

Fig. 1. (*A*) Radiographic image of rotator cuff tear arthropathy, whereby the humeral head is elevated relative to the glenoid and abuts on the undersurface of the acromion. (*B*) Rotator cuff tear arthropathy occurs in the setting of a chronic, massive rotator cuff tear usually involving at least supraspinatus (*arrow*) and infraspinatus tendons.

chronic pathology describe a seemingly innocuous event that triggers an acute worsening of symptoms, known as acute-on-chronic injury.

PATIENT HISTORY

Rotator cuff abnormality usually presents as a dull, aching pain in the anterolateral aspect of the shoulder and lateral deltoid region. The pain peaks toward the end of the day and increases during overhead activities with the arm abducted greater than 90°. A common complaint is night pain and difficulty sleeping on the affected side. While often a reliable harbinger of rotator cuff disorder, pain is by no means ubiquitous. One study demonstrated that up to half of asymptomatic subjects older than 60 years have a full-thickness or partial-thickness rotator cuff tear on magnetic resonance imaging (MRI).[3]

Weakness, especially during arm abduction, is a more variable finding in rotator cuff pathology. Often, the amount of weakness during arm abduction correlates with the extent of abnormality; that is, partial-thickness supraspinatus tendon tears demonstrate more resistive strength than full-thickness massive tears. However, even those with massive cuff tears can have remarkable resistive strength, owing to compensation by the deltoid and other accessory muscles.

Numbness and tingling are only rarely associated with rotator cuff disorder. Therefore if these symptoms are present, an alternative diagnosis of neurologic origin, for example, cervical radiculopathy, should be suspected.

PHYSICAL EXAMINATION

Although much attention has been focused in the literature on the accuracy of specific maneuvers to diagnose various ailments, the physical examination should include the basics of any musculoskeletal evaluation: observation, palpation, range of motion, motor strength, sensation, and pulses. Whenever possible, these findings should be compared with those from the contralateral limb.

Observation of the patient should be performed with full exposure of the affected extremity. The patient should be inspected anteriorly and posteriorly, and any muscle asymmetry, such as wasting within the deltoid or supraspinatus and infraspinatus fossae, or abnormal bulges (**Fig. 2**) should be noted. In cases of massive rotator

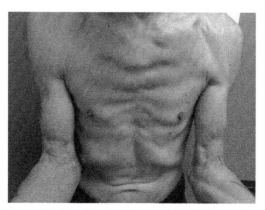

Fig. 2. The classic "Popeye" deformity of a depressed, bulged lateral portion of the biceps (*right*) occurs secondary to a rupture of the long head of the biceps tendon proximally.

cuff tears with humeral head elevation, the humeral head often can be appreciated as a bulge anteriorly within the shoulder. Scapular winging, often seen as protrusion or prominence of the inferomedial border of the scapula, may be present with rotator cuff injury and/or represent an injury to the long thoracic or spinal accessory nerves.

Though not as diagnostically powerful in the shoulder as in other joints, palpation remains a useful tool for diagnosing shoulder injuries. All bony prominences and joints should be palpated for areas of tenderness. Although tenderness along the anterior and posterior glenohumeral joint is elicited in many patients with intra-articular and subacromial injuries, palpation of superficial structures, such as the acromioclavicular joint and the tendon of the long head of the biceps, can pinpoint vague symptoms to a specific location.

Both passive and active range of motion should be performed in each of the 3 planes of motion (flexion-extension, internal-external rotation, abduction-adduction) and compared with findings from the contralateral shoulder. Rotation should be tested at 0° and 90° of shoulder abduction. The normal ranges of shoulder motion are listed in **Table 1**. Overhead athletes can develop physiologic decreases in internal rotation with the arm at 90° of abduction. However, these athletes have an increase in external rotation and, therefore, total arch of motion is preserved. Any limitation of active motion in comparison with passive motion suggests an injury to the musculotendinous unit. If both active and passive ranges of motion are diminished equally, a diagnosis of adhesive capsulitis would be suggested.

Motor testing includes evaluation of specific cervical spine roots (**Table 2**) and shoulder functions. Shoulder abduction strength can be tested by resistance of abduction, either perpendicular to the axial skeleton or parallel to the plane of the scapula (angled 30°–40° anteriorly). The latter position more specifically isolates the supraspinatus muscle. Internal rotation and integrity of the subscapularis tendon are evaluated by the patient's ability to push the hand off the lower back (lift-off test) or bring the elbows forward while the hands are held pressed against the abdomen (belly-press test). With the arm held against the body and the elbow flexed to 90°, strength of external rotation (infraspinatus and teres minor) can be assessed by asking the patient to rotate the arm laterally from a neutral position.

DIAGNOSTIC TESTING

A battery of provocative tests is available for diagnosing various shoulder ailments. Published reports of the effectiveness of these tests in predicting abnormalities are highly variable. **Table 3** lists some of the more commonly used tests for detecting rotator cuff pathology, and their respective sensitivities and specificities.

Table 1 Normal ranges of shoulder motion	
Motion	**Normal Range (Degree)**
Forward flexion	166.7 ± 4.7
Backward extension	62.3 ± 9.5
Internal rotation	68.8 ± 4.6
External rotation	103.7 ± 8.5
Neutral abduction	184.0 ± 7.0

Data from Boone DC, Azen SP. Normal range of motion of joints in male subjects. J Bone Joint Surg Am 1979;61(5):756–9.

Table 2
Evaluation of specific cervical spine roots

Cervical Root	Motor Testing	Sensation Testing
C5	Shoulder abduction	Lateral shoulder
C6	Elbow flexion	Lateral forearm and thumb
C7	Elbow extension, wrist flexion	Middle finger
C8	Wrist extension	Medial 2 digits
T1	Finger abduction	Medial arm

DIAGNOSTIC IMAGING

Physical examination and diagnostic imaging should be performed to determine the stage of disease and identify any abnormality that may be contributory. A thorough shoulder examination should be performed on all patients complaining of shoulder pain, with radiographs and advanced imaging, such as ultrasonography and MRI, reserved for those patients who have either failed a trial of conservative treatment or have a high probability of a rotator cuff tear and wish to proceed with surgical intervention.

A standard impingement series consists of anteroposterior, axillary lateral, and outlet views, which help define the morphology of the anterior acromion (**Fig. 3**). Radiographic imaging can be a less expensive method of ruling out other sources of shoulder pain, such as calcific tendinitis (**Fig. 4**A), glenohumeral arthritis (see **Fig. 4**B), and proximal humerus fractures (see **Fig. 4**C); each can mimic rotator cuff tears.

MRI has become the modality of choice for imaging the soft-tissue structures, such as the rotator cuff tendons. MRI is noninvasive, readily available, and details the entire shoulder region with high accuracy. Several studies report values approaching 100% sensitivity and specificity of MRI for detection of full-thickness supraspinatus tears.[5–7]

Table 3
Commonly used tests for detecting rotator cuff abnormality

Test	Technique	Diagnosis	Sensitivity (%)	Specificity (%)
Neer	Pain with forced forward elevation	Impingement	39–89	31–98
Hawkins	Pain with internal rotation at 90° shoulder abduction	Impingement	72–95	31–78
Jobe (empty can)	Weakness and/or pain with resisted abduction above 90° with the shoulder internally rotated and angled forward 30°	Rotator cuff tear	41–81	50–98
External rotation lag sign	Inability to hold arm in position after passively placed in maximum external rotation with elbow against the body and flexed to 90°	Rotator cuff tear	69–98	72–98

Data from Tennent TD, Beach WR, Meyers JF. A review of the special tests associated with shoulder examination. Part I: the rotator cuff tests. Am J Sports Med 2003;31(1):154–60; and Hegedus EJ, et al. Physical examination tests of the shoulder: a systematic review with meta-analysis of individual tests. Br J Sports Med 2008;42(2):80–92 [discussion: 92].

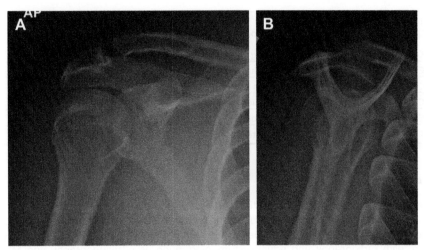

Fig. 3. Radiographs taken in the anteroposterior (AP) (*A*) and outlet (*B*) projections are useful in determining the contour of the acromion, which in this case has a hooked appearance. Acromial morphology, including a curved or hooked contour of the anterior acromion in the sagittal projection, is thought to contribute to rotator cuff abnormality.

The major limitation of MRI is its relatively high cost. Another disadvantage is a higher false-positive rate, particularly in imaging rotator cuff abnormality in older patients.

MRI should be correlated with manual motor testing of shoulder internal rotation (belly-press and lift-off tests), external rotation (external rotation lag test), and abduction (Jobe test) to determine the integrity of the subscapularis, infraspinatus/teres minor, and supraspinatus muscles, respectively. Failure to do so may subject patients to unnecessary and overly aggressive treatment, as studies have demonstrated that rotator cuff abnormalities are detected in up to 35% of MRI[3] and 23% of ultrasonography[8] examinations performed in asymptomatic shoulders.

Ultrasonography is another noninvasive alternative for imaging soft-tissue structures in the shoulder area. Unlike MRI, ultrasonography allows for a dynamic assessment of the rotator cuff tendons. While relatively inexpensive, ultrasonography is limited by the availability and skill of radiologists trained to interpret these studies.

Shoulder arthrography, or imaging of the shoulder following percutaneous injection of a contrast agent into the glenohumeral joint, is generally reserved for cases whereby traditional imaging methods do not clearly delineate suspected abnormality. Administration of a contrast agent, such as gadolinium, outlines normal structures more clearly, and assists in identifying any abnormalities by extravasation of dye into any defects or tears. Magnetic resonance arthrography is particularly useful in assessing partial-thickness rotator cuff tears, which can be overestimated or underestimated on noncontrast images.[5,9–11] Benefits of gadolinium-enhanced MRI should be weighed against potential negative renal consequences.[12]

Computed tomography (CT) can be performed with or without contrast injected into the glenohumeral joint. Though largely supplanted by MRI, contrast-enhanced CT remains a backup technique for visualizing the rotator cuff tendons in those unable to undergo the former procedure and without access to ultrasonography (**Fig. 5**). At least one study confirms that the sensitivity and specificity of CT arthrography are comparable with those of magnetic resonance arthrography in identifying supraspinatus, infraspinatus, and subscapularis tendon tears.[13]

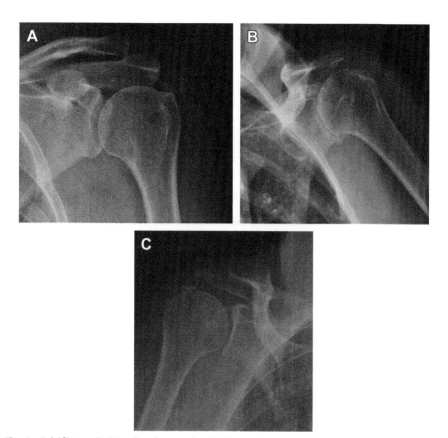

Fig. 4. Calcific tendinitis, glenohumeral arthritis, and proximal humerus fractures can present similarly to rotator cuff tears but are clearly distinguished radiographically. (A) Calcific tendinitis characteristically demonstrates a radio-opacity within the distal portion of the supraspinatus tendon. (B) Narrowing of the glenohumeral joint space is a hallmark finding of glenohumeral arthritis, and is best delineated on true AP or Grashey views. (C) A fracture line and/or displacement involving a tuberosity and/or humeral head are usually seen on radiographs, although occasionally magnetic resonance imaging is required to visualize a nondisplaced fracture.

DIAGNOSTIC DILEMMAS AND DIFFERENTIALS

The cause of shoulder pain is usually confined to the subacromial space, with rotator cuff tendinopathy and impingement involved in 85% and 74%, respectively.[14] Therefore, the tasks of the clinician are to (1) rule out other causes of shoulder pain, and (2) determine the stage of rotator cuff disease (eg, subacromial bursitis, partial-thickness tear, massive retracted tear).

The differential diagnosis of shoulder pain depends largely on the patient's age. In those aged 30 years and younger, the rotator cuff tendons are generally healthy and robust and, unless subjected to repetitive overhead activities, less likely to be the source of symptoms. Although rotator cuff pathology accounts for the vast majority of shoulder pain in patients older than 30 years, adhesive capsulitis and glenohumeral arthritis are not uncommon in this age group.[14] Adhesive capsulitis and glenohumeral osteoarthritis must be differentiated from rotator cuff abnormality because these

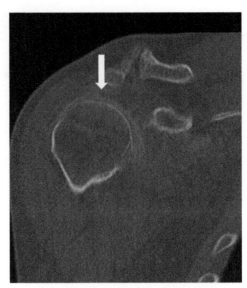

Fig. 5. Though not commonly used, computed tomographic arthrography can provide a clear image of the rotator cuff tendons and adequate characterization of a tear (*arrow*).

entities often change expectations and the course of treatment. Both adhesive capsulitis and glenohumeral osteoarthritis present with asymmetric, limited passive shoulder external rotation, and respond favorably to intra-articular corticosteroid injections. By contrast, those with massive rotator cuff tears with infraspinatus involvement demonstrate active loss of external rotation but maintain passive motion.

The stage of rotator cuff disease is important in developing appropriate treatment strategy. A more surgically aggressive approach may be considered in those with a full-thickness tear than in those suffering from subacromial impingement. The Jobe test is often used to differentiate the two entities: weakness suggests a high-grade partial-thickness or full-thickness supraspinatus tear. However, pain produced by subacromial bursitis can limit patient effort and cause false positives. Advanced imaging such as ultrasonography or MRI is often necessary to elucidate the integrity of the rotator cuff tendons.

Biceps tendinopathy and acromioclavicular joint arthritis can occur in isolation or may be associated with rotator cuff pathology. Given a high association with other diagnoses, the contributions of the biceps tendon and acromioclavicular joint abnormalities to symptoms are difficult diagnostic and treatment dilemmas. Various physical examination tests, such as the Speed and Yergason tests for bicipital tendinopathy and cross-arm adduction for acromioclavicular joint arthritis, have been proposed to delineate the effects of these entities on symptoms (**Table 4**). As for provocative testing for rotator cuff pathology, the sensitivity and specificity of each test are highly variable.[15,16]

PROGNOSIS

Impingement without evidence of rotator cuff injury affects up to 27% adults complaining of shoulder pain,[17] and generally can be successfully managed nonoperatively in 67% with a combination of physical therapy and nonsteroidal

Table 4
Tests associated with biceps tendon and acromioclavicular joint abnormalities

Test	Technique	Sensitivity (%)	Specificity (%)
Speed	Pain in bicipital groove with resisted forward elevation and elbow extended and forearm supinated	6–68	67–98
Yergason	Pain in bicipital groove with resisted elbow supination and elbow flexed to 90°, and forearm pronated	12–43	79–98
Cross-arm adduction	Pain with shoulder maximally adducted across body	77	79

Data from Tennent TD, Beach WR, Meyers JF. A review of the special tests associated with shoulder examination. Part I: the rotator cuff tests. Am J Sports Med 2003;31(1):154–60; and Hegedus EJ, et al. Physical examination tests of the shoulder: a systematic review with meta-analysis of individual tests. Br J Sports Med 2008;42(2):80–92 [discussion: 92].

anti-inflammatory drugs (NSAIDs).[18] Those with impingement symptoms tend to progress to more advanced rotator cuff disease even if acromioplasty is performed.[19] Neither partial-thickness nor full-thickness tears have a propensity to heal spontaneously.[20,21] However, many tears can be asymptomatic: 28% of those older than 60 years have an asymptomatic full-thickness rotator cuff tear confirmed by MRI.[3]

Partial-thickness tears, which can affect either the articular or bursal surface of the tendon, have a more variable prognosis. Because of the presumed, ongoing extrinsic compression of the tendon beneath the acromion, bursal surface partial tears are less likely to respond to nonoperative measures, such as activity modification, physical therapy, and steroid injections, and often require acromioplasty and tendon repair for alleviation of symptoms. Conversely, symptoms produced by articular-sided partial tears, which are 2 to 3 times more common than bursal tears,[22] can be mitigated by a course of physical therapy, a steroid injection, activity modification, and/or medication. There are conflicting reports on partial-thickness tear progression within 2 years: one study reports that only 8% of partial-thickness tears can be expected to increase in size at a minimum of 6 months,[20] whereas another reported 81% of partial tears either increased in size or became full-thickness at a mean of 412 days.[21]

Prognosis of full-thickness tears depends largely on the size and chronicity of the tear. Nearly 50% of those with a full-thickness tear can expect to have an increase in tear size after 18 months.[20] Tear progression is associated with patient age older than 60 years, fatty infiltration, and size of tear.[20] Only 25% of those with small supraspinatus tears experience worsening of the tear within 3.5 years.[23] Pain, especially in those with previously asymptomatic tears, predicts progression of tear size greater than 5 mm.[24] Successful long-term outcomes, especially following surgical repair, are inversely correlated with the size of the tear: the larger the tear, the worse the outcome and the higher chance for retear.[25]

Acute tears, especially if treated within a few months, tend to have more favorable results attributable to increased excursion of the tendon. Fatty infiltration involving greater than 50% of the muscle belly and retraction beyond the glenoid signal a chronic tear and portend a poor prognosis for successful repair.[26] There is evidence to suggest that, even though symptoms may remain stable, a 4-year delay in treatment of a massive tear may render a previously fixable tear irreparable.[27]

MANAGEMENT GOALS

The guiding goals of management are focused on: (1) resolving pain, especially at night and with overhead activity; and (2) restoring function individually defined by range of motion and strength. Each management plan should be tailored to the demands and overall health of each individual. For example, the threshold for surgical intervention is likely considerably lower for a 35-year-old laborer than for an 85-year-old retiree with multiple medical comorbidities. Factors associated with unfavorable outcome following nonoperative treatment include rotator cuff tear size greater than 1 cm, pretreatment symptoms longer than 1 year, and significant functional impairment at the time of initial presentation.[28] In these patients, operative intervention should be considered early in the treatment plan to avoid a prolonged clinical course.[28]

Each care plan should carefully consider the potential consequences of each treatment, such as surgical complications, and expected natural history if no treatment is undertaken. Any patient electing nonoperative management of a full-thickness rotator cuff tear should understand that, if repair is not undertaken, the musculotendinous complex may retract and/or atrophy, or the tear may enlarge and render the tear irreparable or increase the retear rate.

PHARMACOLOGIC STRATEGIES

Whether self-medicated or prescribed by a physician, NSAIDs are often the initial management for those suffering from rotator cuff abnormality.[29] Scientific studies have confirmed a biological mechanism for their efficacy: cyclooxygenase-2 inhibitors can produce a decrease in the levels of stromal cell-derived factor 1, an important cytokine associated with production of bursal inflammation.[30] Although the biological effects of NSAIDs can be beneficial in the nonoperative management of rotator cuff disease, these agents should be avoided in the perioperative period, as NSAIDs have been associated with inhibited healing of tendon to bone.[31] Furthermore, oral NSAIDs, while effective in treating rotator cuff tendinitis, have been shown to produce gains equal (indomethacin) or inferior (diclofenac) in pain reduction, range of motion, and function when compared with subacromial corticosteroid injections (triamcinolone).[32,33]

Subacromial corticosteroid injections are administered to decrease painful inflammation within the subacromial bursa, and thus improve scapulohumeral mechanics[34] and deltoid firing patterns.[35] Studies have demonstrated effectiveness of subacromial corticosteroid/local anesthetic injections in up to 90% of patients within 4 weeks.[36] The beneficial effects of subacromial steroid injections are often short lived: a recent study reported that 40% of patients who underwent a subacromial corticosteroid injection for rotator cuff tendinopathy elected to have surgical intervention within 1 year.[37] Though not reaching significance, the presence of a full-thickness tear portends a higher likelihood of requiring surgery.[37]

Corticosteroids can be injected into the subacromial bursa via several approaches, anterior, lateral, or posterior. In all methods the acromion is palpated, and the needle is directed inferior to the acromial edge and superior to the rotator cuff tendon. Many providers prefer injecting posteriorly beneath the acromion, although at least one study has suggested that injections beneath the lateral acromion may be the ideal route of administration and are accurate in 92%.[38] In the same study, the posterior route was accurate in only 56% and only 38% in females.[38] Other studies have found all methods equally accurate,[39–41] with 66% to 83% of injections reaching the subacromial space.[39–42] Of note, only one study maintained that only accurate injections produce relief of symptoms[43]; the remainder asserted that accuracy of injections does not correlate with clinical improvement.[39–41]

Dosing and timing between injections remain largely empiric and vary between clinicians. Though not clearly elucidated, there appears to be a link between corticosteroid injection and tendon weakening or rupture, especially with repeated injections.[44,45] Tenocytes appear to be particularly sensitive to corticosteroid injections,[46–48] but a single injection in diseased tendon does not appear to be harmful.[49] Most clinicians prefer to avoid performing subacromial injections less than 3 months apart and to limit the total number of injections in each shoulder to 3.[4] Scientific evidence supporting this practice, however, is lacking.[50]

Recently, subacromial injections of local anesthetics, sodium hyaluronate, and NSAIDs have been offered as an alternative to injection of corticosteroid. Subacromial injections of local anesthetics (xylocaine) were performed in similar fashion to corticosteroid injections (betamethasone) in a level I study that examined patients at 2 and 6 weeks after injection.[51] Sodium hyaluronate injected subacromially for 5 consecutive weeks yielded improved clinical outcomes at 6 weeks in comparison with a normal saline placebo injection.[52] Despite early promise on comparison with placebo injections,[53] subacromial injections of NSAIDs (tenoxicam) produced significantly inferior outcomes when compared with subacromial injection of corticosteroid (methylprednisolone) in a prospective, randomized study.[54]

Glyceryl trinitrate patches have gained some recognition as a potentially effective topical agent to treat rotator cuff abnormality.[55] One study did demonstrate positive effects of topical glyceryl trinitrate versus placebo among patients with acute symptoms; however, the study was limited by potential bias.[55] Any excitement over topical glyceryl trinitrate should be tempered by the potential for headaches.[55]

NONPHARMACOLOGIC STRATEGIES

Exercise therapy remains a mainstay of the treatment of rotator cuff abnormality, especially for tendinitis/tendinosis, partial-thickness articular-sided tears, and massive, irreparable tears. The goals of exercise therapy focus on stretching and strengthening intact rotator cuff muscles and periscapular muscles through land-based and/or aquatic-based protocols. For those with massive, irreparable tears, improving strength of the anterior deltoid is paramount to restoration of function.[56]

Initial therapeutic efforts are focused on reducing inflammation and improving the range of motion. During this phase of treatment, modalities such as cryotherapy or massage, or adjuncts such as corticosteroid injections or oral NSAIDs, can be beneficial in reducing painful inflammation. Stretching often involves remedying posterior capsular contracture, a common source of pain. Posterior capsular contracture is manifested as decreased internal rotation with the arm at 90° of abduction, and can often be successfully treated with a series of stretches including horizontal adduction and "sleeper" stretches (**Fig. 6**).[57,58]

Once pain has been managed and motion normalizes, therapeutic efforts shift toward correcting scapulothoracic dyskinesis and weakness with abduction and forward elevation, which have both been proved to lead to pain and loss of function in those with rotator cuff tears.[59] Muscles of the shoulder girdles should be targeted with an array of strengthening exercises to restore normal mechanics. Treatments directed toward improving scapular motor function[60,61] and shoulder abductors[62,63] can produce improvements in self-reported disability and pain control in those suffering from subacromial impingement.[64] Strengthening exercises should be relatively pain free, and can be performed with rubber bands and/or free weights.

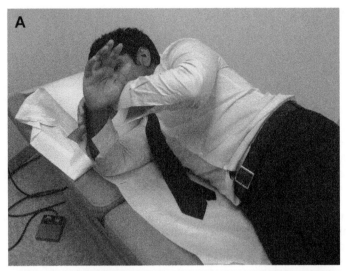

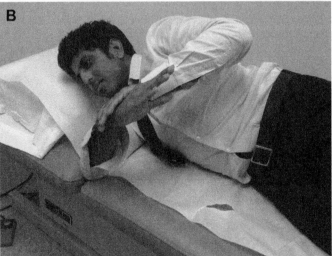

Fig. 6. "Sleeper" stretches, which are useful for stretching the posterior capsule, are performed by lying on the affected side (*A*) and pressing the forearm of the affected shoulder toward the floor (*B*).

Despite there being a dearth of level I studies, evidence suggests that exercise therapy provides at least modest benefit for those with a symptomatic, full-thickness rotator cuff tear.[65] Data guiding specifics of exercise therapy such as timing, duration, and progression of therapy remain inconclusive.[65]

Modalities such as manual therapy, transcutaneous electrical nerve stimulation, low-power laser, and hyperthermia have shown promise in treating rotator cuff pathology.[66–73] However, the precise indications for each remain unknown.

Extracorporeal shock-wave therapy has a potential role in the treatment of calcific tendinitis. Patients with calcific tendinitis experienced increases in range of motion and strength, and decreases pain and size of lesion, after treatment with extracorporeal shock-wave therapy.[74–76]

SELF-MANAGEMENT STRATEGIES

While the benefits of exercise therapy have been well documented, the role of home exercise programs has been less studied. Evidence has suggested significant improvements in pain and function can be attained for those participating in a home exercise program for rotator cuff tendinopathy.[77,78] The effectiveness of home exercise programs versus supervised, clinical programs is less clear.[77–79] Despite success with home programs preoperatively, unsupervised exercise programs following arthroscopic acromioplasty and rotator cuff repairs should be considered with caution. Significant improvements in range of motion, pain, and shoulder function were found at up to 6 months among patients who underwent formal rather than unsupervised postoperative therapy.[80,81]

SURGICAL TECHNIQUE

Despite controversies about specific technical variations (eg, open vs arthroscopic techniques, single-row vs double-row repairs), all surgical techniques that address rotator cuff tears have a common goal: reattachment of the torn tendons to the tuberosity. In the original open techniques, whereby the deltoid origin was detached to expose the underlying rotator cuff tendons, rotator cuff repair was accomplished by passing sutures through the tendon and transosseous through the greater tuberosity and tying over the bone bridge. More modern techniques involve: (1) insertion of suture anchors into the tuberosity; and (2) passage of the sutures from the anchor through the torn tendon (**Fig. 7**).

The development of suture anchors, whereby suture is shuttled through the eyelet of an anchor, and advanced instrumentation have allowed for the emergence of arthroscopic techniques. Although outcomes at 1 year postoperatively are equivalent to those for open techniques involving either detachment or splitting of deltoid muscle fibers,[82–84] arthroscopic techniques are thought to cause less trauma to the overlying deltoid muscle and to allow for more expedient recovery without risks of permanent deltoid dysfunction.[84]

The rotator cuff can be secured to the tuberosity using either a single row or 2 rows of anchors (**Fig. 8**). In a single-row repair, the tendon is "spot-welded" to a single point of fixation, whereas a dual row of anchors (double-row and transosseous equivalent techniques) allows for compression of the torn tendon over a broader surface of the exposed tuberosity. Biomechanical studies have indicated that repairs performed with 2 rows of anchors have higher load to failure[85–87] and lower displacement[88–90] than single-row repairs, and may improve tendon healing.[91–93] However, the biomechanical advantage of a dual-row repair has not been matched clinically: no study has definitively proved that double-row repairs produce clinical outcomes superior to those after single-row repairs.[83,92,94,95] Proponents of single-row repairs argue that double-row repairs are more costly, both financially and temporally, and may cause more difficult revisions.[96]

Acromioplasty and/or biceps tenodesis/tenotomy in the setting of a rotator cuff tear remain controversial, and are often evaluated on a case-by-case basis. The role of acromioplasty, which involves recontouring of the anterior acromion to create a smooth surface that does not impinge on the underlying supraspinatus tendon, has been questioned.[83,97,98] Despite the controversy, most clinicians concur that anterior acromioplasty should be considered in those with a hooked anterior acromion and/or bursal-sided partial-thickness rotator cuff tendon tear. Similarly, biceps abnormality, if present, can be addressed with tenotomy or tenodesis. Tenotomy is generally reserved for those aged 60 years and older, and can be expected to result in 70% of patients with

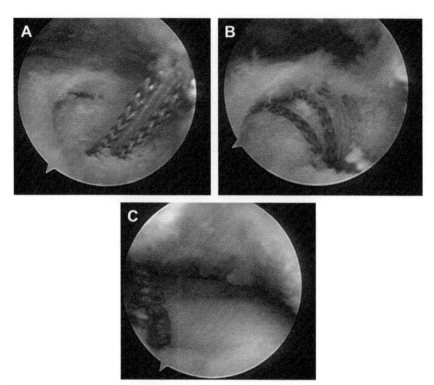

Fig. 7. To perform an arthroscopic rotator cuff repair, an anchor containing sutures is passed into the exposed tuberosity (*A*). Sutures from the anchor are passed through the tendon (*B*) and secured to reapproximate tendon to the tuberosity (*C*).

a "Popeye" sign, 38% complaining of fatigue discomfort with resisted elbow flexion, and none with arm pain at rest.[99] If tenodesis is performed, the long head of the biceps can be reattached to the rotator interval,[100] the short head of biceps tendon,[101] or the proximal humerus, either proximally within or distal to the bicipital groove.[102,103]

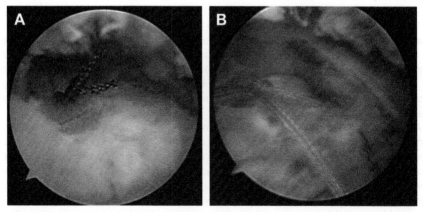

Fig. 8. Arthroscopic repairs are performed using either 1 (*A*) or 2 (*B*) rows of anchors. Though repairs using 2 rows of anchors appear biomechanically stronger, no technique has proved to be clinically superior.

SURGICAL COMPLICATIONS

The overall retear rate among surgically repaired rotator cuff tendons is 19% at 6 months.[25] Large and massive tears account for a significant proportion of these tears.[25] Among patients who underwent repair of a massive rotator cuff tear (ie, a tear involving at least 2 tendons), 37% to 94% suffered a retear.[25,104–106] Despite retear, the overwhelming majority of patients still report improvement of their symptoms, even at long-term follow-up.[104,105,107,108]

Adhesive capsulitis or "frozen shoulder" occurs in roughly 5% of repairs,[109] and is more common among those with type I diabetes, hypothyroidism, long duration of immobilization,[110] old age,[111] and smaller tears. While many patients respond favorably with physical therapy, some require manipulation under anesthesia and/or arthroscopic capsular release.[112]

Infection is rare among those undergoing a rotator cuff repair. Only case reports, mostly superficial infections, are found in the literature.[113–115]

Cerebrovascular accidents caused by cerebral hypoperfusion represent another rare but potentially devastating complication during rotator cuff surgery. Cerebral hypoperfusion has almost exclusively been reported among those undergoing shoulder surgery performed in the beach-chair position, whereby the patient sits upright on the operative table during the procedure.[116,117] This regional hypoperfusion may cause transient ischemia and stroke.

DISCUSSION AND SUMMARY

Most pathology that produces symptoms within the shoulder occurs within the subacromial space, the space between the undersurface of the acromion and the humeral head. Within this space, irritation of the subacromial bursae and pathologic changes of the rotator cuff tendons resulting from a combination of overactivity, narrowing of the subacromial space, and/or age-related degeneration proceed through a sequence of events that may result in a full-thickness rotator cuff tear.

Because the subacromial space is maximally narrowed during shoulder abduction and flexion, most patients suffering from rotator cuff pathology complain of symptoms when performing overhead activities or sleeping, presumably because the humeral head is either directly compressed or positioned in abduction. Provocative tests, such as the Neer, Hawkins, and Jobe, elicit symptoms by decreasing the available subacromial space and/or stressing the supraspinatus tendon.

Determining the severity of rotator cuff abnormality is the foundation for formulating a treatment plan. When bursal inflammation and/or rotator cuff tendinosis is suspected, less aggressive diagnostic imaging and treatment strategies are selected because these conditions often respond to nonoperative therapy, including rest, activity modification, NSAIDs, subacromial corticosteroid injections, and exercise therapy. More advanced disease, such as a full-thickness rotator cuff tear, often require surgical intervention to restore functions. Physical examination and diagnostic imaging, especially MRI, are critical in determining the severity of disease.

Most treatment protocols start with a combination of anti-inflammatory medications given orally and/or injected and exercise therapy. Anti-inflammatory medications are given before initiation of exercise therapy to minimize pain and maximize therapy efforts. Exercise therapy progresses from restoration of motion to periscapular and rotator cuff muscle strengthening. Factors that portend a worse prognosis for successful nonoperative management include a rotator cuff tear greater than 1 cm, pretreatment symptoms lasting longer than 1 year, and functional impairment.[28]

Surgical intervention should be reserved for anyone who has failed conservative methods and/or young and middle-aged patients with a full-thickness rotator cuff tear, functional impairment, and a desire to undergo immediate surgical intervention. Earlier repair of rotator cuff tears may minimize the size of the tendon injury, which can progress.[20]

Surgical procedures consist of repairing the torn rotator cuff tendons and/or anterior acromioplasty (flattening of the anterior acromion) to decrease impingement within the subacromial space. Biceps tenotomy or tenodesis and/or distal clavicle excision can be performed as symptoms warrant. Rotator cuff repairs can be performed using open or arthroscopic techniques, and using a single or dual row of anchors. All techniques consistently reduce pain and increase function. No one surgical method has been definitively proved to be clinically superior to the others, and the benefits and risks of each must be weighed. Retear rates following rotator cuff repair approach 25%[25] and are associated with larger-sized tears.[25,104–106]

REFERENCES

1. Urwin M, Symmons D, Allison T, et al. Estimating the burden of musculoskeletal disorders in the community: the comparative prevalence of symptoms at different anatomical sites, and the relation to social deprivation. Ann Rheum Dis 1998;57(11):649–55.
2. Vecchio P, Kavanagh R, Hazleman BL, et al. Shoulder pain in a community-based rheumatology clinic. Br J Rheumatol 1995;34(5):440–2.
3. Sher JS, Uribe JW, Posada A, et al. Abnormal findings on magnetic resonance images of asymptomatic shoulders. J Bone Joint Surg Am 1995;77(1):10–5.
4. Green A. Chronic massive rotator cuff tears: evaluation and management. J Am Acad Orthop Surg 2003;11(5):321–31.
5. Balich SM, Sheley RC, Brown TR, et al. MR imaging of the rotator cuff tendon: interobserver agreement and analysis of interpretive errors. Radiology 1997; 204(1):191–4.
6. Singson RD, Hoang T, Dan S, et al. MR evaluation of rotator cuff pathology using T2-weighted fast spin-echo technique with and without fat suppression. AJR Am J Roentgenol 1996;166(5):1061–5.
7. Reinus WR, Shady KL, Mirowitz SA, et al. MR diagnosis of rotator cuff tears of the shoulder: value of using T2-weighted fat-saturated images. AJR Am J Roentgenol 1995;164(6):1451–5.
8. Tempelhof S, Rupp S, Seil R. Age-related prevalence of rotator cuff tears in asymptomatic shoulders. J Shoulder Elbow Surg 1999;8(4):296–9.
9. Smith TO, Daniell H, Geere JA, et al. The diagnostic accuracy of MRI for the detection of partial- and full-thickness rotator cuff tears in adults. Magn Reson Imaging 2012;30(3):336–46.
10. Jung JY, Jee WH, Chun HJ, et al. Magnetic resonance arthrography including ABER view in diagnosing partial-thickness tears of the rotator cuff: accuracy, and inter- and intra-observer agreements. Acta Radiol 2010;51(2):194–201.
11. Spencer EE Jr, Dunn WR, Wright RW, et al. Interobserver agreement in the classification of rotator cuff tears using magnetic resonance imaging. Am J Sports Med 2008;36(1):99–103.
12. Steinbach LS, Palmer WE, Schweitzer ME. Special focus session. MR arthrography. Radiographics 2002;22(5):1223–46.
13. Charousset C, Bellaiche L, Duranthon LD, et al. Accuracy of CT arthrography in the assessment of tears of the rotator cuff. J Bone Joint Surg Br 2005;87(6):824–8.

14. Ostor AJ, Richards CA, Prevost AT, et al. Diagnosis and relation to general health of shoulder disorders presenting to primary care. Rheumatology (Oxford) 2005;44(6):800–5.
15. Tennent TD, Beach WR, Meyers JF. A review of the special tests associated with shoulder examination. Part I: the rotator cuff tests. Am J Sports Med 2003;31(1):154–60.
16. Hegedus EJ, Goode A, Campbell S, et al. Physical examination tests of the shoulder: a systematic review with meta-analysis of individual tests. Br J Sports Med 2008;42(2):80–92 [discussion: 92].
17. Pribicevic M, Pollard H, Bonello R. An epidemiologic survey of shoulder pain in chiropractic practice in Australia. J Manipulative Physiol Ther 2009;32(2):107–17.
18. Morrison DS, Frogameni AD, Woodworth P. Non-operative treatment of subacromial impingement syndrome. J Bone Joint Surg Am 1997;79(5):732–7.
19. Hyvonen P, Lohi S, Jalovaara P. Open acromioplasty does not prevent the progression of an impingement syndrome to a tear. Nine-year follow-up of 96 cases. J Bone Joint Surg Br 1998;80(5):813–6.
20. Maman E, Harris C, White L, et al. Outcome of nonoperative treatment of symptomatic rotator cuff tears monitored by magnetic resonance imaging. J Bone Joint Surg Am 2009;91(8):1898–906.
21. Yamanaka K, Matsumoto T. The joint side tear of the rotator cuff. A followup study by arthrography. Clin Orthop Relat Res 1994;(304):68–73.
22. Wolff AB, Sethi P, Sutton KM, et al. Partial-thickness rotator cuff tears. J Am Acad Orthop Surg 2006;14(13):715–25.
23. Fucentese SF, von Roll AL, Pfirrmann CW, et al. Evolution of nonoperatively treated symptomatic isolated full-thickness supraspinatus tears. J Bone Joint Surg Am 2012;94(9):801–8.
24. Mall NA, Kim HM, Keener JD, et al. Symptomatic progression of asymptomatic rotator cuff tears: a prospective study of clinical and sonographic variables. J Bone Joint Surg Am 2010;92(16):2623–33.
25. Wu XL, Briggs L, Murrell GA. Intraoperative determinants of rotator cuff repair integrity: an analysis of 500 consecutive repairs. Am J Sports Med 2012;40(12):2771–6.
26. Meyer DC, Wieser K, Farshad M, et al. Retraction of supraspinatus muscle and tendon as predictors of success of rotator cuff repair. Am J Sports Med 2012;40(10):2242–7.
27. Zingg PO, Jost B, Sukthankar A, et al. Clinical and structural outcomes of nonoperative management of massive rotator cuff tears. J Bone Joint Surg Am 2007;89(9):1928–34.
28. Bartolozzi A, Andreychik D, Ahmad S. Determinants of outcome in the treatment of rotator cuff disease. Clin Orthop Relat Res 1994;(308):90–7.
29. Pedowitz RA, Yamaguchi K, Ahmad CS, et al. American Academy of Orthopaedic Surgeons Clinical Practice Guideline on: optimizing the management of rotator cuff problems. J Bone Joint Surg Am 2012;94(2):163–7.
30. Kim YS, Bigliani LU, Fujisawa M, et al. Stromal cell-derived factor 1 (SDF-1, CXCL12) is increased in subacromial bursitis and downregulated by steroid and nonsteroidal anti-inflammatory agents. J Orthop Res 2006;24(8):1756–64.
31. Cohen DB, Kawamura S, Ehteshami JR, et al. Indomethacin and celecoxib impair rotator cuff tendon-to-bone healing. Am J Sports Med 2006;34(3):362–9.
32. Adebajo AO, Nash P, Hazleman BL. A prospective double blind dummy placebo controlled study comparing triamcinolone hexacetonide injection with

oral diclofenac 50 mg TDS in patients with rotator cuff tendinitis. J Rheumatol 1990;17(9):1207–10.

33. White RH, Paull DM, Fleming KW. Rotator cuff tendinitis: comparison of subacromial injection of a long acting corticosteroid versus oral indomethacin therapy. J Rheumatol 1986;13(3):608–13.

34. Scibek JS, Mell AG, Downie BK, et al. Shoulder kinematics in patients with full-thickness rotator cuff tears after a subacromial injection. J Shoulder Elbow Surg 2008;17(1):172–81.

35. Cordasco FA, Chen NC, Backus SI, et al. Subacromial injection improves deltoid firing in subjects with large rotator cuff tears. HSS J 2010;6(1):30–6.

36. Yu CM, Chen CH, Liu HT, et al. Subacromial injections of corticosteroids and xylocaine for painful subacromial impingement syndrome. Chang Gung Med J 2006;29(5):474–9.

37. Contreras F, Brown HC, Marx RG. Predictors of success of corticosteroid injection for the management of rotator cuff disease. HSS J 2013;9:2–5.

38. Marder RA, Kim SH, Labson JD, et al. Injection of the subacromial bursa in patients with rotator cuff syndrome: a prospective, randomized study comparing the effectiveness of different routes. J Bone Joint Surg Am 2012;94(16):1442–7.

39. Dogu B, Yucel SD, Sag SY, et al. Blind or ultrasound-guided corticosteroid injections and short-term response in subacromial impingement syndrome: a randomized, double-blind, prospective study. Am J Phys Med Rehabil 2012; 91(8):658–65.

40. Kang MN, Rizio L, Prybicien M, et al. The accuracy of subacromial corticosteroid injections: a comparison of multiple methods. J Shoulder Elbow Surg 2008;17(Suppl 1):61S–6S.

41. Yamakado K. The targeting accuracy of subacromial injection to the shoulder: an arthrographic evaluation. Arthroscopy 2002;18(8):887–91.

42. Partington PF, Broome GH. Diagnostic injection around the shoulder: hit and miss? A cadaveric study of injection accuracy. J Shoulder Elbow Surg 1998; 7(2):147–50.

43. Henkus HE, Cobben LP, Coerkamp EG, et al. The accuracy of subacromial injections: a prospective randomized magnetic resonance imaging study. Arthroscopy 2006;22(3):277–82.

44. Tillander B, Franzen LE, Karlsson MH, et al. Effect of steroid injections on the rotator cuff: an experimental study in rats. J Shoulder Elbow Surg 1999;8(3): 271–4.

45. Akpinar S, Hersekli MA, Demirors H, et al. Effects of methylprednisolone and betamethasone injections on the rotator cuff: an experimental study in rats. Adv Ther 2002;19(4):194–201.

46. Tempfer H, Gehwolf R, Lehner C, et al. Effects of crystalline glucocorticoid triamcinolone acetonide on cultured human supraspinatus tendon cells. Acta Orthop 2009;80(3):357–62.

47. Scutt N, Rolf CG, Scutt A. Glucocorticoids inhibit tenocyte proliferation and Tendon progenitor cell recruitment. J Orthop Res 2006;24(2):173–82.

48. Wong MW, Tang YN, Fu SC, et al. Triamcinolone suppresses human tenocyte cellular activity and collagen synthesis. Clin Orthop Relat Res 2004;(421):277–81.

49. Wei AS, Callaci JJ, Juknelis D, et al. The effect of corticosteroid on collagen expression in injured rotator cuff tendon. J Bone Joint Surg Am 2006;88(6):1331–8.

50. Bhatia M, Singh B, Nicolaou N, et al. Correlation between rotator cuff tears and repeated subacromial steroid injections: a case-controlled study. Ann R Coll Surg Engl 2009;91(5):414–6.

51. Alvarez CM, Litchfield R, Jackowski D, et al. A prospective, double-blind, randomized clinical trial comparing subacromial injection of betamethasone and xylocaine to xylocaine alone in chronic rotator cuff tendinosis. Am J Sports Med 2005;33(2):255–62.

52. Chou WY, Ko JY, Wang FS, et al. Effect of sodium hyaluronate treatment on rotator cuff lesions without complete tears: a randomized, double-blind, placebo-controlled study. J Shoulder Elbow Surg 2010;19(4):557–63.

53. Itzkowitch D, Ginsberg F, Leon M, et al. Peri-articular injection of tenoxicam for painful shoulders: a double-blind, placebo controlled trial. Clin Rheumatol 1996; 15(6):604–9.

54. Karthikeyan S, Kwong HT, Upadhyay PK, et al. A double-blind randomised controlled study comparing subacromial injection of tenoxicam or methylprednisolone in patients with subacromial impingement. J Bone Joint Surg Br 2010;92(1):77–82.

55. Cumpston M, Johnston RV, Wengier L, et al. Topical glyceryl trinitrate for rotator cuff disease. Cochrane Database Syst Rev 2009;(3):CD006355.

56. Levy O, Mullett H, Roberts S, et al. The role of anterior deltoid reeducation in patients with massive irreparable degenerative rotator cuff tears. J Shoulder Elbow Surg 2008;17(6):863–70.

57. Bach HG, Goldberg BA. Posterior capsular contracture of the shoulder. J Am Acad Orthop Surg 2006;14(5):265–77.

58. Ticker JB, Beim GM, Warner JJ. Recognition and treatment of refractory posterior capsular contracture of the shoulder. Arthroscopy 2000;16(1):27–34.

59. Harris JD, Pedroza A, Jones GL. Predictors of pain and function in patients with symptomatic, atraumatic full-thickness rotator cuff tears: a time-zero analysis of a prospective patient cohort enrolled in a structured physical therapy program. Am J Sports Med 2012;40(2):359–66.

60. Struyf F, Nijs J, Mollekens S, et al. Scapular-focused treatment in patients with shoulder impingement syndrome: a randomized clinical trial. Clin Rheumatol 2013;32(1):73–85.

61. Baskurt Z, Baskurt F, Gelecek N, et al. The effectiveness of scapular stabilization exercise in the patients with subacromial impingement syndrome. J Back Musculoskelet Rehabil 2011;24(3):173–9.

62. Camargo PR, Avila MA, Alburquerque-Sendin F, et al. Eccentric training for shoulder abductors improves pain, function and isokinetic performance in subjects with shoulder impingement syndrome: a case series. Rev Bras Fisioter 2012;16(1):74–83.

63. Bernhardsson S, Klintberg IH, Wendt GK. Evaluation of an exercise concept focusing on eccentric strength training of the rotator cuff for patients with subacromial impingement syndrome. Clin Rehabil 2011;25(1):69–78.

64. Holmgren T, Bjornsson Hallgren H, et al. Effect of specific exercise strategy on need for surgery in patients with subacromial impingement syndrome: randomised controlled study. BMJ 2012;344:e787.

65. Ainsworth R, Lewis JS. Exercise therapy for the conservative management of full thickness tears of the rotator cuff: a systematic review. Br J Sports Med 2007; 41(4):200–10.

66. Bialoszewski D, Zaborowski G. Usefulness of manual therapy in the rehabilitation of patients with chronic rotator cuff injuries. Preliminary report. Ortop Traumatol Rehabil 2011;13(1):9–20.

67. Tate AR, McClure PW, Young IA, et al. Comprehensive impairment-based exercise and manual therapy intervention for patients with subacromial

impingement syndrome: a case series. J Orthop Sports Phys Ther 2010; 40(8):474–93.

68. Eyigor C, Eyigor S, Kivilcim Korkmaz O. Are intra-articular corticosteroid injections better than conventional TENS in treatment of rotator cuff tendinitis in the short run? A randomized study. Eur J Phys Rehabil Med 2010;46(3):315–24.

69. Razavi M, Jansen GB. Effects of acupuncture and placebo TENS in addition to exercise in treatment of rotator cuff tendinitis. Clin Rehabil 2004;18(8):872–8.

70. Eslamian F, Shakouri SK, Ghojazadeh M, et al. Effects of low-level laser therapy in combination with physiotherapy in the management of rotator cuff tendinitis. Lasers Med Sci 2012;27(5):951–8.

71. Abrisham SM, Kermani-Alghoraishi M, Ghahramani R, et al. Additive effects of low-level laser therapy with exercise on subacromial syndrome: a randomised, double-blind, controlled trial. Clin Rheumatol 2011;30(10):1341–6.

72. Rabini A, Piazzini DB, Bertolini C, et al. Effects of local microwave diathermy on shoulder pain and function in patients with rotator cuff tendinopathy in comparison to subacromial corticosteroid injections: a single-blind randomized trial. J Orthop Sports Phys Ther 2012;42(4):363–70.

73. Di Cesare A, Giombini A, Dragoni S, et al. Calcific tendinopathy of the rotator cuff. Conservative management with 434 Mhz local microwave diathermy (hyperthermia): a case study. Disabil Rehabil 2008;30(20–22):1578–83.

74. Lee SY, Cheng B, Grimmer-Somers K. The midterm effectiveness of extracorporeal shockwave therapy in the management of chronic calcific shoulder tendinitis. J Shoulder Elbow Surg 2011;20(5):845–54.

75. Avancini-Dobrovic V, Frlan-Vrgoc L, Stamenkovic D, et al. Radial extracorporeal shock wave therapy in the treatment of shoulder calcific tendinitis. Coll Antropol 2011;35(Suppl 2):221–5.

76. Sabeti-Aschraf M, Dorotka R, Goll A, et al. Extracorporeal shock wave therapy in the treatment of calcific tendinitis of the rotator cuff. Am J Sports Med 2005; 33(9):1365–8.

77. Senbursa G, Baltaci G, Atay OA. The effectiveness of manual therapy in supraspinatus tendinopathy. Acta Orthop Traumatol Turc 2011;45(3):162–7.

78. Senbursa G, Baltaci G, Atay A. Comparison of conservative treatment with and without manual physical therapy for patients with shoulder impingement syndrome: a prospective, randomized clinical trial. Knee Surg Sports Traumatol Arthrosc 2007;15(7):915–21.

79. Bennell K, Wee E, Coburn S, et al. Efficacy of standardised manual therapy and home exercise programme for chronic rotator cuff disease: randomised placebo controlled trial. BMJ 2010;340:c2756.

80. Lisinski P, Huber J, Wilkosz P, et al. Supervised versus uncontrolled rehabilitation of patients after rotator cuff repair-clinical and neurophysiological comparative study. Int J Artif Organs 2012;35(1):45–54.

81. Holmgren T, Oberg B, Sjoberg I, et al. Supervised strengthening exercises versus home-based movement exercises after arthroscopic acromioplasty: a randomized clinical trial. J Rehabil Med 2012;44(1):12–8.

82. Kasten P, Keil C, Grieser T, et al. Prospective randomised comparison of arthroscopic versus mini-open rotator cuff repair of the supraspinatus tendon. Int Orthop 2011;35(11):1663–70.

83. Seida JC, LeBlanc C, Schouten JR, et al. Systematic review: nonoperative and operative treatments for rotator cuff tears. Ann Intern Med 2010;153(4):246–55.

84. van der Zwaal P, Thomassen BJ, Nieuwenhuijse MJ, et al. Clinical outcome in all-arthroscopic versus mini-open rotator cuff repair in small to medium-sized

tears: a randomized controlled trial in 100 patients with 1-year follow-up. Arthroscopy 2013;29(2):266–73.

85. Gerber C, Schneeberger AG, Beck M, et al. Mechanical strength of repairs of the rotator cuff. J Bone Joint Surg Br 1994;76(3):371–80.

86. Kim DH, Elattrache NS, Tibone JE, et al. Biomechanical comparison of a single-row versus double-row suture anchor technique for rotator cuff repair. Am J Sports Med 2006;34(3):407–14.

87. Meier SW, Meier JD. The effect of double-row fixation on initial repair strength in rotator cuff repair: a biomechanical study. Arthroscopy 2006;22(11):1168–73.

88. Smith CD, Alexander S, Hill AM, et al. A biomechanical comparison of single and double-row fixation in arthroscopic rotator cuff repair. J Bone Joint Surg Am 2006;88(11):2425–31.

89. Milano G, Grasso A, Zarelli D, et al. Comparison between single-row and double-row rotator cuff repair: a biomechanical study. Knee Surg Sports Traumatol Arthrosc 2008;16(1):75–80.

90. Ahmad CS, Kleweno C, Jacir AM, et al. Biomechanical performance of rotator cuff repairs with humeral rotation: a new rotator cuff repair failure model. Am J Sports Med 2008;36(5):888–92.

91. Sugaya H, Maeda K, Matsuki K, et al. Functional and structural outcome after arthroscopic full-thickness rotator cuff repair: single-row versus dual-row fixation. Arthroscopy 2005;21(11):1307–16.

92. Franceschi F, Ruzzini L, Longo UG, et al. Equivalent clinical results of arthroscopic single-row and double-row suture anchor repair for rotator cuff tears: a randomized controlled trial. Am J Sports Med 2007;35(8):1254–60.

93. Charousset C, Grimberg J, Duranthon LD, et al. Can a double-row anchorage technique improve tendon healing in arthroscopic rotator cuff repair?: A prospective, nonrandomized, comparative study of double-row and single-row anchorage techniques with computed tomographic arthrography tendon healing assessment. Am J Sports Med 2007;35(8):1247–53.

94. Koh KH, Kang KC, Lim TK, et al. Prospective randomized clinical trial of single- versus double-row suture anchor repair in 2- to 4-cm rotator cuff tears: clinical and magnetic resonance imaging results. Arthroscopy 2011;27(4):453–62.

95. Nho SJ, Slabaugh MA, Seroyer ST, et al. Does the literature support double-row suture anchor fixation for arthroscopic rotator cuff repair? A systematic review comparing double-row and single-row suture anchor configuration. Arthroscopy 2009;25(11):1319–28.

96. Dines JS, Bedi A, ElAttrache NS, et al. Single-row versus double-row rotator cuff repair: techniques and outcomes. J Am Acad Orthop Surg 2010;18(2):83–93.

97. Gartsman GM, O'Connor DP. Arthroscopic rotator cuff repair with and without arthroscopic subacromial decompression: a prospective, randomized study of one-year outcomes. J Shoulder Elbow Surg 2004;13(4):424–6.

98. Milano G, Grasso A, Salvatore M, et al. Arthroscopic rotator cuff repair with and without subacromial decompression: a prospective randomized study. Arthroscopy 2007;23(1):81–8.

99. Kelly AM, Drakos MC, Fealy S, et al. Arthroscopic release of the long head of the biceps tendon: functional outcome and clinical results. Am J Sports Med 2005;33(2):208–13.

100. Elkousy HA, Fluhme DJ, O'Connor DP, et al. Arthroscopic biceps tenodesis using the percutaneous, intra-articular trans-tendon technique: preliminary results. Orthopedics 2005;28(11):1316–9.

101. Verma NN, Drakos M, O'Brien SJ. Arthroscopic transfer of the long head biceps to the conjoint tendon. Arthroscopy 2005;21(6):764.
102. Provencher MT, LeClere LE, Romeo AA. Subpectoral biceps tenodesis. Sports Med Arthrosc 2008;16(3):170–6.
103. Nho SJ, Strauss EJ, Lenart BA, et al. Long head of the biceps tendinopathy: diagnosis and management. J Am Acad Orthop Surg 2010;18(11):645–56.
104. Galatz LM, Ball CM, Teefey SA, et al. The outcome and repair integrity of completely arthroscopically repaired large and massive rotator cuff tears. J Bone Joint Surg Am 2004;86(2):219–24.
105. Zumstein MA, Jost B, Hempel J, et al. The clinical and structural long-term results of open repair of massive tears of the rotator cuff. J Bone Joint Surg Am 2008;90(11):2423–31.
106. Bartl C, Kouloumentas P, Holzapfel K, et al. Long-term outcome and structural integrity following open repair of massive rotator cuff tears. Int J Shoulder Surg 2012;6(1):1–8.
107. Jost B, Zumstein M, Pfirrmann CW, et al. Long-term outcome after structural failure of rotator cuff repairs. J Bone Joint Surg Am 2006;88(3):472–9.
108. Jost B, Pfirrmann CW, Gerber C, et al. Clinical outcome after structural failure of rotator cuff repairs. J Bone Joint Surg Am 2000;82(3):304–14.
109. Huberty DP, Schoolfield JD, Brady PC, et al. Incidence and treatment of postoperative stiffness following arthroscopic rotator cuff repair. Arthroscopy 2009; 25(8):880–90.
110. Warner JJ. Frozen shoulder: diagnosis and management. J Am Acad Orthop Surg 1997;5(3):130–40.
111. Chung SW, Huong CB, Kim SH, et al. Shoulder stiffness after rotator cuff repair: risk factors and influence on outcome. Arthroscopy 2013;29(2):290–300.
112. Neviaser AS, Neviaser RJ. Adhesive capsulitis of the shoulder. J Am Acad Orthop Surg 2011;19(9):536–42.
113. McBirnie JM, Miniaci A, Miniaci SL. Arthroscopic repair of full-thickness rotator cuff tears using bioabsorbable tacks. Arthroscopy 2005;21(12):1421–7.
114. Krishnan SG, Harkins DC, Schiffern SC, et al. Arthroscopic repair of full-thickness tears of the rotator cuff in patients younger than 40 years. Arthroscopy 2008;24(3):324–8.
115. Randelli P, Spennacchio P, Ragone V, et al. Complications associated with arthroscopic rotator cuff repair: a literature review. Musculoskelet Surg 2012; 96(1):9–16.
116. Moerman AT, De Hert SG, Jacobs TF, et al. Cerebral oxygen desaturation during beach chair position. Eur J Anaesthesiol 2012;29(2):82–7.
117. Jeong H, Lee SH, Jang EA, et al. Haemodynamics and cerebral oxygenation during arthroscopic shoulder surgery in beach chair position under general anaesthesia. Acta Anaesthesiol Scand 2012;56(7):872–9.

Evaluation and Treatment of Sternoclavicular, Clavicular, and Acromioclavicular Injuries

Brenden J. Balcik, MD[a],*, Aaron J. Monseau, MD[a,b],
William Krantz, MD[c]

KEYWORDS

- Clavicle • Sternoclavicular joint • Acromioclavicular joint • Fracture • Dislocation
- Separation

KEY POINTS

- Injuries to the clavicle are relatively common and can occur at any age.
- The mechanism of injury most often involves a direct blow to the shoulder as opposed to a fall on an outstretched hand, as previously thought.
- Diagnosis involves physical examination and imaging. Often, plain radiographs are sufficient (ie, for clavicle fractures and acromioclavicular separations) but certain injuries (ie, sternoclavicular dislocation) require CT imaging for evaluation of underlying structures.
- Management and treatment strategies vary with type of injury, location, and the patient's functional status. Multiple factors must be taken into account when developing a management plan.
- It is important to recognize signs and symptoms of injuries that require orthopedic consultation and early surgical intervention.

INTRODUCTION

Clavicle injuries are common injuries that occur across all age groups.[1,2] Injuries to the clavicle may involve a fracture of the clavicle itself or may involve a sprain, separation, or dislocation of the clavicular joints. The clavicular joints include the sternoclavicular (SC) joint at the medial or proximal end of the clavicle and the acromioclavicular (AC) joint at the lateral or distal end of the clavicle.

The clavicle functions in support and mobility of the upper extremity. It serves as a transition point between the shoulder girdle and the trunk of the body, connecting the

[a] Department of Emergency Medicine, Robert C. Byrd Health Sciences Center, School of Medicine, West Virginia University, PO Box 9149, Morgantown, WV 26506, USA; [b] Department of Orthopedics, Robert C. Byrd Health Sciences Center, West Virginia University, PO Box 9196, Morgantown, WV 26506, USA; [c] Department of Radiology, Robert C. Byrd Health Sciences Center, School of Medicine, West Virginia University, PO Box 9235, Morgantown, WV 26506, USA
* Corresponding author.
E-mail address: bbalcik@hsc.wvu.edu

Prim Care Clin Office Pract 40 (2013) 911–923
http://dx.doi.org/10.1016/j.pop.2013.08.008
0095-4543/13/$ – see front matter © 2013 Elsevier Inc. All rights reserved.

upper extremity to the axial skeleton. In addition to support and mobility, its anatomic location serves to provide protection to underlying mediastinal structures such as the subclavian vessels and brachial plexus.[1–5]

The clavicle has a unique S-shape with the medial (sternal) portion having a cylindrical shape, whereas the lateral (acromial) portion has a flattened shape and is prone to injury due to its anatomic position and structure. The cylindrical nature of the medial portion of the clavicle provides strength to the clavicle, which is needed for protection of the underlying structures. The flattened lateral portion is ideal for attachment of muscles and ligaments. The midportion (or medial third) of the clavicle, where the shape of the bone transitions from the cylindrical form at the medial end to the flattened form at the distal end, is considered relatively weak and at risk for injury.[1–5]

Clavicle Fractures

Fractures of the clavicle are relatively common injuries and may occur at any age. These fractures account for 3% to 5% of all fractures.[2] Although these injuries do not necessarily represent a diagnostic dilemma because most are easily diagnosed by radiography, the management of these injuries can be challenging.

Previously, a fall onto an outstretched hand was thought to be the most common mechanism leading to clavicle fracture. Now, however, a direct blow to the shoulder, whether it is a fall onto the shoulder or a direct impact such as a tackle in football, is considered the most common mechanism. In a direct blow to the shoulder, the compressive force results in buckling of the clavicle, which causes a fracture once the compressive force exceeds the tensile strength of the clavicle. In addition to blows to the shoulder, direct blows to the clavicle resulted in fractures. Falls onto the shoulder account for 87% of clavicle fractures, whereas direct impact to the shoulder accounts for 7% of fractures. Falls onto outstretched hands account for 6% of clavicle fractures.[1,2,4,5]

Clavicle fractures have typically been classified by anatomic location (**Fig. 1**). Allman[6] classifies fractures based on the region of the clavicle in which the fracture lies (**Fig. 2**), as follows:

- Group I: fractures of the midshaft (middle third) of the clavicle; 81.3%
- Group II: fractures of the distal (lateral) third of the clavicle; 16.6%
- Group III: fractures of the medial (proximal) third of the clavicle; 2.1%.

Craig[7] breaks down the Group II fractures even further:

- Type I: fractures lateral to the coracoclavicular (CC) ligaments
- Type II: fractures medial to the CC ligaments

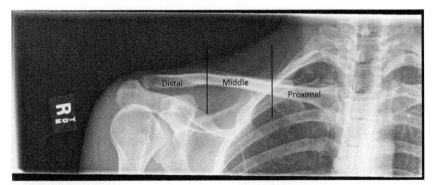

Fig. 1. Regions of the clavicle: proximal, medial, and distal.

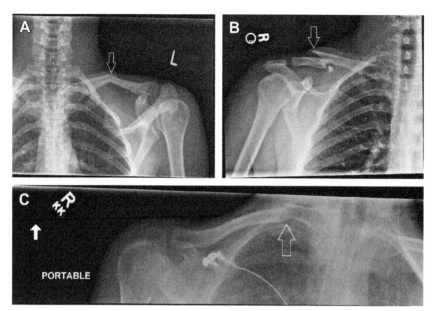

Fig. 2. Clavicle fractures of each third. Fracture lines marked with arrows. (*A*) Fracture of the middle third. (*B*) Fracture of the distal third. (*C*) Fracture of the proximal third.

- Type III: fractures extending into the AC joint
- Type IV: fractures in which the proximal fragment is displaced out of its periosteal tube
- Type V: comminuted fractures in which CC ligaments remain attached to an inferior bone fragment but are not attached to the proximal or distal fragment.

SC Joint Injuries

The SC joint is the most frequently moved, nonaxial joint in the body.[4] This joint is characterized as having the least amount of bony stability of any major joint due to the relatively small articulating surface between the clavicle and the sternum. However, due to the stability afforded by the surrounding ligaments, injuries to this joint are extremely rare, accounting for only 3% of shoulder girdle injuries. Of these, 80% are attributed to motor vehicle collisions (MVCs) or sports-related injuries.[3,8]

Sprains account for most injuries to the SC joint. This is despite the joint's lack of bony articulation. Instead, the SC joint's surrounding ligaments provide a substantial amount of strength preventing dislocation of this joint.

Dislocations of the SC joint are uncommon and comprise only 3% of dislocations around the shoulder girdle.[3–5,8–11] This is primarily due to the strength and integrity provided by the joint's surrounding ligaments. However, when SC joint dislocations do occur, they are typically the result of an MVC or sports-related injury. Of these dislocations, an anterior dislocation is more common than a posterior dislocation. Although an anterior dislocation is more common, a posterior dislocation is the more concerning of the two. This is due to two factors: (1) the amount of force required to dislocate the SC joint posteriorly is more than 1.5 times the force required for anterior dislocation and (2) the chance of damaging underlying mediastinal structures, including the brachial plexus, vascular structures, trachea, and esophagus.[8–12]

Although these types of dislocations are rare, there has been one report of a lethal aortic arch injury following a rugby tackle in which the patient was thought to have sustained a posterior SC joint dislocation.[13] One study reported the structures most often injured during these dislocations are the left and right brachiocephalic veins.[14]

Classification of severity of SC joint injuries is defined as follows[5]:

- Mild: stable joint, ligamentous integrity maintained
- Moderate: joint subluxation, partial ligamentous disruption
- Severe: unstable joint, complete ligamentous disruption.

AC Joint Injuries

The AC joint is a synovial joint with bony articulation between the lateral end of the clavicle with the medial surface of the acromion. Stability of the joint is provided by multiple structures, including fibers of the deltoid and trapezius muscles and the AC and CC ligaments. The AC ligaments provide horizontal stability, whereas the CC ligaments provide vertical stability to the joint. The CC ligament is considered the major suspensory ligament of the upper extremity. Separations of the AC joint account for 9% to 10% of acute injuries to the shoulder girdle in the general population, whereas separations of the AC joint account for 40% of shoulder girdle injuries in athletes.[4,5,15–18]

Classification of AC separations is based on degree of displacement of the distal clavicle. Rockwood and colleagues[19] divide these separations into type I through VI (**Table 1**).

PATIENT HISTORY

When injuries to the clavicle or either of its joints are encountered, the patient typically describes a fall onto the ipsilateral shoulder or some type of direct blow or impact to the shoulder. The mechanism preceding these injuries can often be placed into three main categories: falls, MVCs, or sports injuries.[1–4,10,15]

Table 1
Rockwood and colleagues[19] classification of AC separations

Separation Type	Description	Comments
I	Sprain of AC ligaments	Most common type No joint instability
II	Rupture of AC ligaments Sprain of CC ligaments	Clavicle unstable
III	Rupture of AC ligaments Rupture of CC ligaments Detachment of deltoid and trapezius muscles	Clavicle unstable in vertical and horizontal planes
IV	Rupture of all supporting structures Clavicle displaced in or through trapezius muscle	—
V	Rupture of all supporting structures	More severe form of Type III
VI	Rupture of all supporting structures	Least common Only 3 cases reported

Data from Rockwood CA, Green DP, Bucholz RW. Fractures in adults. 2nd edition. Philadelphia: Lippincott Williams & Wilkins; 1984.

Clavicle Fractures

Fractures of the clavicle are typically the result of a fall onto the shoulder or a direct blow to the clavicle. As described above, falls account for 87% of clavicle fractures.[5] Patients routinely describe a cracking or popping sound or sensation during the injury.[4]

SC Joint Injuries

Patients presenting with SC joint sprains may describe a situation in which their shoulder was hit from behind and forced anteriorly. Patients may also describe a sudden impact on the lateral shoulder in which the force was directed medially.

Patients presenting with SC joint dislocations typically present after MVCs or sports events. Those with anterior dislocations often experience a force directed on the shoulder while the arm was held in an abducted position. Patients presenting with posterior SC joint dislocations often describe an incident in which a force was directed medially with the arm held in adduction and flexed position. These types of injuries are often seen in football players in which the player is "underneath the pile." These dislocations can also be the result of MVCs in which a patient is either run over by a vehicle or pinned against a wall by a vehicle.[4,5,9–12]

AC Joint Injuries

AC joint injuries can be the result of both direct and indirect mechanisms. In the direct mechanism, the patient will describe a fall onto the shoulder, whereas in the indirect mechanism the patient will describe a fall onto an outstretched hand.[4,5,15–17]

PHYSICAL EXAMINATION

When injury of the clavicle or either of its joints is suspected, the physical examination should be performed with the patient in the seated or standing position. Examination should begin with inspection of the shoulder and clavicle. Any asymmetry, swelling, or gross deformities should be noted. Any tenting of the skin should raise concern for significant fracture or dislocation. The shoulder and clavicle should be palpated, noting any irregularities when compared with the noninjured side. Bony defects, crepitus, and point tenderness may be present. Range of motion should be assessed and any pain with movement should be noted. A careful neurologic examination should also be performed because of the proximity of the brachial plexus. The most common nerve injured in midshaft clavicle fracture is the ulnar nerve, so special care should be taken to evaluate this nerve distribution.[2] In evaluating injuries that are the result of high-energy mechanisms, physical examination should also include evaluation of the thorax for additional injuries, such as pneumothorax and hemothorax, especially in patients in whom additional fractures of ribs and scapulae are suspected.[1–5,15,16]

Specific clinical features associated with each type of injury are described below.

Clavicle Fractures

Clavicle fractures can have multiple and variable findings on physical examination.[1–5] Some of the findings described include:

- The ipsilateral arm may be held by the contralateral arm or held in adduction at the side
- There may be swelling overlying the clavicle

- Gross deformity of the clavicle may be visible
- Tenting of the skin may be visible
- Tenderness to palpation (TTP) of the clavicle
- Crepitus may be palpated overlying the fracture site
- There may be a mobile fracture fragment
- A grinding sensation may be felt when evaluating range of motion
- Sensory deficits may be observed (seen most often with fractures of the medial third of the clavicle due to proximity of the brachial plexus).

SC Joint Injuries

Examination of the injured SC joint may reveal severe pain exacerbated by arm motion and lying supine. Inspection of an anterior SC joint dislocation will show a prominent medial clavicle that is palpable anterior relative to the sternum. A posterior SC joint dislocation will reveal a medial clavicle that is less visible and often not palpable. Patients with posterior SC joint dislocations may also show signs of impingement to underlying mediastinal structures such as tachypnea, dyspnea, dysphagia, or venous congestion.[3,4,12,13,20]

AC Joint Injuries

The AC joint should be examined with the upper extremities in a dependent position. This stresses the AC joint and accentuates any deformity that may be present. The characteristic anatomic feature is downward sag of the affect shoulder and arm. Additional features vary with the type of AC separation as described in **Table 2**.[4,5,15,16]

Table 2
Clinical features of AC separations

Separation Type	Examination Findings	Comments
I	No obvious deformity TTP of the AC joint No TTP in the CC interspace No instability Minimal pain with arm movement	—
II	Mild step-off deformity of AC joint with distal clavicle slightly superior to acromion TTP of AC joint TTP in the CC interspace Pain with any arm movement	—
III	Prominent step-off deformity of AC joint Shoulder droop Widening of CC interspace TTP of the AC joint Severe pain with any arm movement	Possible tenting of skin
IV	Posterior displacement of distal clavicle Severe pain with any arm movement	May see tenting of skin in posterior
V	Gross deformity of clavicle Severe pain with movement	—
VI	Shoulder appears flat with prominent acromion Severe swelling	May have associated rib fractures and brachial plexus injury

DIAGNOSTIC IMAGING

Usually, plain radiographs are sufficient for the diagnosis of clavicular injuries.[1–5]

Clavicle Fractures

Clavicle fractures can be routinely identified with standard AP radiographs. However, sometimes overlapping thoracic structures may obscure the suspected fracture. In cases in which questions remain, a view with a 30-degree cephalic tilt may be obtained. This helps eliminate any overlying thoracic structures from obstructing the view. In cases of proximal (medial) third fractures, a serendipity view (40-degree cephalic tilt) can be obtained. Distal third (lateral) fractures may be better visualized using an axillary view or a view with a 15-degree cephalic tilt.

Occasionally, CT imaging maybe required. CT is most often used in fractures of the proximal third of the clavicle.[1–4,8] CT imaging enables the clinician to differentiate between fractures and SC joint dislocations. CT also allows for visualization and evaluation of underlying mediastinal structures.[1]

SC Joint Injuries

Diagnosis of SC joint dislocations often requires additional imaging in conjunction with standard AP radiographs.[3,4,8–12] Standard AP radiographs are often difficult to interpret due to the confluence of bony structures. The serendipity view allows for visualization of the dislocation.

Most clinicians advocate additional CT imaging when an SC joint dislocation is suspected. CT provides a definitive diagnosis for dislocation. In addition, CT imaging shows the dislocation in relation to the underlying mediastinal structures (**Fig. 3**). Intravenous contrast allows for even further evaluation of underlying vascular structures.[3–5,8,10,12,14]

AC Joint Injuries

Typically, plain radiographs are all that are required for diagnosis of AC joint injuries (**Fig. 4**). Specific radiographic findings vary with type of AC joint separation as shown in **Table 3**.[4,5,15,16]

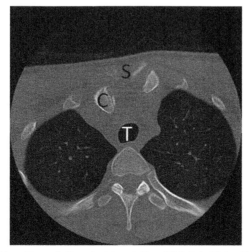

Fig. 3. Posterior dislocation of the clavicle at the SC joint. Note the proximity of the displaced clavicle to the trachea. C, proximal end of the clavicle; S, sternum; T, trachea.

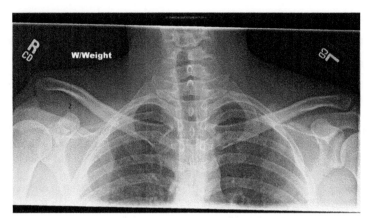

Fig. 4. Radiograph of a type V AC separation. (1) Displacement of the clavicle relative to the acromion. (2) Displacement of the clavicle from the coracoid process. Note the degree of dislocation (>100%) at both junctions.

TREATMENT

The goal of treatment and management of these injuries is to provide adequate pain control, reduce or immobilize (as indicated), address any associated injuries, minimize complications, and refer to appropriate consultants (when required).[1,2,21] Although management of some injuries are widely agreed on (ie, type I AC separations), controversy surrounding the management of other injuries still exist (ie, type III AC separations). The patient's age and functional status are taken into account when deciding on an optimal management plan when standard of care has not clearly been established. In cases such as these, the primary care physician and orthopedist, as well as the patient should be involved in developing the treatment plan. However, it is important to recognize injuries that require early, urgent, or emergent surgical intervention, as shown in **Table 4**.[1,2,5,21,22]

See later discussion on treatment strategies of specific injuries.

Clavicle Fractures

Treatment of clavicle fractures is aimed at minimizing the risk of nonunions and malunion. Nonunion is defined as the absence of clinical or radiographic healing after

Table 3 Radiographic features of AC separations	
Separation Type	**Radiographic Findings**
I	No abnormality
II	Slight AC joint widening Slight elevation (25%–50%) of the distal clavicle relative to the acromion
III	AC joint 100% dislocated
IV	AP radiograph: appears similar to type I and III Axillary view: posterior displacement of clavicle
V	AC joint 100% dislocated CC joint with 100%–300% dislocation
VI	AC joint 100% dislocated Clavicle displaced inferiorly

Table 4	
Indications for early surgical intervention of clavicle injuries	
Injury	**Findings**
Clavicle Fractures	Open fractures
	Skin tenting
	Neurovascular compromise
	Multiple trauma
	Floating shoulder
	Malunion or nonunion
	Shortening (>15–20 mm)
	Displacement (>100%)
	Severe comminution
SC Joint Injuries	Failure of closed reduction
	Any sign of neurovascular compromise
AC Joint Injuries	Any sign of neurovascular compromise
	Types IV, V, VI

4 to 6 months, whereas malunion is associated with angulation, shortening, and poor cosmetic appearance. Historically, it was thought malunion does not affect functional capacity; however, recent studies have found malunion may lead to weakness and fatigability.[1,2,21,22]

In general, most minimally displaced clavicle fractures may be treated nonoperatively with immobilization using either a sling or a figure-of-eight brace. Current studies show little-to-no difference between these two methods of immobilization and the choice should be based on patient comfort and function. However, the sling has been shown to provide more comfort and is associated with fewer complications, such as skin breakdown, because the figure-of-eight brace must be kept in some degree of tension. Additionally, the sling allows for periodic range-of-motion exercises. Regardless of the method of immobilization, some degree of shortening may result. Immobilization is typically maintained for 4 to 6 weeks.

Specific management strategies and caveats exist for fractures depending on anatomic location, degree of displacement, and presence of injuries to associated or underlying structures. In some cases, surgical intervention may be required. Emergent or urgent orthopedic referral is indicated if any of the following are present:

- Open fractures
- Neurovascular compromise
- Skin tenting
- Associated scapular neck fractures
- Severely comminuted or displaced fractures
- Elite athlete status.

Additional management strategies are listed in **Table 5**.

Follow-up evaluation should be performed 1 to 2 weeks after the injury and every 2 to 4 weeks thereafter until clinical and radiographic union have been reached. Fracture union can be verified clinically when there is absence of TTP over the site and full range-of-motion and strength are obtained in the absence of pain. Radiographic union is reached when callus formation is visible on radiograph. A bridging callus is typically identified 6 weeks postinjury.[1] It is important to note that radiographs are not necessary at every follow-up visit because clinical assessment is often all that is required to

Table 5
Management of clavicle fractures

Fracture Location	Nonoperative	Operative	Comments
Middle Third	Typically recommended	Recommended for z-deformity or >1–2 cm shortening	—
Proximal Third	Typically recommended	Consider if underlying injury present	CT imaging recommended if there is concern for underlying neurovascular injury
Distal Third			
Type I and III	Recommended	—	—
Type IV and V	Recommended	—	—
Type II	—	Recommended	High frequency of nonunion[a]

[a] Some investigators contend that nonoperative management can be undertaken if the fracture ends are in contact. In this case, a sling is recommended because a figure-of-eight brace may further displace fragments.
Data from Refs.[1,2,4,5]

monitor healing. However, if healing is not progressing as expected, or additional injury has occurred, radiographs should be obtained for further evaluation.[1,2,21] General timelines for healing are as follows[1,2,4]:

- Middle third: nonoperative management, 6 to 12 weeks
- Distal third: type II, surgical management, 12 weeks
- Distal third: types I and III, nonoperative management, 6 to 8 weeks
- Proximal third: nonoperative management, 6 to 8 weeks.

Because many clavicle fractures are sustained during sports-related activities, it should be no surprise when the athlete patient asks when they can return to play. Special consideration should be given to these cases because multiple factors play a role in management. Factors to consider include the patient's age, sport or activity, location and severity of the fracture, extent and speed of healing, method of treatment (operative vs nonoperative), and any complications encountered during the recovery process.[1,2,21] It is important to ensure both clinical and radiographic healing are obtained before clearance for returning to play. Typically, return to noncontact activity is permitted at 6 weeks after injury and return to contact sports is permitted at 8 to 12 weeks.

For those individuals who need surgical management, an intramedullary pin or external plating may be used. Often, a second procedure is scheduled to remove the hardware after 6 to 8 weeks.[2,4] For athletes considering surgery, the time to return to contact activity is typically a similar 8 to 12 weeks.[1,2] If only one surgery is needed, it will likely be on the shorter end of the range, but return to contact activity will be on the longer end of the range if a second surgery is needed for hardware removal.[2,22]

SC Joint Injuries

Management of SC joint injuries is largely dependent on the degree of injury (mild, moderate, or severe) and the direction of dislocation (anterior vs posterior) as shown in **Table 6**.[4,5,10–14]

Table 6
Management of SC joint injuries

Severity	Management	Comments
Mild	Ice for 24 h Sling immobilization 3–4 d	Return to normal activities as tolerated
Moderate	Ice for 24 h Clavicle splint or figure-eight brace for 1 wk Sling immobilization 4–6 wk	—
Severe		
Anterior	Closed reduction[a] may be attempted but is often unstable and re-dislocated when pressure released Clavicle splint or figure-of-eight brace for 4–6 wk	Orthopedic referral
Posterior	Emergent orthopedic consult Closed reduction[b] often performed in the operating room due to proximity of underlying mediastinal structures and propensity for injury If closed reduction fails, open reduction required Clavicle splint or figure-of-eight brace for 4–6 wk	Cardiothoracic surgery should be available because there may be damage to underlying structures

[a] Closed reduction involves placing the patient in a supine position with a towel roll between the scapulae. The ipsilateral arm is abducted to 90° and traction is applied with slight extension of arm toward the ground. Pressure directed posteriorly is placed over the medial clavicle.
[b] Closed reduction is usually performed under general anesthesia. Patient is placed in a supine position with a towel roll between scapulae. The ipsilateral arm is abducted and extended while traction is applied. The medial clavicle is grasped with a towel clamp and pulled anteriorly.
Data from Refs.[3–5,10,11]

AC Joint Injuries

Management depends on the type of separation[4,5,15–18,21]:

- Type I: sling 1 to 2 weeks, ice and analgesia, early range-of-motion in 1 to 2 weeks
- Type II: sling 1 to 2 weeks, ice, and analgesia, early range-of-motion in 1 to 2 weeks; refrain from heavy activity for 6 weeks
- Type III: controversy exists for optimal treatment with these types of injuries and is largely dependent on the patient and his or her functional status; the current trend is toward nonoperative management; however, there is continued debate and more research is necessary
- Type IV: surgical repair typically required
- Type V: surgical repair required
- Type VI: surgical repair required.

COMPLICATIONS

Complications may be encountered with any clavicle injury. The most serious complications occur when neurovascular structures are compromised. Injuries of this nature must be identified and dealt with immediately. However, less severe complications may also arise.

Table 7		
Complications of clavicle injuries		
Fractures	**SC Joint Injuries**	**AC Joint Injuries**
Poor cosmesis	Poor cosmesis	CC ossification
Nonunion	Pneumothorax	Distal clavicle osteolysis
Malunion	Vascular injury	Arthritis
Neurologic Deficit	Esophageal injury	
	Voice changes	
	Arthritis	

Clavicle fractures may result in malunion. Although this may result in a bony prominence, it rarely results in functional deficit. Nonunion may also be encountered. The incidence of nonunion ranges from 0.1% to 13%.[4] Most nonunion occurs in fractures of the middle third of the clavicle. Risk factors for nonunion have been identified as follows[2,5]:

- Severe trauma (ie, open fracture)
- Significant displacement
- Significant shortening (>2 cm)
- Comminution
- Female
- Elderly
- Inadequate period of immobilization
- Soft-tissue interposition.

Complications involving specific injuries are shown in **Table 7**.[2,10,11,15,16,22]

SUMMARY

Injuries to the clavicle and its joints can occur across all patient demographics. Care must be taken during evaluation to assess for any underlying or associated injuries. When developing a treatment plan, the patient's needs should be taken into account and, often, orthopedic consultation is necessary. Because clavicle injuries are relatively common, there is a high likelihood they will be encountered in the primary care setting. Therefore, the primary care physician should be well versed in the clinical features, evaluation, and treatment modalities available for these injuries.

REFERENCES

1. Pujalte GG, Housner JA. Management of clavicle fractures. Curr Sports Med Rep 2008;7(5):275–80.
2. Jeray KJ. Clavicle shaft fractures. In: Orthopedic knowledge online journal 2009. 8(1). Available at: http://orthoportal.aaos.org/oko/article.aspx?article=OKO_TRA028. Accessed December 21, 2009.
3. Chaudhry FW, Killampalli VV, Chowdhry M, et al. Posterior dislocation of the sternoclavicular joint in a young rugby player. Acta Orthop Traumatol Turc 2011; 45(5):376–8.
4. Rudzinski JP, Pittman LM, Uehara DT. Shoulder and humerus injuries. In: Tintinalli JE, Stapczynski JS, Ma OJ, et al, editors. Tintinalli's emergency medicine: a comprehensive study guide. 7th edition. New York: McGraw Hill; 2011. p. 1830–4.

5. Egol KA, Koval KJ, Zuckerman JD. Clavicle fractures. Acromioclavicular and sternoclavicular joint injuries. In: Orthopedic handbook of fractures. Philadelphia: Lippincott Williams; 2010. p. 143–62.
6. Allman FL Jr. Fractures and ligamentous injuries of the clavicle and its articulation. J Bone Joint Surg Am 1967;49:774–84.
7. Craig EV. Fractures of the clavicle. In: Green DP, Bochwolz RW, Heckman JD, editors. Rockwood and Green's fractures in adults. New York: Lippincott-Raven Publishers; 1996. p. 1109–61.
8. Oikonomou A, Prassopoulos P. CT imaging of blunt chest trauma. Insights Imaging 2011;2(3):281–95.
9. Ferrera PC, Wheeling HM. Sternoclavicular joint injuries. Am J Emerg Med 2000; 18(1):58–61.
10. Philipson MR, Wallwork N. (iii) Traumatic dislocation of the sternoclavicular joint. Orthopaedics and Trauma 2012;26(6):380–4.
11. Thut D, Hergan D, Dukas A, et al. Sternoclavicular Joint Reconstruction: a systematic review. Bull NYU Hosp Jt Dis 2011;69(2):128–35.
12. Garg S, Alshameeri ZA, Wallace WA. Posterior sternoclavicular joint dislocation in a child: a case report with review of literature. J Shoulder Elbow Surg 2012;21(3): e11–6.
13. Shimizu K, Ogura H, Nakagawa Y, et al. Lethal aortic arch injury caused by a rugby tackle. A case report. Am J Sports Med 2008;36(8):1611–4.
14. Ponce BA, Kundukulam JA, Pflugner R, et al. Sternoclavicular joint surgery: how far does danger lurk below? J Shoulder Elbow Surg 2013;22(7):993–9.
15. Petron DJ, Hanson RW. Acromioclavicular joint disorders. Curr Sports Med Rep 2007;6(5):300–6.
16. Mazzocca AD, Arciero RA, Bicos J. Evaluation and treatment of acromioclavicular joint injuries. Am J Sports Med 2007;35(2):316–29.
17. Johansen JA, Grutter PW, McFarland EG, et al. Acromioclavicular joint injuries: indications for treatment and treatment options. J Shoulder Elbow Surg 2011; 20(2):S70–82.
18. Baek SH, Oh CW, Wallace WA, et al. Anterior clavicle dislocation associated with acromioclavicular dislocation in a soccer player: a case report. Am J Sports Med 2007;35(10):1752–5.
19. Rockwood CA, Green DP, Bucholz RW. Fractures in adults. 2nd edition. Philadelphia: Lippincott Williams & Wilkins; 1984.
20. Groh GI, Wirth MA, Rockwood CA. Treatment of traumatic posterior sternoclavicular dislocations. J Shoulder Elbow Surg 2011;20(1):107–13.
21. Lervick GN, Klepps SK. Return to play: shoulder dislocations, clavicle fractures, and acromioclavicular separations. In: Orthopedic knowledge online journal 2011. 9(3). Available at: http://orthoportal.aaos.org/oko/article.aspx?article=OKO_SHO042. Accessed March 1, 2011.
22. Van der Meijden OA, Gaskill TR, Millett PJ. Treatment of clavicle fractures: current concepts review. J Shoulder Elbow Surg 2012;21(3):423–9.

Evaluation and Treatment of Upper Extremity Nerve Entrapment Syndromes

Eric E. Floranda, MD[a],*, Bret C. Jacobs, DO, MA[b,c]

KEYWORDS

- Upper extremity • Neuropathy • Entrapment • Compression • Palsy • Nerve
- Syndrome

KEY POINTS

- A firm knowledge of muscles and the cutaneous distribution of nerve innervates is essential in localizing nerve injury.
- Patients usually present with weakness, pain, and paresthesias in a distribution particular to the nerve and the level of the lesion.
- Tools are available to aid the clinician in the diagnosis and prognostication of nerve injury.
- Conservative management is generally the first-line treatment before surgery is contemplated.

INTRODUCTION

This article describes nerve entrapment syndromes encountered in the upper extremity. These syndromes present with various symptoms and signs corresponding to the site of compression and anatomic distribution supplied by the involved nerve. To make a diagnosis, the clinician must recognize the muscles innervated, sensory distribution, muscle stretch reflex, and compressive sites associated to a particular nerve. Nerves can be purely motor, purely sensory, or mixed. This article starts with the discussion of the proximal nerves of the upper limb and ends with the nerves that can be entrapped both proximally and distally. Learning the anatomy, common areas of injury and associated clinical findings can aid the physician in diagnosing and managing nerve injuries.

[a] The Center for Neuroscience, Calvert Memorial Hospital, Chesapeake Neurology Associates, 130 Hospital Road, Suite 101, Prince Frederick, MD 20678, USA; [b] Department of Family and Community Medicine, Penn State Milton S. Hershey Medical Center, 500 University Drive, Hershey, PA 17033, USA; [c] Department of Orthopaedics and Rehabilitation, Penn State Milton S. Hershey Medical Center, 500 University Drive, Hershey, PA 17033, USA
* Corresponding author.
E-mail address: efloranda@chesapeakeneurologyassociates.com

Prim Care Clin Office Pract 40 (2013) 925–943
http://dx.doi.org/10.1016/j.pop.2013.08.009
0095-4543/13/$ – see front matter © 2013 Elsevier Inc. All rights reserved.

PATHOPHYSIOLOGY

Entrapment neuropathies are caused by structural, mechanical, or dynamic compression at specific locations, which may lead to nerve injury.

Nerve injury is divided into 3 classifications: neuropraxia, axonotmesis, and neurotmesis. Neuropraxia is the mildest form, in which there is myelin sheath injury or ischemia, with sparing of the axon and the connective tissue. It presents with nerve conduction slowing or block on electrodiagnostic studies. Recovery is excellent, in weeks to months.[1] In axonotmesis, there is injury to both axons and their myelin sheaths, but the surrounding connective tissue is relatively intact. Wallerian degeneration follows, with subsequent axonal regrowth. Prognosis is variable and depends on the distance of the nerve to the muscle and integrity of the supporting structures. The most severe form is neurotmesis, in which there is complete disruption of the axon and supporting structures, with no possibility for axonal regrowth. Recovery is poor without surgical intervention.[1]

UPPER EXTREMITY NERVES AND THEIR SYNDROMES
Dorsal Scapular Nerve

Anatomy
The dorsal scapular nerve is a pure motor nerve that arises from the C5 nerve root. It travels through the scalenius medius muscle and innervates the levator scapulae and the rhomboid muscles.[2]

Lesion
An isolated nerve injury can be seen in bodybuilders and in people who require heavy overhead lifting, because the dorsal scapular nerve may become entrapped within the scalenius medius muscle.[3] It is also reported as a complication of the use of a spine brace for idiopathic scoliosis.[4]

History and physical examination
The athlete presents with scapular winging, with lateral displacement of the scapula (**Table 1**). Weakness is shown by having the patient press the elbow backwards against resistance while the hand is on the hip. Weakness is also evident when the patient pushes the palm backwards against resistance, with arms folded behind the back.

Management
Conservative treatment includes physical therapy and antiinflammatory medications. For nerve injuries that lead to scapular winging not responsive to conservative treatment, surgical techniques involving various combinations of fascial graft or transfer of adjacent muscles may be effective.[5]

Long Thoracic Nerve

Anatomy
The long thoracic nerve is a pure motor nerve that emerges from the C5 to C7 roots. It descends inferiorly behind the clavicle and supplies the serratus anterior muscle.[2]

Lesion
The nerve lies superficially in the supraclavicular region, where it is subject to trauma as a result of pressure on the shoulder (eg, rucksack paralysis, automobile accident, playing football, chiropractic manipulation). Activities that involve repetitive stressful movements of the shoulder or those in which the arm is outstretched in an overhead position may cause traction injury (eg, being in the same position for an extended period during general anesthesia). Nerve injury may also occur during surgical procedures around the axilla.

Table 1
Clinical features of upper extremity proximal neuropathies

Nerve Entrapment	Compression Site	Motor Findings	Sensory Findings	Other Findings
Dorsal scapular nerve	Within scalenius medius muscle	Weakness in pressing the elbow backwards against resistance while hand is on the hip or in pushing the palm backward against resistance with arm folded behind the back	—	Scapular winging with lateral displacement; shoulder pain
Long thoracic nerve	Supraclavicular region	Weakness in raising arm above the head	—	Scapular winging when patient pushes arm against the wall while elbow is extended
Suprascapular nerve	Suprascapular notch	Weakness in both abduction and external rotation of arm	—	Deep scapular pain
	Spinoglenoid notch	Weakness of only external rotation of arm	—	Deep scapular pain
Axillary nerve	Lateral aspect of the humerus and quadrilateral space	Weakness of abduction of shoulder between 15° and 90°	Lateral shoulder	Deltoid atrophy
Musculocutaneous neuropathy	At the level of the coracobrachialis	Elbow flexor and forearm supination weakness	Lateral forearm	Proximal forearm pain aggravated by elbow extension; reduced biceps reflex
Lateral antebrachial cutaneous branch	Cubital fossa or forearm	—	Pure sensory deficits along radial aspect of forearm	—

History and physical examination

The player may experience sharp pain in the shoulder, which radiates to the neck and upper arm (see **Table 1**). Weakness of the shoulder and difficulty raising the arm above the head are the primary complaints. Scapular winging is revealed when the patient pushes their arm against the wall while the elbow is extended.[6]

Management

Injury of the nerve caused by repetitive activities and lifting tends to resolve spontaneously within 6 to 24 months.[6,7] Physical therapy and exercise are recommended. An athlete can safely return to play when strength has returned to normal but should try to avoid any precipitating movements and carrying heavy objects across the shoulder. Various combinations of muscle transfers, nerve transfers, and fascial grafts may be considered in patients who do not achieve improvement despite conservative treatment.[6,7]

Suprascapular Nerve

Anatomy

The suprascapular nerve is a branch of the upper trunk of the brachial plexus and is a pure motor nerve. It passes downward through the suprascapular notch. The nerve supplies the supraspinatus muscle, which abducts the humerus and the infraspinatus muscle, which is an external rotator of the upper arm.[2]

Lesion

The nerve may be damaged in acute forceful depression of the shoulder and shoulder dislocation. Nerve entrapment can occur in the suprascapular notch (eg, with ganglia formation, fracture of the suprascapular notch, callus formation from healing fracture), resulting in weakness of both the supraspinatus and infraspinatus muscles. Entrapment at the spinoglenoid notch leads to isolated injury of the branch to the infraspinatus muscle (eg, from ganglia or from a hypertrophied inferior transverse scapular ligament).[8–10]

History and physical examination

The player may present with deep scapular pain aggravated by shoulder movement and overhead activities (see **Table 1**). In lesions at the suprascapular notch, atrophy and weakness of both the supraspinatus and infraspinatus muscles are seen, whereas lesions at the spinoglenoid notch involve only the infraspinatus muscle.

Management

Conservative treatment includes avoidance of precipitating factors to allow recovery, and physical therapy with range-of-motion exercises and strengthening of the shoulder and rotator cuff muscles. Magnetic resonance imaging (MRI) should be considered if there is no improvement. For patients who failed conservative management, surgical release of the transverse scapular ligament and arthroscopic suprascapular nerve decompression may be considered. The presence of a cyst or tumor warrants surgery.[11] An athlete can return to play when muscle strength is appropriate and the sport can be performed safely.

Axillary Nerve

Anatomy

The axillary nerve is a mixed nerve that supplies the deltoid and teres minor muscles (**Fig. 1**). Its sensory branch, the lateral cutaneous nerve of the arm, supplies the skin of the upper lateral aspect of the arm. It passes just below the shoulder joint into the quadrilateral space (bounded by the teres major inferiorly, long head of the triceps

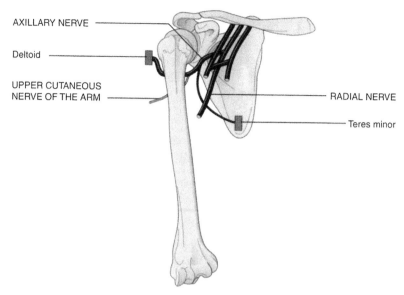

AXILLARY NERVE

Deltoid

UPPER CUTANEOUS
NERVE OF THE ARM

RADIAL NERVE

Teres minor

Fig. 1. Axillary nerve. (*From* O'Brien M. Aids to the examination of the peripheral nervous system. 5th edition. Edinburgh (United Kingdom): Saunders Elsevier; 2010.)

medially, surgical neck of the humerus laterally, and teres minor and subscapularis superiorly).[12] The nerve then winds around the surgical neck of the humerus, accompanied by the posterior circumflex artery.

Lesion
Injury to the nerve most often occurs where the nerve winds around the lateral aspect of the humerus (eg, shoulder dislocation, scapular fracture, humeral fracture and dislocation, shoulder reduction, intrasmuscular shoulder injection, sleeping with arm raised above the head in a prone position).[13,14] Other causes of injury include a fibrous band in the quadrilateral space, trauma in sports (eg, football, skiing, rugby, baseball, ice hockey, soccer, weight lifting, and wrestling), and use of prosthetic devices.[15]

History and physical examination
The athlete presents with deltoid muscle weakness and atrophy, with or without sensory involvement along the outer aspect of the upper arm (see **Table 1**). The examination reveals a problem in abducting, externally rotating, and forward flexing the upper arm against resistance.

Management
Treatment begins with physical therapy, with the goal of preserving shoulder range of motion. Improvement is usually seen by 3 to 4 months with conservative therapy.[13,14] If no improvement is noted after this time, surgery, including nerve grafting, is considered, especially for severe lesions and for those with recurrent shoulder dislocation.[13,14] Return-to-play decisions are individualized based on associated injuries, but typically a player with full shoulder range of motion and normal strength can resume activities without restrictions.

Musculocutaneous Nerve

Anatomy

The musculocutaneous nerve, as the name implies, is a mixed nerve (**Fig. 2**). It supplies the biceps, coracobrachialis, and brachialis muscles. The nerve then continues distally as the lateral cutaneous nerve of the forearm, which supplies sensation to the entire lateral forearm.[2]

Lesion

Nerve injury may result from humeral fractures, osteochondroma of the humerus, and shoulder dislocation. Motor and sensory involvement can occur when the injury occurs as the nerve passes through the coracobrachialis muscle in the upper arm (eg, rowing, weight lifting, football, sleep, general anesthesia). Isolated biceps weakness can also occur with distal motor nerve injury. The lateral cutaneous nerve of the forearm can

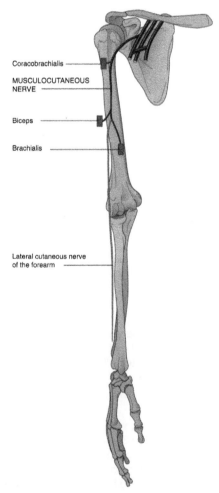

Fig. 2. Musculocutaneous nerve. (*From* O'Brien M. Aids to the examination of the peripheral nervous system. 5th edition. Edinburgh (United Kingdom): Saunders Elsevier; 2010.)

be injured at the cubital fossa or forearm (eg, venipuncture, cut-down procedure, compression), causing a pure sensory syndrome.[16,17]

History and physical examination
The athlete complains of pain in the proximal lateral forearm, often aggravated by elbow extension (see **Table 1**). The patient has elbow flexor weakness and some forearm supination weakness. Biceps atrophy may be noted. Biceps reflex is diminished. Decreased sensation is noted in the radial aspect of the forearm.

Management
Conservative treatment (eg, relative rest, nonsteroidal antiinflammatory drugs, splinting, and physical therapy) is first tried, with consideration of surgical decompression in cases that do not respond. The athlete may return to full activities when muscle weakness is no longer evident.

Median Nerve

Anatomy
The median nerve is a mixed nerve that descends down the medial side of the arm to the cubital fossa in close association with the brachial artery (**Fig. 3**). The median nerve does not supply any muscle until it reaches the elbow. As it passes between the heads of the pronator teres muscle, it supplies the pronator teres, flexor carpi radialis, palmaris longus, and flexor digitorum superficialis muscles. At this level, it also gives off the purely motor anterior interosseus nerve, which supplies the flexor digitorum profundus I and II, flexor pollicis longus, and pronator quadratus muscles. The main branch then continues distally, giving off a palmar cutaneous branch (which supplies skin at the thenar eminence and radial proximal palm) about 5 cm above the wrist, before it courses deep to the flexor retinaculum at the wrist (carpal tunnel) and divides into its terminal branches. The median motor branch innervates the first and second lumbricals, abductor pollicis brevis, opponens pollicis, and flexor pollicis brevis superficial head. The terminal sensory branches supply the thumb to the lateral half of the fourth digit.[2,12]

Lesion
Ligament of Struthers/supracondylar process syndrome A fibrous tunnel may be formed by an osseous spur at the anteromedial surface of the distal humerus (supracondylar process) and a ligament that connects to the medial epicondyle (ligament of Struthers) (**Table 2**). The median nerve can be compressed in this area, and this causes weakness of all muscles innervated by the median nerve, with sensory loss in the distribution of both the palmar cutaneous and palmar digital branches.[18] On plain radiograph, an osseous spur is visible at the anteromedial surface of the distal humerus.[19]

Pronator syndrome The median nerve can be rarely entrapped between the 2 heads of the pronator teres muscle and under the fibrous arch of the flexor digitorum superficialis. Although it may be clinically silent for years, this syndrome can become evident after repetitive pronation and supination. The athlete presents with pain in the proximal forearm aggravated by resisted forearm pronation and resisted wrist flexion. Nocturnal symptoms are not common compared with carpal tunnel syndrome. Patients have tenderness on deep palpation of the pronator teres muscle. Forearm muscles innervated by the median nerve are variably involved, with the pronator teres usually spared. This situation occurs because nerve branches to these muscles may have departed from the main nerve before the site of compression. There is atrophy and weakness

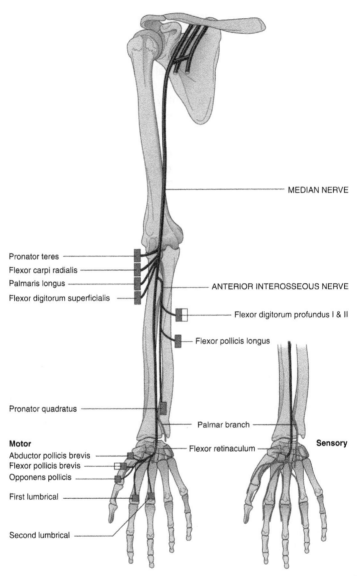

Fig. 3. Median nerve. (*From* O'Brien M. Aids to the examination of the peripheral nervous system. 5th edition. Edinburgh (United Kingdom): Saunders Elsevier; 2010.)

of the thenar muscles supplied by the median nerve. Sensory disturbance is noted in both palmar and digital nerves.[20,21]

Anterior interosseous nerve syndrome A lesion isolated to this nerve can occur as a result of catheterization, venipuncture, fibrous band, exercise, supracondylar fracture, and vascular anomalies.[22] The patient complains of pain in the proximal forearm or arm. It presents as a pure motor syndrome, with weakness of forearm pronation (pronator quadratus), and flexion of the terminal phalanges of second and third digits (flexor digitorum profundus I and II), and flexion of the terminal phalanx of the thumb

Table 2
Clinical features of median neuropathies

Compression Site	Motor Findings	Sensory Findings	Other Findings
Ligament of Struthers	Variable weakness of all median nerve innervated muscles, including the pronator muscle	Thenar eminence and first to lateral fourth digits	Pain in the proximal forearm with forearm supination and elbow extension
Pronator teres muscle	Weakness of the median thenar muscles; variable involvement of the median forearm muscles, with sparing of the pronator muscle	Thenar eminence and first to lateral fourth digits	Pain in the proximal forearm with resistance to forearm pronation and flexion at the wrist
Anterior interosseus nerve (forearm region)	Weakness of forearm pronation, flexion of the terminal phalanges of second and third digits, and flexion of the terminal phalanx of the thumb	—	Pain in the proximal forearm or arm; unable to form an O with thumb and index finger (circle sign)
Wrist (carpal tunnel syndrome)	Thenar atrophy and weakness of thumb abduction	Thumb to lateral half of the fourth digit	Wrist pain; Tinel sign; Phalen sign

(flexor pollicis longus). The patient is unable to form an O with the thumb and index finger (circle sign).[21,23]

Carpal tunnel syndrome Carpal tunnel syndrome is the most common type of nerve injury to the median nerve and is caused by compression of the nerve at the wrist as it passes between the carpal bones and flexor retinaculum. Forceful use of the hands, repetitive use of the hands, and hand-arm vibration are risk factors.[24] Other predisposing factors include obesity, diabetes, pregnancy, hypothyroidism, and connective tissue diseases.[25–27] The athlete presents with pain or paresthesias in the wrist and hand, typically severe at night and relieved with shaking or rubbing the hand. The patient may also complain about dropping things. Examination reveals atrophy and weakness of the thenar eminence with sensory disturbance of the thumb to the lateral half of the fourth digit. Sensation to the thenar eminence and radial palm is spared. The Tinel sign (percussion at the wrist elicits tingling sensation to the fingers innervated by the median nerve) and Phalen sign (flexion of the wrist to 90° for 30–60 seconds aggravates pain and paresthesias) can help confirm the diagnosis.[28–30]

History and physical examination
The athlete presents with atrophy and weakness of the thenar eminence. Numbness of the thumb to the lateral half of the fourth digit may also be a complaint. Weakness of forearm pronation and involvement of other median-innervated forearm muscles indicate a more proximal lesion. Similarly, the presence of numbness in the median palmar aspect indicates a more proximal lesion.

Management

Treatment of Ligament of Struthers/supracondylar process syndrome initially involves activity modification and antiinflammatory drugs. Surgery is often necessary.

Initial treatment of pronator syndrome includes avoiding activities that promote the symptoms (pronation/supination) and nonsteroidal antiinflammatory drugs. Steroid injections into the tender sites of the pronator teres muscle may be beneficial. Decompressing the nerve within the pronator teres muscle should be considered if no improvement is seen despite several months of conservative therapy.[31,32]

Treatment of anterior interosseous nerve syndrome follows conservative management similar to pronator syndrome. Surgery can be considered if symptoms are not improving.

For mild to moderate cases of carpal tunnel syndrome, wrist splinting, especially at night, is first-line therapy. Steroid injection into the wrist is a temporary measure to relieve symptoms. Carpal tunnel release is indicated for cases unresponsive to conservative treatment and for moderate to severe cases. Approximately 70% to 90% of patients have good to excellent long-term outcomes after carpal tunnel release.[33]

Ulnar Nerve

Anatomy

The ulnar nerve is a mixed nerve that descends to the upper arm medial to the brachial artery (**Fig. 4**). At the elbow, it enters the cubital tunnel (the groove between the medial epicondyle and the olecranon with an aponeurosis in between that serves as the roof). Distal to the elbow joint, the ulnar nerve gives off branches to the forearm muscles that it supplies: the flexor carpi ulnaris and flexor digitorum profundus III and IV muscles. At the forearm, it then gives off the dorsal ulnar cutaneous branch (which supplies the dorsal ulnar aspect of the hand, fifth digit, and half of the fourth digit) and the palmar cutaneous branch (which supplies the hypothenar eminence area). The ulnar nerve then enters the wrist lateral to the tendon of the flexor carpi ulnaris muscle and gives off the superficial terminal sensory branches (which supplies the fifth digit and medial aspect of the fourth digit). The ulnar nerve then enters the Guyon canal (formed by the pisiform carpal bone medially and the hook of hamate laterally) as the deep palmar branch. Here, it gives off motor fibers to the 4 hypothenar muscles (abductor digiti minimi, flexor digiti minimi, opponens digiti minimi, and palmaris brevis) and distally to the third and fourth lumbricals, 4 dorsal and 3 palmar interossei, adductor pollicis, and the deep head of the flexor pollicis brevis muscles.[12,34]

Lesion

Ulnar neuropathy at the elbow The most common area of compression for the ulnar nerve is the elbow area (**Table 3**). Ulnar neuropathy at the elbow is the second most common upper extremity compression neuropathy. The ulnar nerve can be compressed at the elbow in the cubital tunnel (cubital tunnel syndrome), which narrows during elbow flexion. The nerve can also be entrapped as a result of the thickening of the humeroulnar aponeurosis or bulging of the medial collateral ligament of the elbow joint. External trauma to the elbow, deformity from elbow injuries, ganglion cyst, fibrous bands, and supracondylar spurs are other causes for injury at the elbow. Pain, when present, may localize to the elbow or radiate to the medial forearm and wrist. During palpation, the ulnar nerve may be enlarged, tender, and undergo subluxation at the medial epicondyle. Applying pressure to the groove behind the medial epicondyle can aggravate paresthesias. Weakness of the flexor digitorum profundus muscle causes flexion weakness of the fourth and fifth fingers. The flexor carpi ulnaris muscle can be spared because of the internal topography of the ulnar nerve, but if

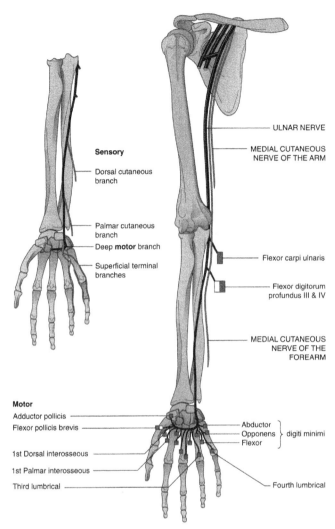

Fig. 4. Ulnar nerve. (*From* O'Brien M. Aids to the examination of the peripheral nervous system. 5th edition. Edinburgh (United Kingdom): Saunders Elsevier; 2010.)

affected leads to weakness of ulnar adduction at the wrist. Ulnar-innervated intrinsic hand muscles are involved, leading to loss of dexterity, and decreased grip and pinch strength. Sensory disturbance involves the fifth and medial fourth digits, medial hand, and dorsal medial hand.[35–37]

Ulnar neuropathy at the forearm Ulnar neuropathy at the forearm can be caused by handcuffs, hypertrophied flexor carpi ulnaris muscles, fibrous bands, hematomas, forearm fractures (eg, Colles fracture), and ischemic neuropathy as a result of an arteriovenous shunt.[38,39]

Ulnar neuropathy at the wrist or hand A lesion at this level can be caused by ganglion formation, laceration, occupational neuropathy, carpal bone fracture, lipoma, rheumatoid cyst, nerve tumor, and external pressure, such as from the use of a screwdriver,

Table 3
Clinical features of ulnar neuropathies

Compression Site	Motor Findings	Sensory Findings	Other Findings
Elbow	Variable weakness of the flexion of the fourth and fifth digits and ulnar adduction at the wrist. Loss of dexterity, decrease grip and pinch strength	Fifth and medial fourth digits, medial hand and dorsal medial hand	Medial elbow pain with tenderness on palpation
Forearm	Loss of dexterity, decreased grip and pinch strength	Fifth and medial fourth digits; variable medial hand and dorsal medial hand	Pain at ulnar forearm
Wrist: 　Proximal canal (main trunk)	Weakness of all ulnar-innervated intrinsic hand muscles	Fifth and medial fourth digits	Ulnar wrist pain
Hypothenar and deep palmar motor branch	Weakness of all ulnar-innervated intrinsic hand muscles	—	
Distal deep palmar motor branch	Weakness of the lumbricals, interossei, and adductor pollicis muscles; intact hypothenar strength	—	
Branch to first dorsal interosseus and adductor pollicis muscles	Weakness of the first dorsal interosseous and adductor pollicis muscles	—	
Sensory fibers to the fourth and fifth digits	—	Fifth and medial fourth digits	

bicycle (handlebar palsy), wheelchair, and walker. Pingree and colleagues[40] reported a case of delayed ulnar neuropathy at the wrist after open carpal tunnel release caused by translocation of the carpal tunnel contents. Ulnar neuropathy at or distal to the wrist can be divided into 5 types[41–44]:

- Proximal canal lesion: motor and sensory involvement (proximal canal lesion affecting main trunk). The patient has weakness of all ulnar hand muscles, with numbness to the medial fourth and fifth digits.
- Proximal deep palmar motor lesion: pure motor lesion affecting the hypothenar motor branches and the deep palmar motor branch. The patient has weakness of all ulnar hand muscles but has intact sensation.
- Distal deep palmar motor lesion: pure motor, affecting only the distal deep palmar motor branch. The patient has weakness of the ulnar hand muscles except the hypothenar muscles.
- More distal deep palmar motor lesion: pure motor, affecting the proximal to motor branch of the first dorsal interosseous and adductor pollicis muscles.
- Pure sensory lesion: the patient has pure sensory symptoms involving the sensory fibers to the fourth and fifth digits.

History and physical examination

Typically, the patient comes in with fourth and fifth finger numbness associated with ulnar distribution wrist and hand muscle weakness. They may have either medial elbow pain or medial wrist pain. Examination reveals tenderness at the elbow or wrist area. The presence of sensory loss at the dorsal ulnar aspect of the hand implies a lesion proximal to the wrist. The sparing of the flexor carpi ulnaris and flexor digitorum profundus III and IV muscles suggests a lesion at the wrist. In moderate or advanced cases, examination often shows the following:

- Benediction posture/ulnar claw hand: the fourth and fifth digits have a clawed appearance, with the metacarpophalangeal joints hyperextended and the proximal and distal interphalangeal joins flexed, and the fingers and thumb are held slightly abducted.
- Wartenberg sign: the fifth finger is passively abducted as a result of weakness of the third palmar interosseous muscle. The patient notes that the little finger often gets caught when they put their hand in the pocket.
- Froment sign: the thumb and indexed finger have a flexed posture when the patient is asked to pinch a paper or an object.

Management

For ulnar neuropathy at the elbow, keeping the elbow straight at night (with the use of extension splints or wrapping the elbow with a thick towel), avoiding leaning on the elbow, and use of elbow pads are recommended. For ulnar neuropathy at the wrist, the use of a wrist splint and activity modification may be sufficient. Surgery should be considered in cases unresponsive to conservative treatment, or when weakness or a compressive lesion is noted. Athletes should closely examine their biomechanics (eg, throwing motion, bike fit) before return to sport, in order to alleviate possible causes of injury.

Radial Nerve

Anatomy

The radial nerve is a mixed nerve (**Fig. 5**). After descending from the axilla, it gives rise to the posterior cutaneous nerve of the arm (which supplies posterior aspect of the arm), lower lateral cutaneous nerve of the arm (which supplies the lower lateral aspect of the arm), and the posterior cutaneous nerve of the forearm (which supplies the extensor aspect of the arm and forearm). It then gives off motor branches to the triceps and anconeus muscles before coursing around the spiral groove. The nerve then descends to the front of the lateral condyle, where it supplies the brachialis, brachioradialis, and extensor carpi radialis longus muscles. At the elbow level, it divides into the superficial branch and the deep branches. The superficial branch descends to the forearm to become the superficial radial sensory nerve (which supplies the lateral dorsum of the hands, dorsal thumb, and dorsal proximal phalanges of the second to fourth digits). The deep branch enters the supinator muscle under the arcade of Frohse and becomes the posterior interosseous nerve, which supplies the supinator, extensor carpi radialis brevis, extensor digitorum, extensor digiti minimi, extensor carpi ulnaris, abductor pollicis longus, extensor pollicis longus, extensor pollicis brevis, and extensor indicis proprius muscles.[12,45,46]

Lesions

Radial neuropathy at the spiral groove Radial nerve injury most commonly occurs at the spiral groove (**Table 4**). This condition can be caused by compression, humeral fracture, or lacerations.[47] Other circumstances include prolonged kneeling in a shooting

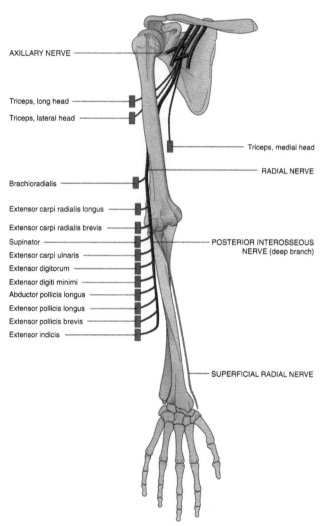

AXILLARY NERVE

Triceps, long head
Triceps, lateral head

Triceps, medial head

RADIAL NERVE

Brachioradialis

Extensor carpi radialis longus

Extensor carpi radialis brevis
Supinator
Extensor carpi ulnaris
Extensor digitorum
Extensor digiti minimi
Abductor pollicis longus
Extensor pollicis longus
Extensor pollicis brevis
Extensor indicis

POSTERIOR INTEROSSEOUS
NERVE (deep branch)

SUPERFICIAL RADIAL NERVE

Fig. 5. Radial nerve. (*From* O'Brien M. Aids to the examination of the peripheral nervous system. 5th edition. Edinburgh (United Kingdom): Saunders Elsevier; 2010.)

position in the military, wheelchair use, windmill pitching motion in softball, and repetitive sudden forceful contraction and stretching of the arm muscles.[48] Saturday night palsy is a radial nerve injury caused by prolonged compression of the radial nerve at the spiral groove after a night of deep sleep, typically associated with alcohol use. The patient presents with wrist drop, finger drop, and mild weakness of supination and elbow flexion, with sparing of the triceps muscle. Sensory disturbance is present in the lateral dorsum of the hand, thumb, and dorsal proximal part of the second and fourth digits.

Posterior interosseus nerve palsy The posterior interosseus nerve may become entrapped at the sharp edge of the extensor carpi radialis brevis muscle, arcade of Frohse, substance of supinator muscle, and constricting band at the radiohumeral joint capsule. Other causes of injury at the level include gunshot wounds, lacerations,

Table 4
Clinical features of radial neuropathies

Compression Site	Motor Findings	Sensory Findings	Other Findings
Spiral groove	Wrist drop with weakness of all radial innervated muscles except the triceps and anconeus	Lateral dorsum of the hand, dorsal thumb, and dorsal proximal phalanges of the second to fourth digits	Tenderness at spiral groove
Posterior interosseous nerve (proximal forearm)	Wrist drop with sparing of the triceps, anconeus, brachioradialis, extensor carpi radialis longus and supinator muscles	—	Wrist deviates radially when patient attempts to make a fist because of weakness of the extensor carpi ulnaris muscle
Superficial radial cutaneous branch (forearm)	—	Lateral dorsum of the hand, dorsal thumb, and dorsal proximal phalanges of the second to fourth digits	Radial forearm pain and tenderness

fractures of the proximal radius, repeated supination, and local mass lesion. The patient has wrist drop and finger drop, but the triceps, supinator, anconeus, brachioradialis, and extensor carpi radialis longus muscles are spared. The wrist deviates radially when the patient attempts to make a fist as a result of weakness of the extensor carpi ulnaris muscle, with sparing of the extensor carpi radialis muscle. There is no sensory deficit, because the superficial radial sensory nerve is also spared.[49,50]

Superficial radial neuropathy The superficial radial cutaneous branch may be injured in the forearm because of its superficial location (eg, crushing or twisting injuries, compression from handcuffs, wrist watch, ropes, bracelets, lacerations, and local nerve tumors). The patient presents with a pure sensory syndrome affecting the radial dorsum of the hand and thumb to half of the fourth digit.[51,52]

History and examination
The athlete complains of a wrist drop. There may be variable paresthesias and sensory loss on the extensor surface of the arm, forearm, and radial dorsum of the hand. Depending on the level of lesion, the athlete has weakness of elbow extension, supination, wrist extension, metacarpophalangeal joint extension, and extension and abduction of the thumb. Triceps and brachioradialis reflexes may be reduced.

Management
A trial of nonsurgical treatment (eg, antiinflammatory medications, physical therapy, cortisone injection) is warranted in all cases of radial neuropathy, except for cases with progressive motor weakness or if a compressive lesion is identified. Arnold and colleagues[53] reported that almost all patients with compressive radial neuropathy at the spiral groove experienced complete recovery, with mean time to complete recovery of 3.4 months. Patients who do not respond or continue to progress despite conservative treatment are candidates for surgical decompression.

DIAGNOSTICS
Electrodiagnostic Study

Electrodiagnostic study involves a nerve conduction study and needle examination of muscles (electromyography [EMG]). EMG is one of the main tools for diagnosing and prognosticating peripheral nerve injury. However, it is important to understand when to order the test, because optimal timing of an electrodiagnostic study varies according to the clinical situation. At 7 to 10 days after injury, electrodiagnostic study is useful at localization and separating conduction block from axonotmesis. However, if the study is performed at 3 to 4 weeks after injury, needle examination changes are evident to permit more diagnostic information. To document interval recovery or worsening of the nerve, a study 3 to 6 months from initial testing may be repeated.[1]

Imaging Studies

Plain radiography can be ordered to exclude fractures and abnormal bony formations that can compress nerves. MRI is most useful in looking for a ganglion cyst, synovial hypertrophy, muscle hypertrophy, vascular disease, and nerve changes. On MRI, normal nerve signal intensity is of intermediate to low on T1-weighted sequences, becoming slightly higher on T2-weighted and other fluid-sensitive sequences with no contrast enhancement. Abnormal MRI findings include nerve enlargement with increased T2 signal, fatty infiltration, muscle edema, and muscle atrophy.[12] MRI study for carpal tunnel syndrome has low sensitivity and specificity (sensitivity, 23%–96%; specificity, 39%–87%), but has value when looking for other structural causes of compression (eg, neoplasm, arthritis, congenital anomaly, postoperative wrist).[19]

Nerve Ultrasonography

With improving resolution, wider access, and increased portability of ultrasound instruments, nerve ultrasonography is becoming a valuable tool for assessing compressive neuropathies. The user measures the cross-sectional area (CSA) and longitudinal diameter of the nerve and looks for compressive lesions. Pathologic findings include nerve hypoechogenicity and increased CSA.[54–56] Median nerve ultrasonography can be used as a screening tool for carpal tunnel syndrome, with high sensitivity for electrodiagnostic abnormality, but it cannot determine severity.[57]

SUMMARY

By understanding the anatomy and having a firm knowledge of muscles and the cutaneous distribution that a nerve innervates, a clinician is able to localize a nerve injury. Patients usually present with weakness, pain, and paresthesias in a distribution particular to the nerve and the level of the lesion. Diagnostic tools are available to aid the clinician in the diagnosis and prognostication. Conservative management is generally attempted first before surgery is contemplated. Return to play for the athlete depends on the specific condition. In most cases, athletes can return when they attain full range of motion and full strength.

REFERENCES

1. Robinson L. Traumatic injury to peripheral nerves. Muscle Nerve 2000;23: 863–73.
2. Brazis P, Masdeu J, Jose B. Localization in clinical neurology. 4th edition. Philadelphia: Lippincott Williams & Wilkins; 2001.

3. Akgun K, Aktas I, Terzi Y. Winged scapula caused by a dorsal scapular nerve lesion: a case report. Arch Phys Med Rehabil 2008;89(10):2017–20.
4. Deeber P, Van Den EE, Moens P. Scapular winging: an unusual complication of bracing in idiopathic scoliosis. Clin Orthop Relat Res 2007;461:258–61.
5. Galano G, Bigliani L, Ahmad C, et al. Surgical treatment of winged scapula. Clin Orthop Relat Res 2008;466(3):652–60.
6. Wiater J, Flatow E. Long thoracic nerve injury. Clin Orthop Relat Res 1999;368: 17–27.
7. Neal S, Fields K. Peripheral nerve entrapment and injury in the upper extremity. Am Fam Physician 2010;81(2):147–55.
8. Boykin R, Friedman D, Higgine L. Suprascapular neuropathy. J Bone Joint Surg Am 2010;92(13):2348–64.
9. Piasecki D. Suprascapular neuropathy. J Am Acad Orthop Surg 2009;17(11): 665–76.
10. Moen T. Suprascapular neuropathy: what does the literature show? J Shoulder Elbow Surg 2012;21(6):835–46.
11. Shah A, Butler R, Sung SY, et al. Clinical outcomes of suprascapular nerve decompression. J Shoulder Elbow Surg 2011;20(6):975–82.
12. Dong Q, Jacobson J, Jamadar D, et al. Entrapment neuropathies in the upper and lower limbs: anatomy and MRI features. Radiol Res Pract 2012;2012:230679.
13. Steinmann S, Moran E. Axillary nerve injury: diagnosis and treatment. J Am Acad Orthop Surg 2011;9(5):328–35.
14. Perlmutter G. Axillary nerve injury. Clin Orthop Relat Res 1999;368:28–36.
15. Lee S, Saetia K, Saha S, et al. Axillary nerve injury associated with sports. Neurosurg Focus 2011;31(5):E10.
16. Besleaga D, Castellano V, Lutz C, et al. Musculocutaneous neuropathy: case report and discussion. HSS J 2010;6(1):112–6.
17. Stevens R, Mahadevan V, Moss A. Injury to the lateral cutaneous nerve of forearm after venous cannulation: a case report and literature review. Clin Anat 2012;25(5):659–62.
18. Pecina M, Boric I, Anticevic D. Intraoperatively proven anomalous Struthers' ligament diagnosed by MRI. Skeletal Radiol 2002;31(9):532–5.
19. Andreisek G, Crook D, Marincek B, et al. Peripheral neuropathies of the median, radial, and ulnar nerves: MR imaging features. Radiographics 2006;26(5):1267–87.
20. Rehak D. Pronator syndrome. Clin Sports Med 2001;20(3):531–40.
21. Dang A, Rodner C. Unusual compression neuropathies of the forearm, part II: median nerve. J Hand Surg Am 2009;34(10):1915–20.
22. Brennan T, Cupler E. Anterior interosseous nerve syndrome following peripheral catheterization: magnetic resonance imaging and electromyography correlation. Muscle Nerve 2011;43(5):758–60.
23. Spinner R, Amadio P. Compressive neuropathies of the upper extremity. Clin Plast Surg 2003;30(2):155–73.
24. Herbert R, Frederick G, Dropkin J. Clinical evaluation and management of work-related carpal tunnel syndrome. Am J Ind Med 2000;37(1):62–74.
25. Padua L, Pasqualle AD, Pazzaglia C, et al. Systematic review of pregnancy-related carpal tunnel syndrome. Muscle Nerve 2010;42(5):697–702.
26. Bland JD. The relationship of obesity, age, and carpal tunnel syndrome: more complex than was thought? Muscle Nerve 2005;32(4):527–32.
27. Van Djik M, Reitsma J, Fischer J, et al. Indications for requesting laboratory tests for concurrent diseases in patients with carpal tunnel syndrome: a systematic review. Clin Chem 2003;49(9):1437–44.

28. Ibrahim I, Khan W, Goddard N, et al. Carpal tunnel syndrome: a review of recent literature. Open Orthop J 2012;6:69–76.

29. Aroori S, Spence R. Carpal tunnel syndrome. Ulster Med J 2008;77(1):6–17.

30. MacDermid J, Wessel J. Clinical diagnosis of carpal tunnel syndrome: a systematic review. J Hand Ther 2004;17(2):309–19.

31. Lee A, Khorsandi M, Nurbhai N, et al. Endoscopically assisted decompression for pronator syndrome. J Hand Surg 2012;37(6):1173–9.

32. Zancolli E III, Zancolli E IV, Perotto C. New mini-invasive decompression for pronator teres syndrome. J Hand Surg 2012;37(8):1706–10.

33. Turner A, Kimble F, Gulyas K. Can the outcome of open carpal tunnel release be predicted?: a review of the literature. ANZ J Surg 2010;80(1–2):50–4.

34. Karatas A, Apaydin N, Uz A, et al. Regional anatomic structures of the elbow that may potentially compress the ulnar nerve. J Shoulder Elbow Surg 2009; 18(4):627–31.

35. Assmus H, Antoniadis G, Hoffman R, et al. Cubital tunnel syndrome–a review and management guidelines. Cent Eur Neurosurg 2011;72(2):90–8.

36. Palmer B, Hught T. Cubital tunnel syndrome. J Hand Surg 2010;35(1):153–63.

37. Gonzalez M, Lotfi P, Bendre A, et al. The ulnar nerve at the elbow and its local branching: an anatomic study. J Hand Surg Br 2001;26(2):142–4.

38. Hirasawa H, Sakai A, Toba N, et al. Bony entrapment of ulnar nerve after closed forearm fracture: a case report. J Orthop Surg (Hong Kong) 2004;12(1):122–5.

39. Campbell W. Ulnar neuropathy at the distal forearm. Muscle Nerve 1989;12: 347–52.

40. Pingree M, Bosch P, Liu P, et al. Delayed ulnar neuropathy at the wrist following open carpal tunnel release. Muscle Nerve 2005;31(3):394–7.

41. Akuthota V, Plastaras C, Lindberg K, et al. The effect of long-distance bicycling on ulnar and median nerves: an electrophysiologic evaluation of cyclist palsy. Am J Sports Med 2005;33(8):1224–30.

42. Capitani D, Beer S. Handlebar palsy–a compression syndrome of the deep terminal (motor) branch of the ulnar nerve in biking. J Neurol 2002;249(10): 1441–5.

43. Karam C, Quinn C, Panganoni S, et al. Teaching neuroimages: ganglion cyst causing pure sensory ulnar neuropathy at the wrist. Neurology 2012;79(8):e76.

44. Pearce C, Feinberg J, Wolfe S. Ulnar neuropathy at the wrist. HSS J 2009;5(2): 178–85.

45. Thomas S, Yakin D, Parry B, et al. The anatomical relationship between the posterior interosseous nerve and the supinator muscle. J Hand Surg 2000;25(5): 936–41.

46. Konjenbang M, Elangbam J. Radial nerve in the radial tunnel: anatomic sites of entrapment neuropathy. Clin Anat 2004;17(1):21–5.

47. Shao Y, Harwood P, Grotz M, et al. Radial nerve palsy associated with fractures of the shaft of the humerus: a systematic review. J Bone Joint Surg Br 2005; 87(12):1647–52.

48. Moore F. Radial neuropathies in wheelchair users. Am J Phys Med Rehabil 2009; 88(12):1017–9.

49. Naam N, Sajjan N. Radial tunnel syndrome. Orthop Clin North Am 2012;43(4): 529–36.

50. Krishnan G, Winston T, Seshadri V. Posterior interosseous nerve palsy due to intermuscular lipoma. Surg Neurol 2006;65(5):495–6.

51. Robson A, See M, Ellis H. Applied anatomy of the superficial branch of the radial nerve. Clin Anat 2008;21(1):38–45.

52. Balakrishnan C, Bachusz R, Balakrishan A, et al. Intraneural lipoma of the radial nerve presenting as Wartenberg syndrome: a case report and review of literature. Can J Plast Surg 2009;17(4):e39–41.
53. Arnold DW, Krishna V, Freimer M, et al. Prognosis of acute compressive radial neuropathy. Muscle Nerve 2012;45(6):893–5.
54. Impink B, Gagnon D, Collinger J, et al. Repeatability of ultrasonographic median nerve measures. Muscle Nerve 2010;41(6):767–73.
55. Padua L, Liotta G, Pasquale D. Contribution of ultrasound in the assessment of nerve diseases. Eur J Neurol 2012;19(1):47–54.
56. Martinoli C, Bianchi S, Pugliese F. Sonography of entrapment neuropathies in the upper limb (wrist excluded). J Clin Ultrasound 2004;32(9):438–50.
57. Mhoon J, Juel V, Hobson-Webb L. Median nerve ultrasound as a screening tool in carpal tunnel syndrome: correlation of cross-sectional area measures with electrodiagnostic abnormality. Muscle Nerve 2012;46(6):871–8.

Complementary and Alternative Treatments in Sports Medicine

Michael A. Malone, MD, ABIHM[a],*, Kathryn Gloyer, MD, CAQSM[a,b]

KEYWORDS

- Sports medicine • Pain • Musculoskeletal • Integrative • Holistic
- Complementary and alternative medicine • Acupuncture

KEY POINTS

- Complementary and alternative medicine (CAM) treatments are commonly used by patients for a variety of musculoskeletal conditions.
- There is a scarcity in both the quantity and quality of CAM treatments for specific musculoskeletal conditions.
- Acupuncture may be useful for multiple musculoskeletal conditions, although studies on acupuncture for these conditions often show conflicting results.
- Multiple CAM treatments exist for the treatment of osteoarthritis (OA) and may play an important role in reducing inflammation, pain, and even joint destruction related to OA.
- Data from small studies are encouraging for the possible treatment of concussion with omega-3 fatty acids, although more clinical data are needed.
- Vitamin D may be useful in preventing sports injuries, particularly stress fractures, although more studies are needed in this area.
- Functional medicine and mind-body medicine are treatment approaches that may be useful in multiple musculoskeletal conditions.

INTRODUCTION

Many patients suffering from pain and dysfunction attributable to musculoskeletal conditions will use some form of complementary and alternative medicine (CAM). Unfortunately, there is a paucity of both the quantity and quality of CAM treatments for specific musculoskeletal conditions. Many CAM treatments are used for a variety of musculoskeletal conditions, but may be more commonly used for specific conditions. This article first addresses the use of CAM for specific musculoskeletal conditions, followed by a

[a] Department of Family and Community Medicine, Penn State Milton S. Hershey Medical Center, 500 University Drive, Hershey, PA 17033, USA; [b] Department of Orthopaedics and Rehabilitation, Penn State Orthopaedics, 1850 East Park Avenue, Suite 112, State College, PA 16803, USA
* Corresponding author.
E-mail address: mmalone@hmc.psu.edu

Prim Care Clin Office Pract 40 (2013) 945–968
http://dx.doi.org/10.1016/j.pop.2013.08.010   **primarycare.theclinics.com**
0095-4543/13/$ – see front matter © 2013 Elsevier Inc. All rights reserved.

review of other CAM treatments and their potential indications for a multitude of conditions, based on the current medical literature and traditional use.

LATERAL EPICONDYLITIS
Acupuncture

Acupuncture does have evidence for efficacy in lateral epicondylitis. A placebo-controlled, single-blind trial of 45 people with tennis elbow compared the effectiveness of real and sham acupuncture given twice weekly for 10 weeks. The results showed significant improvement in pain intensity and ability to use the elbow among those who received real acupuncture.[1] Good results were also seen in a placebo-controlled study of 48 people with tennis elbow.[2] A systematic review concluded: "There is strong evidence suggesting that acupuncture is effective in the short-term relief of lateral epicondyle pain."[3] However, another study showed only temporary efficacy and was ineffective compared with placebo at 3 months.[4]

Laser acupuncture has not been shown to be an adequate substitute for needle acupuncture. A double-blind study of 49 people with tennis elbow failed to find 10 treatments with laser acupuncture to be more effective than the same number of treatments using fake laser acupuncture.[5] Another study of 58 patients with the same condition found laser acupuncture to be no more effective than ultrasound treatments or wearing a brace.[6]

Leech Therapy

Based on a small randomized trial, leech therapy (applying leeches to the painful area) may provide better short-term pain relief for people with tennis elbow in comparison with topical diclofenac.[7]

TENDONITIS
Rotator Cuff Tendonitis

Acupuncture has been found to be effective for the treatment of rotator cuff tendonitis. A trial of 52 people with rotator cuff tendonitis found acupuncture to be more effective than a similar therapeutic setting with placebo needling in the treatment of pain.[8] In another study, 117 people with rotator cuff injury (including tendonitis) were randomized to receive corticosteroid injections plus exercise or 10 acupuncture treatments plus exercise. Both groups experienced similar improvements in shoulder function and pain.[9]

In a sizable randomized trial, 425 patients receiving physical therapy for their persistent shoulder pain were divided into two groups: one received single-point acupuncture while the other received a sham treatment for 3 weeks. The acupuncture group showed significant improvement over the control group 1 week after treatment.[10] However, not all studies have been positive. In a small trial of 32 patients with rotator cuff tendonitis, acupuncture was no better than placebo transcutaneous electrical nerve stimulation (TENS) when added to exercise.[11]

Tendonitis (of All Types) Treatments

A form of massage called deep transverse friction massage has shown some promise for tendonitis, but as yet the research record is too weak for conclusions to be drawn.[12]

The herb white willow contains a substance called salicin, which is similar in some respects to aspirin. It seems likely that appropriate doses of the herb might offer some symptomatic relief for tendonitis.

OSTEOARTHRITIS

Osteoarthritis (OA) is a progressive degenerative joint disease that has a major impact on joint function and quality of life. Multiple CAM treatments exist for the treatment of OA, and may play an important role in reducing inflammation, pain, and even joint destruction related to OA.

Acupuncture

A meta-analysis of 14 randomized controlled trials (RCTs) involving 3835 patients evaluated short-term pain, long-term pain, and functional measures. The study concluded that acupuncture provided significantly better relief from knee OA pain and a larger improvement in function than sham acupuncture, standard care treatment, or waiting for further treatment.[13]

A Cochrane review of acupuncture for OA concluded:

Sham-controlled trials show statistically significant benefits; however, these benefits are small, do not meet our pre-defined thresholds for clinical relevance, and are probably due at least partially to placebo effects from incomplete blinding. Waiting list-controlled trials of acupuncture for peripheral joint OA suggest statistically significant and clinically relevant benefits, much of which may be due to expectation or placebo effects.[14]

S-Adenosylmethionine

S-Adenosylmethionine (SAMe) is a naturally occurring compound found in almost every tissue and fluid in the body. SAMe plays a role in the immune system, maintains cell membranes, and helps produce and breakdown central nervous system neurotransmitters, such as serotonin, melatonin, and dopamine. It was discovered in 1952 and has been used intravenously to treat medical conditions in Europe since the 1970s. More stable enteric forms were developed during the 1990s, which is also when SAMe became available in the United States.[15]

Medical literature on efficacy
A review of 11 studies reported that "SAMe appears to be as effective as NSAIDs [nonsteroidal anti-inflammatories] in reducing pain and improving limitations in patients with OA, without the adverse effects often associated with NSAIDs."[16] More recently, a 16-week randomized, double-blind, crossover study of 61 patients comparing SAMe 1200 mg with celoxicam 200 mg showed no significant difference between the two groups ($P<.01$). The end points of the study included pain, functional health, mood status, isometric joint function tests, and side effects.[17] A 2009 Cochrane review, however, identified 4 trials (N = 656) comparing SAMe with placebo or no intervention and was inconclusive, hampered by the inclusion of mainly small trials of questionable quality.[18]

Dosage and forms
A typical dose in OA is 400 to 1200 mg per day, in 2 to 3 divided doses. There are 2 chemical forms of SAMe available on the market. There is a 1,4-butane disulfonate form (controlled studies done mostly with this form), and a tosylate (toluene sulfonate) form that is not well studied. SAMe use is limited by its high costs and product quality issues. SAMe biochemically is an unstable compound, therefore it is unclear as to how much active ingredient remains after a product sits on the store shelf for weeks or months.[19]

Side effects
SAMe is also used as an antidepressant, and may induce mania in patients with bipolar disorder.[20]

Taking SAMe at the same time as selective serotonin reuptake inhibitors may increase the risk of serotonin syndrome.

Pregnant and breastfeeding women should not take SAMe, as it interacts with folic acid.

Aquamin

This mineral-rich supplement is derived from Lithothamnion coralloides, a (sustainably harvested) form of red algae. In a 12-week pilot RCT of 22 men and women with moderate to severe knee OA, those randomized to 2400 mg daily of Aquamin showed significant increases in passive and active extension, and an increased 6-minute walk distance (but with no differences in pain or joint mobility scores). There was a 50% reduction in use of nonsteroidal anti-inflammatory drugs (NSAIDs) in the Aquamin group.[21]

Avocado-Soybean Unsaponifiables

This supplement is proposed to increase collagen production and suppress inflammatory cytokines. Avocado-soybean unsaponifiables (ASU) have been available for many years in France as the prescription drug Piascledine.

Medical literature on efficacy

A 2003 systematic review was inconclusive, stating that:

> The majority of rigorous trial data available to date suggest that ASU is effective for the symptomatic treatment of OA and more research seems warranted. However, the only real long-term trial yielded a largely negative result.[22]

A 2008 systematic review of 4 trials (all supported by the manufacturer) concluded that:

> Based on the available evidence, patients may be recommended to give ASU a chance for about 3 months. Meta-analysis data support better chances of success in patients with knee OA than in those with hip OA.[23]

Boswellia

This herb is commonly used in Ayurvedic medicine, which is native to the Indian subcontinent, and as a form of alternative medicine in the United States.

Medical literature on efficacy

Benefit was seen in an 8-week RCT of 30 subjects with knee OA, but the article did not discuss the randomization process.[24] A more recent 90-day, double-blind, randomized, placebo-controlled study on 60 patients with OA showed statistically significant improvements in pain scores and physical function scores with Boswellia in comparison with placebo.[25]

In a 6-month controlled study of knee OA published in 2013, Ayurvedic formulations (extracts of Tinospora cordifolia, Zingiber officinale, Emblica officinalis, Boswellia serrata) significantly reduced knee pain and improved knee function, and were equivalent to glucosamine and celecoxib. However, unexpected liver abnormalities were found (see later discussion).[26]

Boswellia serrata was found to be the most promising anti-inflammatory supplement in a recent review of natural anti-inflammatories.[27]

Safety

A significant proportion of Ayurvedic medicines (such as Boswellia) contain heavy metals, and there are numerous reports of heavy metal poisoning, particularly lead poisoning, related to use of these products.[28]

In the 2013 trial showing efficacy of Ayurvedic formulations for knee OA, there was an unexpected increase in alanine aminotransferase (with otherwise normal liver function tests), which requires further safety assessment.[26]

Bromelain

Bromelain is a proteolytic enzyme present in the stem and fruit of pineapple. A 2004 review of the current literature concluded that evidence of benefit is promising for the treatment of OA, but that more definitive studies are needed. A follow-up double-blind RCT of 47 subjects in 2006 by the same lead author concluded that bromelain was not efficacious as an adjunctive treatment of moderate to severe OA.[29,30]

BSP 201 (Shea-Nut Extract)

BSP 201 is a high-triterpene shea-nut extract, containing 70% triterpenes. Shea nuts have been used in food and traditional African medicine for generations, particularly in West Africa.[31,32]

A 15-week RCT in 117 patients with clinical and radiographic evidence of hip or knee OA showed significant reductions in biomarkers of inflammation, including tumor necrosis factor α, interleukin (IL)-6, C-reactive protein (CRP), and C-telopeptide of type II collagen.[31]

Cat's Claw (Uncaria tomentosa)

Cat's claw, which derives its name from its claw-shaped thorns, is a woody vine found in the tropical jungles of South and Central America. Benefit was shown in a 4-week RCT with 45 men, using 100 mg of a freeze-dried extract, with some responding in as little as 1 week, and with a reduction in prostaglandin E_2 observed in the treatment group.[32] Another review of the efficacy of Uncaria for OA concluded that "cat's claw is an effective treatment for osteoarthritis."[32] A more recent 2012 review, however, concluded that: "Cat's claw has not been rigorously tested to determine its antiarthritic potential in in vitro and in vivo models. High-quality clinical trials are needed to determine its effectiveness."[33]

Turmeric (Genus Cercuma)

This Ayurvedic anti-inflammatory herb, whose active ingredient is curcumin, has been used for 4000 years to treat a variety of conditions. Turmeric is widely used in cooking, and gives Indian curry its flavor and yellow color. The best characterized constituent is curcumin.

Medical literature on efficacy

In a 6-week RCT of 107 patients with symptomatic primary OA of the knee, those randomized to Curcuma domestica extract, 500 mg 4 times a day, showed significant improvement in pain and function from baseline, similar in magnitude to the group randomized to ibuprofen 400 mg twice a day.[34]

Meriva is a brand-name product designed to enhance absorption of curcumin and increase resistance of curcumin to degradation. In a 90-day RCT of 50 patients with radiographically confirmed OA, those randomized to 1 g daily of Meriva showed a 58% improvement in WOMAC (Western Ontario and McMaster Universities Arthritis Index) scores and a marked decrease in CRP levels.[35] In a subsequent 8-month trial of 100 patients with OA of one or both knees, those randomized to 1 g daily of Meriva showed a significant increase in treadmill distance, significant improvement in inflammatory markers, a 63% decrease in NSAID and painkiller usage, and significant improvement in functional, social, and emotional parameters.[36]

Ginger

Ginger is an anti-inflammatory herb native to Asia. It has been used as a cooking spice for thousands of years and has been used as a medicine in Asian, Indian, and Arabic herbal traditions since ancient times.

Benefit was reported with brand-name ginger extract EV.EXT 77 in a 6-week, manufacturer-sponsored multicenter RCT of 261 patients with knee OA.[37] In a 3-month double-blind, placebo-controlled crossover trial in 29 patients with debilitating knee OA, patients experienced less pain while taking ginger.[38] However, no benefit was seen in a previous crossover trial.[39]

A 6-week, double-blind RCT with 50 subjects looked at the efficacy of a combination 4% ginger and plai extract gel compared with 1% diclofenac gel for the treatment of OA of the knee. Both the combination ginger and plai extract gel relieved joint pain, improved problematic symptoms, and improved the quality of life in knee OA during a 6-week treatment regimen, with no differences from the 1% diclofenac gel group.[40]

Side effects

Side effects from ginger are rare, but if taken in high doses the herb may cause mild heartburn, diarrhea, and irritation of the mouth.[15]

Niacinamide

Niacinamide is a potent inhibitor of poly(ADP)-ribose synthase (PARS), and thus suppresses cytokine-mediated induction of nitric oxide synthase (NOS). Niacinamide 500 mg in combination with N-acetylcysteine 200 mg and vitamin C 100 mg is available as the proprietary product Alapars (Metagenics), with suggested dosing of 1 tablet 3 times a day.

In a 12-week double-blind pilot study of 72 patients, niacinamide 500 mg 6 times a day was effective for OA.[41]

Pine Bark Extract (Pycnogenol)

Pine bark is an antioxidant with several proposed medical uses, including cardiovascular and musculoskeletal. Pycnogenol is a standardized extract of French maritime pine bark. In a 3-month RCT of 100 patients with stages I and II OA of the knee, those treated with Pycnogenol 50 mg 3 times a day showed significant improvement on the WOMAC, significant alleviation of pain by visual analog scale (VAS), and less use of analgesics.[42]

In an RCT of 156 OA patients with high-sensitivity (hs)-CRP greater than 3 mg/L, those treated with Pycnogenol 100 mg/d showed a significantly greater decrease in the hs-CRP, as well as a reduction in pain and stiffness.[43]

Side effects

No major side effects were noted in these studies or in other recent studies on pine bark extract.[44]

Rose Hips

Rose hips are the round portion of the rose flower just below the petals, and have been a popular medicinal treatment for many years in Scandinavia. The standardized product used in the published studies is Hyben Vital, also known as LitoZin, marketed in the United States through EuroPharma in Green Bay, Wisconsin. This fruit is rich in vitamin C, but much of the vitamin C in rose hips is destroyed during drying and processing and also declines rapidly during storage. For this reason, many rose hip–derived "natural" vitamin C products have actually been fortified with laboratory-made vitamin C, but their labels may not always say so.[45]

Medical literature on efficacy

A manufacturer-sponsored 4-month RCT of 100 patients on a waiting list for a hip or knee replacement and using 5 g/d rose hips powder and a primary outcome of hip or knee mobility showed a significant benefit of treatment.[46] A second manufacturer-sponsored 3-month crossover RCT of 112 patients, average age 64 years, using 5 g/d rose hips powder and a primary outcome of pain and stiffness, showed significant benefit of treatment.[47] A third manufacturer-sponsored 3-month RCT of 94 patients with OA using 5 g/d rose hips powder showed significant improvement in WOMAC scores at 3 weeks, but no significant difference in WOMAC scores at 3 months. There was a 40% reduction in the use of rescue analgesics in the treatment group.[48]

Vitamin D

Framingham data in 556 subjects showed that the risk of progression of knee OA was increased about 3-fold in those in the middle and lowest tertiles for vitamin D intake, as well as those in the lowest and middle tertiles for serum 25-hydroxyvitamin D (25(OH) D) levels.[49] Although a review concluded that "the findings indicate that vitamin D status is unrelated to the risk of joint space or cartilage," a more recent 2013 systematic review concluded that data are currently insufficient to determine the association between vitamin D and OA.[50,51]

White Willow Bark

White willow bark is the plant from which aspirin is derived. Therefore, it does not have significant theoretical benefit over aspirin. However, pain relief with the herb is reported to be more gradual in onset and longer lasting than that with aspirin. Benefit was seen in a 2-week trial in 78 hospitalized patients,[52] which concluded that the willow bark extract showed a moderate analgesic effect in OA and appeared to be well tolerated. The typical dose is 2 400-mg tablets (15% salicin) daily.

Vitamin C

Framingham data show that higher intake is associated with slower progression of OA symptoms.[53] Vitamin C is required for the synthesis of collagen, and this may be the basis of benefit associated with higher intake.

Tai Chi

An RCT of 72 patients examining the implementation of 12 forms of Tai Chi exercise for 12 weeks documented safety and efficacy, although there was a 42% dropout rate.[54] A systematic review article of 5 RCTs and 7 controlled clinical trials concludes that Tai Chi may be effective for pain control in patients with knee OA, but the evidence is not convincing for improvement in physical function.[55]

Magnetic Bracelets

Magnetic bracelets of 170- to 200-mT strength appeared to be effective in a 12-week RCT of 194 individuals with knee or hip OA, based on changes in WOMAC and VAS pain scores.[56] A small RCT of 29 subjects in which the experimental subjects received either high-strength magnetic (active) or placebo-magnetic (placebo) knee-sleeve treatment for 4 hours in a monitored setting and self-treatment 6 hours daily for 6 weeks also showed statistically significant evidence of efficacy for the magnetic sleeve.[57]

However, results from a randomized, double-blind, placebo-controlled crossover trial of 45 patients for 16 weeks indicate that magnetic and copper bracelets are generally ineffective for managing pain, stiffness, and physical function in OA, and concluded that therapeutic benefits are most likely attributable to nonspecific placebo effects. However, such devices have no major adverse effects and may provide hope.[58]

Limbrel

Limbrel is a proprietary mixture (>90% standardized blend) of 2 specific flavonoids (baicalcin and catechin) shown to have inhibitory effects on cyclooxygenase (COX)-1, COX-2, and 5-lipoxygenase.[59] Limbrel is marketed as a medical food and is available only by prescription. In a 4-week pilot RCT of 103 individuals with grade 2 or 3 OA of the knee, those who received Limbrel 500 mg twice a day showed improvement similar in magnitude to those who received naproxen 500 mg twice a day. In each group, the reduction in signs and symptoms from baseline was approximately 85% ($P<.001$).[60]

Side effects
Limbrel can cause clinically significant liver injury, which seems to resolve within weeks after cessation.[61]

Glucosamine with Chondroitin

Historically, glucosamine and chondroitin have been available in Europe and other countries since the 1980s, often available only by prescription. These supplements were not widely available in the United States until the late 1990s, but have become very popular for the treatment of OA.

Medical literature on efficacy
Results have been conflicting for glucosamine. A 3-year study of 202 Czech subjects with OA of the knee who received 1500 mg glucosamine sulfate daily (Rotta Pharmaceuticals preparation) showed a statistically significant mean reduction of 26% in WOMAC scores, compared with a mean reduction of 16% in WOMAC scores in the placebo group. The study concluded that "long-term treatment with glucosamine sulfate retarded the progression of knee OA, possibly determining disease modification."[62]

A meta-analysis of 7 RCTs (N = 703) of chondroitin sulfate monotherapy for OA of the hip or knee showed a 20% improvement in pain scores with placebo, compared with a 60% improvement in pain scores with chondroitin sulfate, a statistically significant difference. Global assessments by physicians and patients also consistently favored chondroitin over placebo. These trials were all conducted in Europe, and most were 3 to 6 months in duration.[63] However, a more recent meta-analysis of chondroitin sulfate that examined 20 trials (N = 3846) concluded that only 3 trials that were large and methodologically rigorous enough, and analysis of these 3 trials failed to show significant symptomatic benefit associated with the use of supplemental chondroitin sulfate.[64]

In 2006, the Glucosamine/Chondroitin Arthritis Intervention Trial (GAIT) trial, a double-blinded placebo and celecoxib-controlled trial, was published in the *New England Journal of Medicine*. The results of this trial, which failed to show benefit from glucosamine and chondroitin, were widely publicized in the lay press. This 6-month trial examined differences in pain and function in 1583 patients suffering from primary OA of the knee. Subjects (mean age 59 years) were stratified at baseline based on symptom severity. Acetaminophen (Tylenol) 500 mg in doses up to 4 g per 24 hours was available to all groups as rescue medicine for pain. The 4 arms of the trial included glucosamine HCl

500 mg 3 times a day (manufactured by Ferro-Pfanisteihl, Germany), chondroitin sulfate 400 mg 3 times a day (manufactured by Bioberica, Spain), glucosamine HCl 500 mg 3 times a day plus chondroitin sulfate 400 mg 3 times a day, celecoxib (Celebrex) 200 mg daily, and placebo. The only group in which the primary outcome measure was statistically different from placebo was the celecoxib group (70.1% vs 60.1% in the placebo arm). The response rate was 64% in the glucosamine arm, 65.4% in the chondroitin arm, and 66.6% in the glucosamine plus chondroitin arm, all statistically comparable with placebo.[65]

Data since the GAIT trial, however, have been conflicting. In support of efficacy, a 6-month trial of 318 patients with moderately severe knee OA published in 2007 compared the efficacy of oral glucosamine sulfate 1500 mg once daily, acetaminophen 3 g/d, and placebo. The study found that glucosamine sulfate was more effective than placebo in treating knee OA symptoms. Although acetaminophen also had a higher response rate than placebo, it failed to show significant effects on the algofunctional indexes (Lequesne index and WOMAC).[66]

A 2005 Cochrane review concluded that "pooled results from studies using a non-Rotta preparation or adequate allocation concealment failed to show benefit in pain and WOMAC function while those studies evaluating the Rotta preparation showed that glucosamine was superior to placebo in the treatment of pain and functional impairment resulting from symptomatic OA." A 2009 update of this Cochrane review came to the same conclusion.[67] However, a network meta-analysis of 10 RCTs (N = 3803), with 8 trials of the knee, 1 of the hip, and 1 of the knee and hip, concluded that glucosamine and chondroitin, alone or in combination, do not clinically improve joint pain in the knee or hip.[68]

Side effects

Although shellfish allergy is considered by some as a relative contraindication to glucosamine, there are no published reports of reactions to glucosamine in those with shellfish allergy.[69] For those individuals with shellfish allergy who are concerned about taking glucosamine, Regenasure is a glucosamine product manufactured from corn instead of shellfish. Moreover, although there are case reports of bleeding or bruising in patients on warfarin who take glucosamine, most individuals in the case reports were taking much higher doses than the recommended dose of 1500 mg/d.

Most chondroitin is derived from bovine cartilage. Although there is a theoretical concern that lax manufacturing practices could allow for cross-contamination of the bovine cartilage with bovine tissue known to cause bovine encephalopathy, there are no published case reports of bovine encephalopathy attributed to consumption of bovine cartilage.

Guided Imagery

Guided imagery is a therapeutic modality whereby directed thoughts and suggestions are used to guide imagination toward a relaxed, focused state. A facilitator, tapes, or scripts can be used to guide the body to respond the imagined state as though it were real. A small 12-week RCT of 28 older women with OA reported significant reduction in pain and mobility scores with 12 weeks of treatment.[70]

Exercise

This treatment could be considered "alternative" or "complementary," as it is often something most patients do not want to do, and is an activity that physicians may fail to emphasize in the treatment of OA.

Medical literature: knee OA and exercise

A systematic review of 3 RCTs, 8 to 24 weeks in duration, found that an aerobic walking program was more effective than placebo in reducing pain and improving function in those with knee OA.[71] A Cochrane review of land-based therapeutic exercise for OA of the knee identified 32 studies (N = 3616 for pain and N = 3719 for physical function), and reported that while there was marked variability across the studies, the studies using more rigorous methodologies did report benefit. The investigators concluded:

> There is platinum level evidence that land-based therapeutic exercise has at least short term benefit in terms of reduced knee pain and improved physical function for people with knee OA. The magnitude of the treatment effect would be considered small, but comparable to estimates reported for nonsteroidal anti-inflammatory drugs.[72]

High-Heeled Shoes

Avoiding the chronic use of high-heeled shoes may reduce the risk for developing degenerative changes, as a small study showed increased force across the patellofemoral joint and a greater compressive force on the medial compartment of the knee (average 23% greater forces) during walking in high heels than when barefoot. The altered forces at the knee caused by walking in high heels may predispose to degenerative changes in the joint.[73]

Yoga

A small 8-week RCT showed that yoga in conjunction with patient education and group support improved pain and tenderness in patients with hand OA.[74] Yoga also appeared to attenuate peak muscle soreness in women following a bout of eccentric exercise. These findings may have implications for coaches, athletes, and the exercising public who may wish to implement yoga training as a preseason regimen or supplemental activity to lessen the symptoms associated with muscle soreness.[75]

CONCUSSION/MILD TRAUMATIC BRAIN INJURY

Concussion, also known as mild traumatic brain injury (TBI), is defined as a complex pathophysiologic process affecting the brain, induced by biomechanical forces. The subsequent pathologic cascade that ensues is due to inflammatory responses, excitotoxicity, and oxidative stress. The clinical changes largely reflect a functional disturbance rather than a structural injury.[76]

Omega-3 Fatty Acids

There are recent promising data (mostly animal models) supporting the use of nutritional support, mainly omega-3 fatty acids (O3FAs), for both prevention and treatment of the effects of mild TBI. There have not been any human clinical trials published involving supplementation in individuals sustaining this type of injury, but laboratory data are favorable.

Docosahexaenoic acid (DHA) and eicosapentaenoic acid (EPA) are the most important O3FAs for potential benefit in concussion and TBI. These acids must be obtained from the diet, and humans need to supplement dietary intake. There are many other proposed mechanisms of action of O3FAs within the brain. O3FAs are essential for maintenance of cellular membrane fluidity, which affects the neurotransmission speed. DHA and EPA can also regulate voltage-gated ion channels such as K^+ channels. Dietary supplementation of DHA and EPA has been shown to decrease reactive oxygen species and to improve cognitive function in vivo.[77]

A study found that supplementation with O3FAs 30 days after injury reduces the number of damaged axons to levels similar to those of uninjured animals.[78] The same laboratory also published another study showing that giving supplemental O3FAs 30 days before TBI reduces the injury response, as measured by axonal injury counts, markers for cellular injury and apoptosis, and memory assessment by water-maze testing.[79] Another study demonstrated that fish oil can attenuate TBI-induced deficits in evoked dopamine release in the striatum, which may have implications for behavioral impairments.[80] Case studies have reported remarkable improvement in function and status after high doses of DHA and EPA were given after TBI.[81]

More studies need to be done to investigate how these O3FAs respond in humans with both mild TBI and TBI. O3FAs are readily available, highly safe, and well tolerated, making them an enticing potential option for treatment.

COMPLEMENTARY AND ALTERNATIVE TREATMENTS USEFUL IN A MULTITUDE OF MUSCULOSKELETAL CONDITIONS
Procedural Treatments

Acupuncture
History of acupuncture Acupuncture originated in China approximately 2000 to 5000 years ago, and is one of the oldest medical procedures in the world. The word "acupuncture" is derived from the Latin words *acus* (needle) and *punctura* (penetration).

Use of acupuncture in the United States In the 1980s and 1990s, less than 1% of Americans had tried acupuncture. Despite an overall decrease in visits to CAM providers in 2007 compared with 1997, visits to acupuncturists increased over this same period, with 17.6 million visits estimated for 2007 (79.2 visits per 1000 adults), or 3 times that observed in 1997 (27.2 visits per 1000 adults). The most commonly treated conditions were back pain, neck pain, joint pain, and headache.[82]

Types of acupuncture There are multiple types of acupuncture, including traditional Chinese, French, hand, auricular, and scalp acupuncture. The needles can be heated with moxa (made from dried mugwort). Elecroacupuncture is a technique used to augment acupuncture, whereby a small electric current is used to stimulate the acupuncture needles.

Possible complications Although acupuncture is considered to be low risk for complications, the following have been reported:

- Bleeding
- Infection
- Vasovagal syncope (to prevent this, the patient should be lying down, particularly for the first time that the patient has the procedure performed)
- Lightheaded/dizziness
- Nausea
- Damage to underlying nerves, blood vessels, and organs
- Pneumothorax

Postprocedural care The patient is monitored until not lightheaded or nauseous.

Current controversies There are ongoing controversies regarding the placebo used in acupuncture studies. Many of the "placebos" used may be effective treatments for pain. This aspect becomes particularly problematic in systematic reviews of acupuncture for pain in which different placebos from multiple studies are combined.

A recent article reviewing this controversy concluded:

Experimental and clinical studies have shown that the acupuncture placebo procedures applied are not inert, (from a psycho-physiological perspective) and should therefore not be interpreted as placebo controls in RCTs for the test of efficacy, that is, the present research trial design (placebo acupuncture vs acupuncture) may be questioned. Instead of reducing bias, it introduces a bias against the findings of the acupuncture treatment. The introduction of the placebo needle was a brilliant idea, however, it is up to the user to determine what its use may reflect and how its effect should be interpreted in an evidenced-based medicine perspective.[83]

Literature review

Acupuncture for back pain Most of the meta-analyses on acupuncture for pain are inconclusive, owing to the significant effect of "sham acupuncture." However, a meta-analysis of 33 RCTs of acupuncture for acute or chronic back pain was performed. For the primary outcome of short-term relief of chronic pain, the meta-analysis showed that acupuncture is significantly more effective than sham treatment (standardized mean difference, 0.54 [95% confidence interval, 0.35–0.73]; 7 trials) and no additional treatment (standardized mean difference, 0.69 [95% confidence interval, 0.40–0.98]; 8 trials). For patients with acute low back pain, data were sparse and inconclusive. Data were insufficient for drawing conclusions about acupuncture's short-term effectiveness in comparison with most other therapies.[84]

An RCT compared acupuncture, simulated acupuncture, and usual care for chronic low back pain. At 8 weeks and 1 year, there was significant improvement in the acupuncture group compared with the usual-care group. However, the improvement was not statistically different from the improvement obtained with simulated acupuncture.[85]

A 2010 systematic review of 50 years of medical literature on acupuncture for back pain concluded that "most of the published articles about acupuncture for LBP [low back pain] in the biomedical literature consist of case reports, case series, or intervention studies with designs inadequate to assess its efficacy."[86]

Electroacupuncture has been shown to improve pain and posttreatment function to a greater extent than sham percutaneous electrical nerve stimulation, TENS, and exercise ($P<.05$). Compared with the other 3 modalities, 91% of the patients reported that electroacupuncture was the most effective in decreasing their low back pain.[87] Another study showed that electroacupuncture in combination with general conditioning and aerobic exercise was more effective than either treatment alone.[88]

Functional ankle instability A study of 50 athletes with functional ankle instability who were treated for 8 weeks with electroacupuncture or physiotherapy evaluated the effect on proprioception. The study concluded that electroacupuncture can effectively improve the proprioception of athletes with functional ankle instability, and achieves efficacy superior to that of conventional physiotherapy.[89]

Exercise recovery A Chinese study investigated the effects of auricular acupuncture on 24 male elite basketball athletes' recovery abilities after exercise. The data of heart rate (HR_{max}), oxygen consumption (VO_{2max}), and blood lactic acid were measured at 4 points of time: during the rest period, after warm-ups, and at the 5th, 30th and 60th minutes after exercise, respectively. The results showed that both HR_{max} and blood lactic acid in auricular acupuncture were significantly lower in the athletes who received auricular acupuncture when compared with controls who did not. The investigators concluded that their data suggest that auricular acupuncture can enhance athletes' recovery abilities after aggressive exercise.[90]

A field test was performed on 3 groups of runners of different performance levels preparing for a marathon. The first group was given acupuncture and the second a placebo, with the third being the control group. After their maximum pulse rates were recorded, the runners were asked to run 5000 m 4 times in 4 weeks at 75% of their maximum pulse rate. Their pulse rates were measured for each runner at the finish of the run, and subsequently 1, 2, and 5 minutes after the run. Based on these data, the complexity factor (running time multiplied by the respective pulse rate) was calculated for all 4 recorded pulse rates for each run and each runner. All groups showed statistically significant enhancements in their running times and their complexity factors, but in the case of the runners treated with acupuncture, the improvements were highly significant. The field test showed that acupuncture has a significant impact on the performance of the athletes in endurance sports.[91]

Plantar fasciitis A study of 38 male subjects with plantar fasciitis randomly allocated subjects to two different groups of 19 male participants in each group. One group was treated with ice, NSAID medication, and a stretching and a strengthening program, while a second group received the same therapeutic procedures as group 1, reinforced by acupuncture treatment. The study concluded that "acupuncture should be considered as a major therapeutic instrument for the decrease of heel pain, combined with traditional medical approaches."[92]

Achilles tendonitis An RCT at 2 centers of 64 randomized patients aged 18 to 70 years with chronic Achilles tendinopathy concluded that acupuncture intervention could improve pain and activity in patients with chronic Achilles tendinopathy, in comparison with eccentric exercises.[93]

For rotator cuff tendonitis, OA, and epicondylitis, see the sections on each individual condition.

Massage therapy
Since ancient times, massage, together with olive oil rub, has been used to reduce muscle fatigue and to prevent the occurrence of sports injuries. The therapeutic use of oil massage in the ancient world was fully recognized. As a result, Athenian athlothetes (sponsors of sporting events) provided free oil to all sports facilities, where athletes could make free use of it.[94]

Benefit was seen with massage therapy in an RCT of 68 subjects with knee OA.[95] An RCT of Chinese massage combined with herbal ointment also showed benefit for nonspecific low back pain in 110 subjects. After 4 weeks, the experimental group experienced significant improvements in pain and in local muscle stiffness compared with the control group. No adverse events were observed. Findings suggested that Chinese massage combined with herbal ointment may be a beneficial CAM therapy for athletes with nonspecific low back pain.[96] A Cochrane review of massage for low back pain concluded that "massage might be beneficial for patients with subacute and chronic nonspecific low back pain, especially when combined with exercises and education."[97]

Tai Chi
The ancient health art of Tai Chi contributes to chronic pain management in 3 major areas: adaptive exercise, mind-body interaction, and meditation. Trials examining the health benefit of Tai Chi in chronic pain conditions are mostly of low quality. A

review of Tai Chi for pain conditions concluded that Tai Chi appears to be an effective intervention in OA, low back pain, and fibromyalgia.[98]

Manipulative therapies

A prospective, single-blinded, placebo-controlled study of spinal manipulative therapy (SMT) for chronic, nonspecific low back pain concluded that maintenance SMT (12 times in the first month, then 2 times per month) was effective at 10 months. Treatment benefit, however, was not maintained if manipulative therapy was discontinued after the first month.[99]

Energy medicine

Therapies such as healing touch, Reiki, and Jin shin jyutsu may be beneficial for musculoskeletal conditions, although there are few high-quality data in the literature.

Therapeutic touch Therapeutic touch (TT) is a technique, developed in the 1970s, whereby the hands are used to direct human energy for healing purposes. There is usually no actual physical contact. The intent of the practitioner is to balance and modulate the energy flow through and around the body of the patient. Evidence is scarce in the medical literature, but a pilot study of 20 elderly patients with chronic pain showed some improvement in pain scores with 7 TT treatment sessions.[100] Improvement in function and pain was also documented in a single-blinded RCT in 25 patients with knee OA.[101]

Magnet therapy

A systematic review of 9 randomized, placebo-controlled trials of static magnets for reduction in pain concluded that "the evidence does not support the use of static magnets for pain relief, and therefore magnets cannot be recommended as an effective treatment."[102]

Medication Treatments

Capsaicin cream

Capsaicin is a crystalline alkaloid found in chili peppers (*Capsicum frutescens*). It stimulates the release of substance P such that eventually the nerve terminals become depleted of substance P. There have been small RCTs showing efficacy, and a 2007 Cochrane systematic review on herbal medications for low back pain noted that "*Capsicum frutescens* seems to reduce pain more than placebo."[103] However, a 2012 Cochrane review noted that there were insufficient data from which to draw any conclusions about the efficacy of low-concentration (<1%) capsaicin cream in the treatment of neuropathic pain. The Cochrane review noted:

> The information we have suggests that low-concentration topical capsaicin is without meaningful effect beyond that found in placebo creams; given the potential for bias from small study size, this makes it unlikely that low-concentration topical capsaicin has any meaningful use in clinical practice. Local skin irritation, which was often mild and transient but may lead to withdrawal, was common. Systemic adverse effects were rare.[104]

There has been some concern that capsaicin's depletion of substance P could delay and prolong tendon healing. However, a placebo-controlled crossover study was performed in 19 healthy male athletes, 18 to 20 years old, to investigate the influence of oral capsaicin on performance of, and the IL-6 response to, repeated sprints. Results did not show that capsaicin influenced repeated sprint performance or the IL-6 response, but it did cause significant gastrointestinal discomfort.[105]

Devil's claw (Harpagophytum procumbens)

There is evidence of effectiveness of Devil's claw in low back pain, based on a Cochrane review of herbal medications for back pain. The presumed mechanism of action is inhibition of COX-2 and 5-lipoxygenase. Possible side effects include diarrhea, abdominal pain, and skin reactions.[103] However, a systematic review noted that efficacy cannot be determined based on the current evidence, stating that "the methodological quality of the existing clinical trials is generally poor, and although they provide some support, there are a considerable number of methodologic caveats that make further clinical investigations warranted."[106]

Menthol (mint)

Menthol is an organic compound made synthetically or obtained from cornmint, peppermint, or other mint oils. Menthol's ability to chemically trigger the cold-sensitive TRPM8 receptors in the skin is responsible for the well-known cooling sensation it provokes when inhaled, eaten, or applied to the skin.[107] Menthol is endowed with analgesic properties mediated through a selective activation of κ-opioid receptors.[108] There are multiple menthol-containing over-the-counter preparations available, including Bengay, Icy-Hot, and Tiger-Balm.

The findings of a recent study indicate that topical applications of various doses of menthol to the thigh results in a significant decrease in local and generalized blood flow following a maximum voluntary muscle contraction. The study concluded that these findings may indicate that menthol affects blood flow through inhibiting local NOS and NO, and increasing systemic A_{2c} adrenergic tone. The investigators also concluded that "clinicians may apply the findings of this study to support using topical menthol gels or wipes to decrease local blood flow and attenuate the inflammation process following a soft tissue injury." Finally, the local and generalized effect of menthol on blood flow reported in this study warrants further investigation, to identify the mechanisms of action and to determine the effect of topical menthol on muscle performance.[109] Another study looked at the ability of menthol to decrease muscle soreness after strenuous physical activity. The study concluded that, compared with ice, the topical menthol-based analgesic decreased perceived discomfort to a greater extent and permitted greater tetanic forces to be produced.[110]

The effect of peppermint was studied in 12 healthy male students, who took peppermint essential oil orally for 10 days. Blood pressure, heart rate, and spirometry parameters were determined 1 day before, and after the supplementation period. Participants underwent a treadmill-based exercise test with metabolic gas analysis and ventilation measurement testing. Spirometry results significantly changed after 10 days of supplementation. Exercise performance significantly increased ($P<.001$), and the results of respiratory gas analysis showed a significant difference in the treatment group. The results of the experiment supported the use of peppermint essential oil in improving exercise performance, gas analysis, spirometry parameters, blood pressure, and respiratory rate in the young male students.[111]

Vitamin D

There are multiple studies on vitamin D supplementation in athletes, but the evidence does not appear conclusive. A literature review of the medical evidence on vitamin D's effects on physical and athletic performance concluded that vitamin D may improve athletic performance, but only in vitamin D–deficient athletes. This study noted that peak athletic performance may occur when 25(OH)D levels approach those obtained by natural, full-body, summer sun exposure, which is at least 50 nmol/L.[112] A more recent study assessed the effects of vitamin D_3 supplementation on serum 25(OH)D concentrations and physical performance. Serum vitamin D levels and muscle function (bench press, leg press, and vertical jump height) were measured presupplementation and both 6 and 12 weeks postsupplementation. Supplementation with both 20,000 and 40,000 IU vitamin D_3 over a 6-week period elevated serum 25(OH)D concentrations to higher than 50 nmol/L, but did not improve measures of physical performance.[113]

A 6-month randomized, placebo-controlled trial of 45 athletes, randomized to 4000 IU vitamin D or placebo, looked at the effect of season-long (September–March) vitamin D supplementation on changes in vitamin D status (measured as 25(OH)D), body composition, inflammation, injury, and frequency of illness. In this study, 25(OH)D levels did not correlate with changes in bone turnover markers or inflammatory cytokines. Illness and injury were not related to 25(OH)D; however, 77% of injuries coincided with decreases in vitamin D levels. The study concluded that 4000 IU vitamin D supplementation is an inexpensive intervention that effectively increased vitamin D levels, which was positively correlated with bone measures in the proximal dual femur and maximum femoral length. The study concluded that future studies with larger sample sizes and improved supplement compliance were needed to expand our understanding of the effects of vitamin D supplementation in athletes.[114]

Vitamin D and stress fracture Because of the role of vitamin D in the maintenance of bone density, supplementation with vitamin D has been studied as a possible method for reducing stress fractures. A prospective study examined serum 25(OH) D concentration, body mass index (BMI), and smoking, and their correlation with bone stress fractures in 756 military recruits. Twenty-two recruits with stress fracture were identified (2.9%). The average serum 25(OH)D concentration was significantly lower in the group with fracture, suggesting a relationship between vitamin D and fatigue bone stress fracture. No significant associations between BMI ($P = .255$), age ($P = .216$), or smoking ($P = .851$) and bone stress fracture were found in this study population.[115]

A review of the published studies on vitamin D and calcium on stress fractures noted that the literature is conflicting as to the role of these nutrients in young athletes aged 18 to 35 years, for both bone development and the prevention of bone overuse injuries. Evidence regarding the relationship of vitamin D intake with the prevention of fractures in athletes was also noted to be limited. The review concluded that more studies are needed to evaluate the role of calcium and vitamin D intake in prevention of stress-fracture injuries in both male and female adolescent athletes, particularly those participating in sports with greater incidences of stress fracture injury.[116]

Vitamin C

The effect of vitamin C (in combination with quercetin) on exercise performance was investigated in a placebo-controlled, double-blind study of male students supplemented with quercetin and vitamin C for 8 weeks. The study concluded that supplementation did not improve exercise performance, but did reduce muscle damage and percentage of body fat in healthy subjects.[117]

Other Treatment Approaches (Nonprocedural or Medical)

Functional medicine

Functional medicine is a combination of Eastern medicine, Western medicine, and scientific research. It combines the philosophy of balance and the knowledge of biochemistry and physiology with scientific research about how genetics, environment, and lifestyle all interact with each other. Functional medicine focuses assessment and intervention at the root levels of metabolic imbalance, and is focused on prevention. It is less concerned with making a diagnosis and more concerned with the underlying imbalances, which are the mechanisms of the disease process. This approach is focused on prevention and aims to address imbalances before the onset of pathologic conditions.[118]

The clinical approach examines imbalances at the root of disease conditions, including:

- Gastrointestinal function
- Immune surveillance
- Inflammatory process
- Oxidative stress
- Detoxification and biotransformation
- Hormonal and neurotransmitter regulation
- Structural imbalance
- Mind and spirit

Mind-body medicine

Mind-body medicine focuses on the interactions between the brain, the rest of the body, and behavior. The concept of the mind influencing physical health dates back to ancient times. The role of mind and belief in health and illness began to re-enter Western health care in the twentieth century, led by discoveries about pain control via the placebo effect and effects of stress on health. Mind-body medicine includes emotional, mental, social, spiritual, and behavioral factors that can influence health.[119]

Mind-body therapy has been shown to be effective for multiple conditions. A systematic review of Mind-body therapy concluded that "there is now considerable evidence that an array of mind-body therapies can be used as effective adjuncts to conventional medical treatment for several common clinical conditions."[115] Mind-body therapies for pain in adolescents, including cognitive-behavioral therapy, relaxation therapy, and biofeedback, all produced significant and positive effects on pain reduction.[120]

Examples of mind-body therapies

Patient and family education A double-blind RCT concluded that "A 30-min educational session on pain physiology imparts a better understanding of pain and brings about less rumination in the short term. Pain physiology education can be an important therapeutic modality."[121] A 2012 Cochrane review also concluded that "there is good evidence for the effectiveness of including parents in psychological (mind-body) therapies that reduce pain in children with painful conditions."[122]

Biofeedback The effectiveness of biofeedback in limiting pain may be related to muscular relaxation associated with decreased oxidative stress accompanied by psychological well-being.[123]

Relaxation and imagery techniques
Progressive muscle relaxation
Deep breathing exercises[124]
Meditation
Hypnosis
Cognitive distraction and reframing
Psychotherapy and structured support
Pastoral counseling/spirituality
Support groups

SUMMARY

Complementary and alternative treatments are commonly used by patients for a variety of musculoskeletal conditions.

There is a scarcity in both the quantity and quality of CAM treatments for specific musculoskeletal conditions.

Acupuncture may be useful for multiple musculoskeletal conditions, although studies on acupuncture for these conditions often show conflicting results.

Multiple CAM treatments exist for the treatment of OA, and may play an important role in reducing inflammation, pain, and even joint destruction related to OA.

Data from small studies are encouraging for possible treatment of concussion with O3FAs, although more clinical data are needed.

Vitamin D may be useful in preventing sports injuries, particularly stress fractures, although more studies are needed in this area.

Functional medicine and mind-body medicine are treatment approaches that may be useful in multiple musculoskeletal conditions.

REFERENCES

1. Fink M, Wolkenstein E, Karst M, et al. Acupuncture in chronic epicondylitis: a randomized controlled trial. Rheumatology 2002;41:205–9.
2. Molsberger A, Hille E. The analgesic effect of acupuncture in chronic tennis elbow pain. Br J Rheumatol 1994;33:1162–5.
3. Trinh KV, Phillips SD, Ho E, et al. Acupuncture for the alleviation of lateral epicondyle pain: a systematic review. Rheumatology (Oxford) 2004;43(9):1085–90.
4. Haker E, Lundeberg T. Acupuncture treatment in epicondylalgia: a comparative study of two acupuncture techniques. Clin J Pain 1990;6:221–6.
5. Haker E, Lundeberg T. Laser treatment applied to acupuncture points in lateral humeral epicondylalgia. A double-blind study. Pain 1990;43:243–7.
6. Oken O, Kahraman Y, Ayhan F, et al. The short-term efficacy of laser, brace, and ultrasound treatment in lateral epicondylitis: a prospective, randomized, controlled trial. J Hand Ther 2008;21:63–8.
7. Bäcker M, Lüdtke R, Afra D, et al. Effectiveness of leech therapy in chronic lateral epicondylitis: a randomized controlled trial. Clin J Pain 2011;27(5):442–7.
8. Kleinhenz J, Streitberger K, Windeler J, et al. Randomised clinical trial comparing the effects of acupuncture and a newly designed placebo needle in rotator cuff tendinitis. Pain 1999;83(2):235–41.
9. Johansson K, Bergström A, Schröder K, et al. Subacromial corticosteroid injection or acupuncture with home exercises when treating patients with subacromial impingement in primary care—a randomized clinical trial. Fam Pract 2011;28(4):355–65.
10. Razavi M, Jansen GB. Effects of acupuncture and placebo TENS in addition to exercise in treatment of rotator cuff tendinitis. Clin Rehabil 2004;18:872–8.
11. Vas J, Ortega C, Olmo V, et al. Single-point acupuncture and physiotherapy for the treatment of painful shoulder: a multicentre randomized controlled trial. Rheumatology (Oxford) 2008;47(6):887–93.
12. Brosseau L, Casimiro L, Milne S, et al. Deep transverse friction massage for treating tendinitis. Cochrane Database Syst Rev 2002;(1):CD003528.
13. Cao L, Zhang XL, Gao YS, et al. Needle acupuncture for osteoarthritis of the knee. A systematic review and updated meta-analysis. Saudi Med J 2012; 33(5):526–32.

14. Manheimer E, Cheng K, Linde K, et al. Acupuncture for peripheral joint osteoarthritis. Cochrane Database Syst Rev 2010;(1):CD001977. http://dx.doi.org/10.1002/14651858.CD001977.pub2.

15. University of Maryland web site. Available at: http://www.umm.edu/altmed/. Accessed March 2013.

16. Soeken K, Lee WL, Bausell B, et al. Safety and efficacy of S-adenosylmethionine (SAMe) for osteoarthritis, a systematic review. J Fam Pract 2002;51:425–30.

17. Najm WI, Reinsch S, Hoehler F, et al. S-Adenosyl methionine (SAMe) versus celecoxib for the treatment of osteoarthritis symptoms: a double-blind cross-over trial. BMC Musculoskelet Disord 2004;5:6.

18. Rutjes AW, Nüesch E, Reichenbach S, et al. S-Adenosylmethionine for osteoarthritis of the knee or hip. Cochrane Database Syst Rev 2009;(4):CD007321.

19. Gregory PJ, Sperry M, Wilson AF. Dietary supplements for osteoarthritis. Am Fam Physician 2008;77(2):177–84.

20. Janicak PG, Lipinski J, Davis JM, et al. Parenteral S-adenosyl-methionine (SAMe) in depression: literature review and preliminary data. Psychopharmacol Bull 1989;25(2):238–42 PMID 2690166.

21. Frestedt JL, Kuskowski MA, Zenk JL. A natural seaweed derived mineral supplement (Aquamin F) for knee osteoarthritis: a randomised, placebo controlled pilot study. Nutr J 2009;8:7.

22. Ernst E. Avocado-soybean unsaponifiables (ASU) for osteoarthritis—a systematic review. Clin Rheumatol 2003;22:285–8.

23. Christensen R, Bartels EM, Astrup A, et al. Symptomatic efficacy of avocado-soybean unsaponifiables (ASU) in osteoarthritis (OA) patients: a meta-analysis of randomized controlled trials. Osteoarthritis Cartilage 2008;16(4):399–408.

24. Kimmatkar N, Thawani V, Hingorani L, et al. Efficacy and tolerability of *Boswellia serrata* extract in treatment of osteoarthritis of knee—a randomized double blind placebo controlled trial. Phytomedicine 2003;10(1):3–7.

25. Sengupta K, Krishnaraju AV, Vishal AA, et al. Comparative efficacy and tolerability of 5-Loxin and Aflapin against osteoarthritis of the knee: a double blind, randomized, placebo controlled clinical study. Int J Med Sci 2010;7(6):366–77.

26. Chopra A, Saluja M, Tillu G, et al. Ayurvedic medicine offers a good alternative to glucosamine and celecoxib in the treatment of symptomatic knee osteoarthritis: a randomized, double-blind, controlled equivalence drug trial. Rheumatology (Oxford) 2013;52(8):1408–17.

27. Di Lorenzo C, Dell'agli M, Badea M, et al. Plant food supplements with anti-inflammatory properties: a systematic review. Crit Rev Food Sci Nutr 2013; 53(5):507–16.

28. Dargan P. Heavy metal poisoning from Ayurvedic traditional medicines: an emerging problem? Int J Environ Health 2008;2(3/4):463.

29. Brien S, Lewith G, Walker A, et al. Bromelain as a treatment for osteoarthritis: a review of clinical studies. Evid Based Complement Alternat Med 2004;1(3):251–7.

30. Brien S, Lewith G, Walker AF, et al. Bromelain as an adjunctive treatment for moderate-to-severe osteoarthritis of the knee: a randomized placebo-controlled pilot study. QJM 2006;99(12):841–50.

31. Cheras PA, Myers SP, Outerbridge K, et al. Randomised placebo controlled trial on the safety and efficacy of BSP-201 in osteoarthritis. Australian Centre for Complementary Medicine Education and Research [ACCMER]; 2007.

32. Piscoya J, Rodriguez Z, Bustamante SA, et al. Efficacy and safety of freeze-dried cat's claw in osteoarthritis of the knee: mechanisms of action of the species *Uncaria guianensis*. Inflamm Res 2001;50(9):442–8.

33. Akhtar N, Haqqi TM. Current nutraceuticals in the management of osteoarthritis: a review. Ther Adv Musculoskelet Dis 2012;4(3):181–207.

34. Kuptniratsaikul V, Thanakhumtorn S, Chinswangwatanakul P, et al. Efficacy and safety of *Curcuma domestica* extracts in patients with knee osteoarthritis. J Altern Complement Med 2009;15:891–7.

35. Belcaro G, Cesarone MR, Dugall M, et al. Product-evaluation registry of Meriva®, a curcumin-phosphatidylcholine complex, for the complementary management of osteoarthritis. Panminerva Med 2010;52:55–62.

36. Belcaro G, Cesarone MR, Dugall M, et al. Efficacy and safety of Meriva®, a curcumin-phosphatidylcholine complex, during extended administration in osteoarthritis patients. Altern Med Rev 2010;15:337–44.

37. Altman RD, Marcussen KC. Effects of a ginger extract on knee pain in patients with osteoarthritis. Arthritis Rheum 2001;44:2531–8.

38. Wigler I, Grotto I, Caspi D, et al. The effects of Zintona EC (a ginger extract) on symptomatic gonarthritis. Osteoarthritis Cartilage 2003;11:783–9.

39. Bliddal H, Rosetzsky A, Schlichting P, et al. A randomized, placebo-controlled, cross-over study of ginger extracts and ibuprofen in osteoarthritis. Osteoarthritis Cartilage 2000;8:9–12.

40. Niempoog S, Siriarchavatana P, Kajsongkram T. The efficacy of Plygersic gel for use in the treatment of osteoarthritis of the knee. J Med Assoc Thai 2012; 95(Suppl 10):S113–9.

41. Jonas WB, Rapoza CP, Blair WF. The effect of niacinamide on osteoarthritis: a pilot study. Inflamm Res 1996;45:330–4.

42. Cisár P, Jány R, Waczulíková I, et al. Effect of pine bark extract (Pycnogenol) on symptoms of knee osteoarthritis. Phytother Res 2008;22:1087–92.

43. Belcaro G, Cesarone MR, Errichi S, et al. Variations in C-reactive protein, plasma free radicals and fibrinogen values in patients with osteoarthritis treated with Pycnogenol. Redox Rep 2008;13:271–6.

44. Drieling RL, Gardner CD, Ma J, et al. No beneficial effects of pine bark extract on cardiovascular disease risk factors. Arch Intern Med 2010;170:1541–7.

45. Litozin web site. Available at: http://litozin.com. Accessed March 1, 2013.

46. Warholm O, Skaar S, Hedman E, et al. The effect of a standardized herbal remedy made from a subtype of *Rosa canina* in patients with osteoarthritis: a double-blind, randomized, placebo-controlled clinical trial. Curr Ther Res 2003;64:21–31.

47. Rein E, Kharazmi A, Winther K. A herbal remedy, Hyben Vital (stand. powder of a subspecies of *Rosa canina* fruits), reduces pain and improves general well-being in patients with osteoarthritis—a double-blind, placebo-controlled, randomised trial. Phytomedicine 2004;11:383–91.

48. Winther K, Apel K, Thamsborg G. A powder made from seeds and shells of a rose-hip subspecies (*Rosa canina*) reduces symptoms of knee and hip osteoarthritis: a randomized, double-blind, placebo-controlled clinical trial. Scand J Rheumatol 2005;34:302–8.

49. McAlindon TE, Felson DT, Zhang Y, et al. Relation of dietary intake and serum levels of vitamin D to progression of osteoarthritis of the knee among participants in the Framingham Study. Ann Intern Med 1996;125(5):353–9.

50. Felson DT, Niu J, Clancy M, et al. Low levels of vitamin D and worsening of knee osteoarthritis: results of two longitudinal studies. Arthritis Rheum 2007;56(1):129–36.

51. Cao Y, Winzenberg T, Nguo K, et al. Association between serum levels of 25-hydroxyvitamin D and osteoarthritis: a systematic review. Rheumatology (Oxford) 2013;52(7):1323–34.

52. Schmid B, Lüdtke R, Selbmann HK, et al. Efficacy and tolerability of a standardized willow bark extract in patients with osteoarthritis: randomized placebo-controlled, double blind clinical trial. Phytother Res 2001;15:344–50.

53. McAlindon TE, Jacques P, Zhang Y, et al. Do antioxidant micronutrients protect against the development and progression of knee osteoarthritis? Arthritis Rheum 1996;39(4):648–56.

54. Song R, Lee EO, Lam P, et al. Effects of tai chi exercise on pain, balance, muscle strength, and perceived difficulties in physical functioning in older women with osteoarthritis: a randomized clinical trial. J Rheumatol 2003;30:2039–44.

55. Lee MS, Pittler MH, Ernst E. Tai chi for osteoarthritis: a systematic review. Clin Rheumatol 2007;19:139–46.

56. Harlow T, Greaves C, White A, et al. Randomised controlled trial of magnetic bracelets for relieving pain in osteoarthritis of the hip and knee. BMJ 2004; 329:1450–4.

57. Wolsko PM, Eisenberg DM, Simon LS, et al. Double-blind placebo-controlled trial of static magnets for the treatment of osteoarthritis of the knee: results of a pilot study. Altern Ther Health Med 2004;10(2):36–43.

58. Richmond SJ, Brown SR, Campion PD, et al. Therapeutic effects of magnetic and copper bracelets in osteoarthritis: a randomised placebo-controlled crossover trial. Complement Ther Med 2009;17(5–6):249–56. http://dx.doi.org/10.1016/j.ctim.2009.07.002.

59. Altavilla D, Squadrito F, Bitto A, et al. Flavocoxid, a dual inhibitor of cyclooxygenase and 5-lipoxygenase, blunts pro-inflammatory phenotype activation in endotoxin-stimulated macrophages. Br J Pharmacol 2009;157(8):1410–8.

60. Levy RM, Saikovsky R, Shmidt E, et al. Flavocoxid is as effective as naproxen for managing the signs and symptoms of osteoarthritis of the knee in humans: a short-term randomized, double-blind pilot study. Nutr Res 2009;29:298–304.

61. Chalasani N, Vuppalanchi R, Navarro V, et al. Acute liver injury due to flavocoxid (Limbrel), a medical food for osteoarthritis: a case series. Ann Intern Med 2012; 156(12):857–60. http://dx.doi.org/10.7326/0003-4819-156-12-201206190-00006 W297–300.

62. Pavelká K, Gatterová J, Olejarová M, et al. Glucosamine sulfate use and delay of progression of knee osteoarthritis: a 3-year, randomized, placebo-controlled, double-blind study. Arch Intern Med 2002;162:2113–23.

63. Leeb BF, Schweitzer H, Montag K, et al. A meta-analysis of chondroitin sulfate in the treatment of osteoarthritis. J Rheumatol 2000;27:205–11.

64. Reichenbach S, Sterchi R, Scherer M, et al. Meta-analysis: chondroitin for osteoarthritis of the knee or hip. Ann Intern Med 2007;146:580–90.

65. Clegg DO, Reda DJ, Harris CL, et al. Glucosamine, chondroitin sulfate, and the two in combination for painful knee osteoarthritis. N Engl J Med 2006;354(8): 795–808.

66. Herrero-Beaumont G, Ivorra JA, Del Carmen Trabado M, et al. Glucosamine sulfate in the treatment of knee osteoarthritis symptoms: a randomized, double-blind, placebo-controlled study using acetaminophen as a side comparator. Arthritis Rheum 2007;56(2):555–67.

67. Towheed T, Maxwell L, Anastassiades TP, et al. Glucosamine therapy for treating osteoarthritis. Cochrane Database Syst Rev 2005;(2):CD002946.

68. Giacovelli G, Rovati LC. Glucosamine and osteoarthritis. Conclusions not supported by methods and results. BMJ 2010;341:c4675.

69. Gray HC, Hutcheson PS, Slavin RG. Is glucosamine safe in patients with seafood allergy? J Allergy Clin Immunol 2004;114(2):459–60.

70. Baird CL, Sands L. A pilot study of the effectiveness of guided imagery with progressive muscle relaxation to reduce chronic pain and mobility difficulties of osteoarthritis. Pain Manag Nurs 2004;5(3):97–104.

71. Roddy E, Zhang W, Doherty M. Aerobic walking or strengthening exercise for osteoarthritis of the knee? A systematic review. Ann Rheum Dis 2005;64:544–8.

72. Fransen M, McConnell S. Exercise for osteoarthritis of the knee. Cochrane Database Syst Rev 2008;(4):CD004376.

73. Kerrigan DC, Todd MK, Riley PO. Knee osteoarthritis and high-heeled shoes. Lancet 1998;351(9113):1399–401.

74. Garfinkel MS, Schumacher HR Jr, Husain A, et al. Evaluation of a yoga based regimen for treatment of osteoarthritis of the hands. J Rheumatol 1994;21: 2341–3.

75. Boyle CA, Sayers SP, Jensen BE, et al. The effects of yoga training and a single bout of yoga on delayed onset muscle soreness in the lower extremity. J Strength Cond Res 2004;18(4):723–9.

76. McCrory P, Meeuwisse W, Aubry M, et al. Consensus statement on concussion in sport: The 4th International Conference on Concussion in Sport held in Zurich, November 2012. BMJ 2013.

77. Hasadsri L, Wang BH, Lee JV, et al. Omega-3 fatty acids for treatment of traumatic brain injury. J Neurotrauma 2013;30(11):897–906.

78. Mills JD, Bailes JE, Sedney CL, et al. Omega-3 fatty acid supplementation and reduction of traumatic axonal injury in a rodent head injury model. J Neurosurg 2011;114(1):77–84. http://dx.doi.org/10.3171/2010.5.JNS08914.

79. Mills JD, Hadley K, Bailes JE. Dietary supplementation with the omega-3 fatty acid docosahexaenoic acid in traumatic brain injury. Neurosurgery 2011;68(2): 474–81. http://dx.doi.org/10.1227/NEU.0b013e3181ff692b [discussion: 481].

80. Shin SS, Dixon CE. Oral fish oil restores striatal dopamine release after traumatic brain injury. Neurosci Lett 2011;496(3):168–71. http://dx.doi.org/10.1016/j.neulet.2011.04.009.

81. Lewis M, Ghassemi P, Hibbeln J. Therapeutic use of omega-3 fatty acids in severe head trauma. Am J Emerg Med 2013;31(1):273.e5–8. http://dx.doi.org/10.1016/j.ajem.2012.05.014.

82. Richard L, Nahin R, Barnes P, et al. Costs of complementary and alternative medicine (CAM) and frequency of visits to CAM practitioners: United States, 2007. Natl Health Stat Report 2009;(18):1–14.

83. Lundeberg T, Lund I, Sing A, et al. Is placebo acupuncture what it is intended to be? Evid Based Complement Alternat Med 2011;2011:932407.

84. Manheimer E, White A, Berman B, et al. Meta-analysis: acupuncture for low back pain. Ann Intern Med 2005;142(8):651–63.

85. Cherkin D, Sherman K, Avins A, et al. A randomized trial comparing acupuncture, simulated acupuncture, and usual care for chronic low back pain. Arch Intern Med 2009;169(9):858–66.

86. Lewis K, Abdi S. Acupuncture for lower back pain: a review. Clin J Pain 2010; 26(1):60–9.

87. Ghoname EA, Craig WF, White PF, et al. Percutaneous electrical nerve stimulation for low back pain a randomized crossover study. JAMA 1999;281:818–23.

88. Weiner D, Perera S, Rudy T, et al. Efficacy of percutaneous electrical nerve stimulation and therapeutic exercise for older adults with chronic low back pain: a randomized controlled trial. Pain 2008;140(2):344–57.

89. Zhu Y, Qiu ML, Ding Y, et al. Effects of electroacupuncture on the proprioception of athletes with functional ankle instability. Zhongguo Zhen Jiu 2012;32(6):503–6.

90. Lin ZP, Chen YH, Fan C, et al. Effects of auricular acupuncture on heart rate, oxygen consumption and blood lactic acid for elite basketball athletes. Am J Chin Med 2011;39(6):1131–8.

91. Benner S, Benner K. Improved performance in endurance sports through acupuncture. Sportverletz Sportschaden 2010;24(3):140–3. http://dx.doi.org/10.1055/s-0029-1245406.

92. Karagounis P, Tsironi M, Prionas G, et al. Treatment of plantar fasciitis in recreational athletes: two different therapeutic protocols. Foot Ankle Spec 2011;4(4):226–34. http://dx.doi.org/10.1177/1938640011407320.

93. Zhang BM, Zhong LW, Xu SW, et al. Acupuncture for chronic Achilles tendinopathy: a randomized controlled study. Chin J Integr Med 2012 [Epub ahead of print].

94. Nomikos NN, Nomikos GN, Kores DS. The use of deep friction massage with olive oil as a means of prevention and treatment of sports injuries in ancient times. Arch Med Sci 2010;6(5):642–5. http://dx.doi.org/10.5114/aoms.2010.17074.

95. Perlman AI, Sabina A, Williams AL, et al. Massage therapy for osteoarthritis of the knee: a randomized controlled trial. Arch Intern Med 2006;166:2533–8.

96. Kong LJ, Fang M, Zhan HS, et al. Chinese massage combined with herbal ointment for athletes with nonspecific low back pain: a randomized controlled trial. Evid Based Complement Alternat Med 2012;2012:695726.

97. Furlan AD, Imamura M, Dryden T, et al. Massage for low-back pain. Cochrane Database Syst Rev 2008;(4):CD001929. http://dx.doi.org/10.1002/14651858.CD001929.pub2.

98. Peng PW. Tai chi and chronic pain. Reg Anesth Pain Med 2012;37(4):372–82.

99. Senna MK, Machaly SA. Does maintained spinal manipulation therapy for chronic non-specific low back pain result in better long term outcome? Spine (Phila Pa 1976) 2011;36(18):1427–37.

100. Decker S, Wardell DW, Cron SG. Using a healing touch intervention in older adults with persistent pain: a feasibility study. J Holist Nurs 2012;30(3):205–13.

101. Gordon A, Merenstein JH, D'Amico F, et al. The effects of therapeutic touch on patients with osteoarthritis of the knee. J Fam Pract 1998;47(4):271–7.

102. Pittler MH, Brown EM, Ernst E. Static magnets for reducing pain: systematic review and meta-analysis of randomized trials. CMAJ 2007;177(7):736–42.

103. Gagnier JJ, van Tulder MW, Berman B, et al. Herbal medicine for low back pain: a Cochrane review. Spine (Phila Pa 1976) 2007;32(1):82–92.

104. Derry S, Moore RA. Topical capsaicin (low concentration) for chronic neuropathic pain in adults. Cochrane Database Syst Rev 2012;(9):CD010111.

105. Opheim MN, Rankin JW. Effect of capsaicin supplementation on repeated sprinting performance. J Strength Cond Res 2012;26(2):319–26. http://dx.doi.org/10.1519/JSC.0b013e3182429ae5.

106. Brien S, Lewith GT, McGregor G. Devil's claw (*Harpagophytum procumbens*) as a treatment for osteoarthritis: a review of efficacy and safety. J Altern Complement Med 2006;12(10):981–93.

107. Eccles R. Menthol and related cooling compounds. J Pharm Pharmacol 1994;46(8):618–30 PMID 7529306.

108. Galeotti N, Di Cesare Mannelli L, Mazzanti G, et al. Menthol: a natural analgesic compound. Neurosci Lett 2002;322(3):145–8.

109. Topp R, Winchester L, Schilero J, et al. Effect of topical menthol on ipsilateral and contralateral superficial blood flow following a bout of maximum voluntary muscle contraction. Int J Sports Phys Ther 2011;6(2):83–91 PMCID: PMC3109898.

110. Johar P, Grover V, Topp R, et al. A comparison of topical menthol to ice on pain, evoked tetanic and voluntary force during delayed onset muscle soreness. Int J Sports Phys Ther 2012;7(3):314–22.

111. Meamarbashi A, Rajabi A. The effects of peppermint on exercise performance. J Int Soc Sports Nutr 2013;10(1):15.

112. Cannell JJ, Hollis BW, Sorenson MB, et al. Athletic performance and vitamin D. Med Sci Sports Exerc 2009;41(5):1102–10.

113. Close GL, Leckey J, Patterson M, et al. The effects of vitamin D3 supplementation on serum total 25[OH]D concentration and physical performance: a randomised dose-response study. Br J Sports Med 2013;47(11):692–6.

114. Lewis RM, Redzic M, Thomas DT. The effects of season-long vitamin D supplementation on collegiate swimmers and divers. Int J Sport Nutr Exerc Metab 2013. [Epub ahead of print].

115. Ruohola JP, Laaksi I, Ylikomi T, et al. Association between serum 25(OH)D concentrations and bone stress fractures in Finnish young men. J Bone Miner Res 2006;21(9):1483–8.

116. Tenforde AS, Sayres LC, Sainani KL, et al. Evaluating the relationship of calcium and vitamin D in the prevention of stress fracture injuries in the young athlete: a review of the literature. PM R 2010;2(10):945–9. http://dx.doi.org/10.1016/j.pmrj. 2010.05.006.

117. Askari G, Ghiasvand R, Karimian J, et al. Does quercetin and vitamin C improve exercise performance, muscle damage, and body composition in male athletes? J Res Med Sci 2012;17(4):328–31.

118. Institute for Functional Medicine web site. Available at: http://www. functionalmedicine.org/. Accessed March 15, 2013.

119. Astin JA, Shapiro SL, Eisenberg DM, et al. Mind-body medicine: state of the science, implications for practice. J Am Board Fam Pract 2003;16(2):131–47.

120. Palermo TM, Eccleston C, Lewandowski AS, et al. Randomized controlled trials of psychological therapies for management of chronic pain in children and adolescents: an updated meta-analytic review. Pain 2010;148(3):387–97.

121. Meeus M, Nijs J, Van Oosterwijck J, et al. Pain physiology education improves pain beliefs in patients with chronic fatigue syndrome compared with pacing and self-management education: a double-blind randomized controlled trial. Arch Phys Med Rehabil 2010;91(8):1153–9.

122. Eccleston C, Palermo TM, Fisher E, et al. Psychological interventions for parents of children and adolescents with chronic illness. Cochrane Database Syst Rev 2012;(8):CD009660. http://dx.doi.org/10.1002/14651858.CD009660.pub2.

123. Ciancarelli I, Tozzi-Ciancarelli MG, Spacca G, et al. Relationship between biofeedback and oxidative stress in patients with chronic migraine. Cephalalgia 2007;27(10):1136–41.

124. Mehling WE, Hamel KA, Acree M, et al. Randomized, controlled trial of breath therapy for patients with chronic low-back pain. Altern Ther Health Med 2005; 11(4):44–52.

Evaluation and Treatment of Biking and Running Injuries

Sean M. Oser, MD, MPH[a], Tamara K. Oser, MD[a],
Matthew L. Silvis, MD[a,b],*

KEYWORDS

- Running • Cycling • Biking • Injuries

KEY POINTS

- As more individuals participate in running-related and cycling-related activities, physicians must be increasingly aware of the common injuries encountered in these pursuits.
- Training errors lead to most running and biking injuries.
- History and physical examination are often adequate for proper diagnosis and management of running-related and cycling-related injuries.
- Imaging can sometimes help assist in differentiating among diagnoses with similar clinical presentations or to determine degree of injury.
- Correct ergonomics, including bike fit and equipment, and training/technique should be emphasized, and errors in these areas should be corrected when treating injured cyclists.

INTRODUCTION

Exercise is universally recognized as a key feature for maintaining good health. Likewise, lack of physical activity is a major risk factor for chronic disease and disability, an especially important fact considering our rapidly aging population.[1]

Obesity has become a major health problem facing the US population. Approximately 36% of adults in the United States are obese, with an additional 33% overweight and therefore at increased risk for becoming obese.[2] More than 1 in 6 US adolescents are obese, and less than 50% of children meet exercise guidelines recommended by the American Academy of Pediatrics.[3]

Physicians are increasingly recommending cardioaerobic fitness activities for their health benefits. The popularity of aerobic exercise, including running and biking, has

---

[a] Department of Family and Community Medicine, Penn State Milton S. Hershey Medical Center, 500 University Drive, Hershey, PA 17033, USA; [b] Primary Care Sports Medicine, Department of Orthopedics and Rehabilitation, Penn State Milton S. Hershey Medical Center, H154, 500 University Drive, Hershey, PA 17033, USA
* Corresponding author. Penn State Milton S. Hershey Medical Center, H154, 500 University Drive, Hershey, PA 17033.
E-mail address: msilvis@hmc.psu.edu

Prim Care Clin Office Pract 40 (2013) 969–986
http://dx.doi.org/10.1016/j.pop.2013.08.011   **primarycare.theclinics.com**

increased significantly over the past 4 decades.[4] Running is a particularly popular choice for many, because it can be performed virtually anywhere without special equipment. Cycling has long been a common pastime and is increasing in popularity for numerous reasons, including not only its exercise benefits but also as a less expensive and greener mode of transportation.

The American College of Sports Medicine recommends that all healthy adults 18 to 65 years of age participate in moderate-intensity aerobic (endurance) physical activity for a minimum of 30 minutes on 5 days each week or vigorous-intensity aerobic physical activity for a minimum of 20 minutes on 3 days each week.[4] These recommendations are similar for adults older than 65 years, but intensity should take into account aerobic fitness level. Flexibility and balance exercises are also recommended for older adults.[5]

As more individuals participate in running-related and cycling-related activities, physicians must be increasingly aware of the common injuries encountered in these pursuits. This review focuses on the evaluation and management of common running-related and biking-related injuries.

RUNNING
Introduction

In the United States, in the past, running was mostly considered an elite, fringe sporting activity for competitive men.[6] In the late 1960s to the 1970s, 3 historical events brought running into mainstream American life.[7] Dr Kenneth Cooper's 1968 book, *Aerobics*,[8] advanced the theory of how people could most efficiently reach high levels of physical fitness based on his work with the US Air Force. In 1972, American Frank Shorter won the Olympic gold medal in marathon in Munich. In 1977, Jim Fixx published *The Complete Book of Running*,[9] the first self-help guide for individuals beginning a running program; it became a bestseller. The 1970s running boom that followed has yet to plateau. There were more than 13 million road race finishers in 2010 in the United States.[10]

The benefits of running are numerous and include lower risks of early death, coronary artery disease, cerebrovascular disease, hypertension, adverse lipid profile, type 2 diabetes mellitus, metabolic syndrome, colon cancer, and breast cancer. Other benefits include prevention of weight gain, acceleration of weight loss, prevention of falls, and reduced risk of depression.[11] Vigorous exercise in middle and older ages has been associated with reduced disability in later life and notable survival advantage.[12]

Running can be hazardous. Between 37% and 56% of recreational runners sustain running-related injuries each year.[13] Most injuries are caused by overuse. The onset is insidious, with no specific traumatic event. Risk factors for running-related injury fall into 4 broad categories (**Box 1**).[5]

Known predictors of lower extremity running injury include running more than 64.4 km (40 miles) per week and history of previous lower extremity injury.[14–16] A

Box 1	
Risk factors for running-related injury	
Systemic	Gender, weight, knee alignment, arch type, flexibility
Running/training related	Training frequency, alterations, terrain, race distance, running experience, shoe age, pace
Health	Previous injuries, medical problems
Lifestyle	Alcohol, tobacco, cross-training

recent systematic review found that most leg injuries in runners were caused by knee pain, lower leg pain, foot pain, or thigh pain.[17] The differential diagnosis for leg pain in a runner is broad (**Table 1**).[18] In a study of more than 2000 running-related injuries,[19] the most common leg injuries included the following:

- Medial tibial stress syndrome (MTSS)
- Achilles tendinopathy
- Tibial stress fractures

Evaluation

History
Evaluation of an injured runner should include details such as location, duration, onset, course, quality, and intensity of symptoms. Asking a runner when they experience symptoms is also a critical part of the assessment: at rest or during or after the run. Previous treatments should be explored as well as exacerbating or relieving factors.

Training errors lead to most running injuries. "Too much, too far, and too often" is often to blame. Asking questions in regard to weekly running mileage, changes in duration/intensity of training, changes in the type of running surface, surface grade, age of footwear, and recent changes in gait, footwear, or orthotics can often help to determine the underlying cause for the injury.

Physical examination
Physical examination of the injured runner should include a detailed examination of the injured area. However, the examination must reach beyond the site of injury. Most runners arrive in clinic already knowing their diagnosis from previous experiences or from reading running magazines/Web sites. The more important and difficult aspect of the examination is determining what potential biomechanical factors may have led to the injury.[20]

Examination typically begins with a screening gait evaluation and then observing the injured runner while standing, sitting, lying supine, lying prone, and lying on 1 side. A thorough site-specific examination is performed on the injured region.[20]

Gait analysis
A runner's gait can be evaluated in several ways. Observational gait analysis (eg, patient walking in a hallway) can provide useful information. However, multiplanar videotape observational gait analysis, when available, provides the truest picture of

Table 1	
Differential diagnosis of leg pain in runners	
Body System	**Possible Specific Diagnoses**
Skeletal	Medial tibial stress syndrome, stress fracture
Musculotendinous	Tendinopathy, myopathy
Vascular	Exertional compartment syndrome, venous thrombosis, popliteal artery entrapment syndrome, claudication
Neurologic	Nerve entrapment, lumbosacral radiculopathy, neurogenic claudication
Infectious	
Neoplastic	

Data from Gallo R, Plakke M, Silvis M. Common leg injuries of long-distance runners: anatomical and biomechanical approach. Sports Health 2012;4(6):485–95.

running form.[20] Although gait analysis may help identify underlying biomechanical abnormalities, it is not clear whether correction of these factors helps prevent or treat running injuries.

In developed countries, most runners wear running shoes and heel strike. In its simplest form, running gait begins with lateral heel strike, followed by foot pronation during midstance and foot supination during liftoff.[21,22] Proper gait is critical for a runner to absorb the impact of foot strike, because ground reaction forces can reach 1.5 to 3 times the runner's weight.[23] The rear foot strike pattern of most runners is aided by the elevated and cushioned heels of modern running shoes. Modern running shoes are typically recommended based on arch and foot type, but although these shoes are popular, recent studies have not found this approach to be successful in reducing injury rates.[24–27]

Recently, biomechanical research and popular books such as *Born to Run*[28] have led to an interest in barefoot running.[29–31] Barefoot runners land on the forefoot or midfoot instead of the heel, resulting in smaller impact forces on foot strike. No clinical studies have shown that this running style reduces risk of injury.[29,30]

Imaging and additional testing

History and physical examination are often adequate for proper diagnosis and management of running-related injuries. However, imaging can sometimes help assist in differentiating among diagnoses with similar clinical presentations or to determine degree of injury.[32] Imaging modalities and ancillary tests are discussed later in this review in regard to specific running-related injuries.

BIKING
Introduction

Participation in cycling is increasing across the United States, especially among those seeking a low-impact alternative to running and other aerobic activities. Although road cycling decreased slightly in 2010, there were significant increases in BMX bicycling, mountain biking, and triathlon participation when compared with previous years. Adults older than 25 years averaged 50.5 outings per year, whereas youth aged 6 to 24 years averaged 66.7 outings per year, for a total of 2.4 billion bike outings combined.[33]

Benefits of cycling are similar to those of running or other forms of cardioaerobic exercise.

Cycling-related injuries are also increasing as more people participate. Most reported cycling injuries are related to overuse,[34] with gradual onset and without specific traumatic event, because of the repetitive nature of the activity.[35,36] If most cyclists average between 50 and 120 revolutions/min, that translates into 3000 to more than 7000 revolutions in 1 hour. In addition to overuse, important contributors to cycling injury are improper bike fit and improper technique/training.[37] The most commons sites for nontraumatic cycling-related injuries include the knee, leg, hand/wrist, neck/shoulder, back, and perineum.[35,38,39]

Prevention

Bicycle safety helmet use has been associated with decreased risk of head, brain, facial, and fatal injury,[40] and legislation requiring helmet use in children has also been associated with lower rates of injury.[41] Correct ergonomics, including bike fit and equipment, and training/technique should be emphasized, and errors in these areas should be corrected.[34–36,39]

Evaluation

History
The history is crucial in evaluating the injured cyclist; as in much of medicine, the history helps guide additional evaluation and approach to therapy. Clinicians should enquire about recent changes in riding position, equipment (saddle, handlebars, shoes, cleats), and training (schedule, distance, terrain).[34,36] Evaluation of an injured cyclist should include details such as location, duration, onset, course, quality, and intensity of pain. Previous treatments should be explored as well as exacerbating and relieving factors.

Physical examination
Physical examination of the injured cyclist should begin with a detailed examination of the injured area. However, the examination must reach beyond the site of injury. The more important and difficult aspect of the examination is determining what potential biomechanical factors may have led to the injury, including the role of the cyclist's bike fit.

Road bicycle fit
Specific adjustments (**Table 2**) may resolve a patient's symptoms in many cases or prevent their recurrence after an appropriate period of rest. Among the most helpful tools in addressing underlying factors leading to nontraumatic cycling injuries is observation of the cyclist on their bike using a trainer stand, although this may be beyond the scope of most primary care physicians. Silberman and colleagues[35] have published a concise illustrated guide to road bicycle fitting.

Imaging and additional testing
History and physical examination are often adequate for proper diagnosis and management of cycling-related injuries, similar to injured runners. Likewise, imaging can be helpful in assisting in differentiating among diagnoses with similar clinical presentations or in determining degree of injury.

SPECIFIC ORTHOPEDIC CONDITIONS ENCOUNTERED IN RUNNING AND/OR BIKING, PRESENTED ALPHABETICALLY
Achilles Tendinopathy (Running, Biking)

Introduction
Achilles tendinopathy is common in runners, with an incidence of approximately 10%,[42] and may occur in cyclists as well, although less frequently. Diagnosis is based on the history and physical examination. Imaging is used to exclude other causes and to confirm an Achilles rupture.

Cause
Achilles disorders are especially common in middle-aged athletes.[34] During running, the Achilles tendon experiences loading 12.5 times body weight.[18] Achilles tendinopathy is affected by both intrinsic and extrinsic risk factors (**Box 2**).[18,35,43]

Clinical presentation
Achilles tendinopathy presents as gradual pain of insidious onset. Patients with milder injury experience mild pain during exercise only, whereas more severe cases can affect normal daily activities. Acute injury with the sudden sensation of being struck in the back of the heel suggests Achilles rupture.

Physical examination
Achilles tendinopathy is suggested by tenderness to palpation 2 to 6 cm proximal to the tendon insertion over the posterior calcaneus. Tendon thickening and presence of

Table 2
Location of symptoms and suggested bicycle adjustments in cyclists with pain or numbness

Location of Symptoms	Suggested Adjustment(s)
Neck or scapula	Adopt more upright riding position Raise stem (handlebar) height Shorten stem length Ride with hands on upper handlebar position or on top of handlebars
Hand(s), especially ulnar	Use padded gloves Add/increase handlebar padding Change hand position every few minutes Raise stem height Move saddle backward Level saddle if tilted down
Low back pain	Adopt more upright riding position Raise stem height Shorten stem length
Shin	Lower saddle height
Heel	Adjust saddle height (may be too high or too low)
Foot	Move cleat back (or more rarely forward) Check sole for wear Check for inward cleat bolt pressure Use wider shoes Loosen shoe straps/buckles
Perineum	Lower saddle height Reduce saddle tilt Use saddle with cutaway midline section (for men) Use wider saddle (especially for women)
Knee, anterior	Raise saddle height Move saddle backward Reduce climbing Increase cadence, decrease resistance (use smaller gears) Shorten cranks
Knee, medial	Reduce outward toe-pointing Reduce tension needed to exit clipless shoe-pedal system Ride with feet closer together
Knee, lateral	Reduce inward toe-pointing Ride with feet further apart
Knee, posterior	Lower saddle height Move saddle forward

Data from Silberman MR, Webner D, Collina S, et al. Road bicycle fit. Clin J Sport Med 2005;15(4):271–76; and Wanich T, Hodgkins C, Columbier JA, et al. Cycling injuries of the lower extremity. J Am Acad Orthop Surg 2007;15(12):748–56.

a nodule may be noted. Crepitus over the tendon suggests acute tenosynovitis. The Thompson test should be performed if Achilles rupture is suspected; loss of passive ankle plantar-flexion with a calf squeeze is a positive test.

Treatment
Relative rest, ice, and nonsteroidal antiinflammatory drugs (NSAIDs) reduce pain from inflammation in the acute phase. Physical therapy and heel lifts can help correct underlying biomechanical abnormalities predisposing to this injury. Running and biking are usually avoided during the acute phase. Light loading of the Achilles tendon

---

Box 2
Intrinsic and extrinsic risk factors affecting Achilles tendinopathy

Intrinsic Risk Factors	Extrinsic Risk Factors
• Regional hypovascularity	• Overuse
• Endocrine/metabolic disorders	• Poor flexibility
• Genetic factors	• Training errors
	• Excessive lateral heel strike
	• Hip muscle weakness
	• Cycling position
	• Incorrect bike fit

---

is recommended after the acute phase while the tendon is remodeling.[18] Raising saddle height may reduce symptoms for cyclists,[43,44] as may properly aligning an incorrectly rotated foot, or placing the foot further forward on the pedal.[43] Eccentric calf strength training has been shown to help runners with Achilles tendinopathy and forms the cornerstone of treatment.[45] Shock wave therapy is an unproven treatment, corticosteroid injections should be avoided, and other injections (eg, platelet-rich plasma injections) are considered experimental. Although several surgical techniques are described for persistent Achilles tendinopathy, most injuries resolve with conservative care, and operative management is therefore rarely necessary.[18]

Chronic Exertional Compartment Syndrome (Running, Biking)

Introduction
Chronic exertional compartment syndrome (CECS) is a common complaint, reported in 22% to 33% of runners with leg pain,[46,47] and is often overlooked as a source of pain in cyclists.[43] There are 4 compartments in the leg, with specific structures enclosed within each defined space (**Box 3**).[48]

Cause
CECS results from increased pressure, resulting in reversible ischemia within a closed fibro-osseous space.[43,48] This situation leads to decreased blood flow, with resultant ischemic pain. Although multiple predisposing factors have been investigated, data are limited on specific risk factors.[18]

Clinical presentation
Runners with CECS typically report recurrent pain that occurs at a well-defined point during running and that quickly disappears with cessation of running. Cyclists experience pain from shortly after the start of a ride until several minutes after its end. The pain is commonly described as a dull ache or burning sensation over the involved compartment. Symptoms are bilateral in most athletes. The length of the rest period required before resolution of symptoms increases over time with continued exercise, resulting in consultation.

Physical examination
CECS is diagnosed best by history, because physical examination findings are frequently normal at rest. After an exercise challenge, the involved compartment(s)

Box 3
Specific structures enclosed within compartments in the leg

Anterior (45% of cases)	• Tibialis anterior muscle
	• Extensor hallucis longus muscle
	• Extensor digitorum longus muscle
	• Peroneus tertius muscle
	• Deep peroneal nerve
	• Anterior tibial artery and vein
Posterior, deep (40%)	• Tibialis posterior muscle
	• Flexor hallucis longus muscle
	• Flexor digitorum longus muscle
	• Posterior tibial nerve
	• Posterior tibial artery and vein
Posterior, superficial (5%)	• Gastrocnemius muscle
	• Soleus muscle
	• Sural nerve
Lateral (10%)	• Peroneus longus muscle
	• Peroneus brevis muscle
	• Superficial peroneal nerve

---

may become tender and swollen. Occasionally, a soft tissue bulge occurs with muscle contraction, representing muscle herniation.

Compartment pressure testing is used by sports medicine specialists to confirm the diagnosis of CECS.[49,50] Near-infrared spectroscopy and magnetic resonance imaging (MRI) are being studied as alternative, noninvasive methods of measuring intracompartmental pressures.[48]

Treatment

Conservative treatment is typically attempted for 6 to 12 weeks. Conservative measures include reduction/cessation of running, NSAIDs, stretching, and orthotics. A recent study reported on successful treatment of anterior compartment syndrome with alteration of running gait to barefoot running.[51]

For most runners who wish to continue running, definitive treatment is surgical. Subcutaneous fasciotomy of the involved compartment(s) provides effective, long-lasting relief of symptoms.

Iliotibial Band Syndrome (Running, Biking)

Introduction

Iliotibial band syndrome (ITBS) is the most common lateral knee injury in runners, with an incidence between 5% and 14%,[52] and is common in cyclists as well. The iliotibial (IT) band is a confluence of proximal fascia of the hip flexors, extensors, and abductors. It originates at the lateral iliac crest and extends distally to the patella, tibia, and biceps femoris tendon.

Cause
Several suggested causes include friction of the IT band against the lateral femoral epicondyle, compression of the fat and connective tissue deep to the IT band, and chronic inflammation of the IT band bursa.[53] Although likely multifactorial, associated factors include excessive mileage, sudden increase in mileage, little running experience, leg length discrepancy, genu varum, high arches, hip abductor weakness, banked running surfaces, and hip inflexibility.[54,55] Diagnosis is based on the history and physical examination. Imaging is used to exclude other causes.

Clinical presentation
Diffuse lateral knee pain is the primary initial complaint, most often during running or cycling. Often pain begins several minutes into activity, or even after completion. As ITBS worsens, symptoms present earlier in exercise or even at rest. Patients may be unable to localize 1 specific area of pain but indicate pain over the entire lateral aspect of the thigh and knee. If the precipitating activity continues, the initial achiness progresses to a sharp and localized pain over the lateral femoral epicondyle or lateral tibial tubercle. Lateral knee snapping is also a common complaint in runners with ITBS. Running down hills often worsens the pain, as does sitting for extended periods with the knee in flexion.[52,53]

Physical examination
Patients often have lateral knee tenderness to palpation 2 cm above the joint line. Tenderness is often more pronounced when the patient is standing with the knee flexed at 30°. Patients may have weakness in the knee extensors, knee flexors, and hip abductors. The Ober test can be used to assess tightness of the IT band. The patient is asked to lie on the unaffected side, with the unaffected hip and knee both flexed at 90°. While stabilizing the pelvis, the affected leg is abducted and extended until aligned with the rest of the body. The affected leg is then lowered into adduction. If there is tightness of the IT band, the leg remains abducted and the patient experiences lateral knee pain.[52]

Treatment
Prognosis for ITBS is generally good. The initial goal of treatment is to reduce inflammation. NSAIDs and ice may be used. Patients should avoid activities that require repeated knee flexion and extension. The triggering activity is typically discontinued until symptoms improve. A stretching and strengthening regimen focused on the IT band should then be prescribed; physical therapy can be helpful. IT band flexibility can be increased by overhand arm extension while performing a standing IT band stretch.[55] Foam roll bars are commonly recommended to improve IT band flexibility.

When a runner can resume strength exercises without pain, running can be resumed at a gradual pace on a level surface and slowly increased over 3 to 6 weeks. Addressing underlying biomechanical conditions or training errors reduces risk of recurrence.

Cyclists may find relief from adjusting cycling position, saddle height, or their pedal/cleat system.[34]

Rarely, corticosteroids or surgery may be indicated if patients do not respond to conservative management.[52,53]

MTSS (Running)

Introduction
MTSS is defined as exercise-related leg pain over the mid to distal posteromedial tibia. With an incidence of 4% to 33% in military personnel and athletes,[56] MTSS commonly affects runners.

Cause

Numerous theories relate functional anatomy and pathologic biomechanics to MTSS. Historically, periosteal inflammation has been attributed to MTSS caused by abnormal traction of the calf muscles (eg, soleus),[57] but recent histologic reviews contradict this theory. Mismatch between bone formation and resorption causing overloading of the tibial cortex is the most likely cause.[56] MTSS is associated with the following risk factors[18,56]:

- Imbalance of foot pressure
- Excessive pronation
- Female sex
- Higher body mass index
- Previous MTSS
- Sudden increases in training intensity and duration
- Uneven running surfaces

Clinical presentation

Runners with mild MTSS typically describe mid to distal posteromedial tibial pain, which begins with initiation of running and which subsides with continued exercise. Severe MTSS is present throughout exercise and at rest and should heighten suspicion for stress fracture.

Physical examination

Accurate location of symptoms, risk factor evaluation, and elimination of other conditions associated with leg pain in runners form the basis of the physical examination. Diffuse tenderness to palpation over the mid to distal posteromedial tibia is the most sensitive finding.[58] Focal tenderness should heighten suspicion for stress fracture. The diagnosis of MTSS is clinical. Imaging should be obtained if the diagnosis is unclear.

Treatment

MTSS is treated with activity modification, stretching, ice, and NSAIDs. Calf muscle strengthening, antipronation insoles, massage, aerobic fitness, electrotherapy, and acupuncture are commonly recommended, but randomized controlled trials and case series supporting their use are lacking.[56]

Patellofemoral Pain Syndrome (Running, Biking)

Introduction

As discussed earlier, most injuries during running and cycling lead to knee pain, and patellofemoral pain syndrome is responsible for nearly 25% of injuries to the knee.[59] The patella articulates with the patellofemoral groove in the femur. As the patella moves up and down, tilts, and rotates, there are numerous points of contact between its undersurface and the femur.

Cause

Although the cause of patellofemoral pain syndrome is not fully understood, it is most commonly hypothesized that increased stress on the patellofemoral joint leads to wear of the articular cartilage.[59] Possible predisposing factors include anatomic variations that precipitate patellar malalignment and instability, lower extremity malalignment from foot hyperpronation or other causes, and imbalances in muscle and soft tissue (eg, between the medial and lateral quadriceps muscles).

Clinical presentation

Patients present with anterior knee pain, which can have insidious onset, typically occurring with exercise, and worsening when squatting, descending steps or hills, or after prolonged sitting.[34,59,60] Pain is usually achy, sometimes sharp, and may occur in 1 or both knees. Gross effusions are rare, but mild swelling may be present. There may be perceived instability, which should be distinguished from instability caused by patellar dislocation, subluxation, or ligamentous injury of the knee.

Physical examination
Inspection may reveal vastus medialis oblique muscle atrophy or abnormalities in alignment such as the J sign (curvilinear lateral tracking of the patella with quadriceps contraction) or a Q angle, caused by excessive lateral insertion of the patellar tendon. Despite abnormal patellar tracking, there should be no decrease in range of motion. Crepitus is common with active extension. Tenderness is common along the femoral condyles and patellar facets, as is tenderness behind the patella with light patellar compression. It is important to consider radiography with a history of trauma or dislocation or with lack of improvement after several weeks of conservative therapy.

Treatment
The first stage of a comprehensive treatment plan is symptom control. This goal may be achieved through activity modification, NSAIDs, ice, and patellar taping or bracing with a rubber sleeve with a patellar hole. Total inactivity should be avoided, because it promotes deconditioning, which may increase susceptibility to stress injury when resuming normal activity. Cyclists may benefit from adjusting their cycling position, saddle height, or pedal/cleat system. Physical therapy is often helpful and should focus on quadriceps strengthening and correction of any issues of hip and ankle strength and control. Proprioceptive control training can be helpful as well, especially in patients with alignment issues and excessive laxity. Most athletes respond to nonoperative treatment.

Plantar Fasciitis (Running, Biking)

Introduction
Plantar fasciitis is common, with between 1 and 2 million people in the United States affected each year, and is the most common cause of plantar heel pain.[61,62] Plantar fasciitis affects both active and sedentary populations, with peak incidence between 40 and 60 years of age.[62] Most patients seek care from their primary care provider. Plantar fasciitis is diagnosis is based on the history and physical examination.

Cause
Plantar fasciitis is now believed to be a degenerative process, rather than an acute inflammatory process. It likely results from repetitive microscopic trauma at the origin of the plantar fascia. Prolonged standing or running can contribute to the biomechanical overuse associated with plantar fasciitis.[61,62] Incorrect saddle height may be contributory in cyclists.[44] Heel spurs can occur with plantar fasciitis, but they are not the cause. Risk factors include excessive running, obesity, and prolonged standing. Excessive foot pronation can contribute as well.

Clinical presentation
Patients report posterior heel pain, which developed gradually. It is usually worst with the first step in the morning or after prolonged sitting. The pain usually improves gradually with activity, but may be worse at the end of the day if the patient continues to walk or stand for extended periods.[62] Walking barefoot, on toes, or up stairs may increase pain.[63] Plantar fasciitis pain does not often radiate and is not associated with nerve paresthesias. Constant pain or pain that wakes the patient from sleep should prompt evaluation for other causes.[62]

Physical examination

The foot and ankle should be inspected with the patient standing and walking. Pes planus (flat foot) or pes cavus (high arch) foot deformity may be present, because these can increase loading of the plantar fascia. There is often tenderness with passive dorsiflexion, as well as tenderness to palpation over the medial plantar calcaneal tuberosity at the origin of the plantar fascia, although tenderness anywhere along the plantar fascia may be present.[62]

Treatment

Most cases of plantar fasciitis respond to nonsurgical modalities, with response most often within 1 year, regardless of treatment; conservative therapy has been reported to be successful in up to 90% of cases.[61] Patients should be counseled that pain may often persist for 6 to 12 months before resolving. Relative rest, ice, massage, and NSAIDs are common initial recommendations. Prefabricated foot orthotics can be used, as can night splints, which stretch the plantar fascia during sleep.[34,61–63] Progressive plantar fascia and intrinsic foot muscle stretching techniques have been shown to reduce plantar fasciitis pain and should be performed multiple times daily; these are more effective than calf stretching.[63] Helpful adjustments for cyclists may include raising saddle height, increasing cadence, and decreasing resistance.[43] Corticosteroid injections can be used, and if symptoms persist longer than expected despite these measures, extracorporeal shock wave therapy or plantar fasciotomy may be considered.[61]

Pudendal (Bicycle Seat) Neuropathy (Biking)

Introduction

Although rarer among cyclists compared with upper or lower extremity symptoms, pelvic/pudendal symptoms can occur. Because they are less common, they may be less suspect and therefore more difficult to link initially to the cycling activity.

Cause

Symptoms may arise from pudendal nerve compression between the saddle and the pubic symphysis, or from cavernous nerve compression.[44] This situation may be caused by a saddle position that is too high or excessively tilted (either up or down). In addition, the saddle may not be wide enough to support the ischial tuberosities.[35]

Clinical presentation

Male and female patients may present with perineal numbness and tingling. Men may experience these in the penis or scrotum, and impotence may be present, although this is less common.[44]

Physical examination

Decreased sensation in the affected area helps confirm the diagnosis. Inspection may yield additional clues, such as skin irritation or calluses.[44]

Treatment

Affected cyclists should not resume cycling until symptoms resolve, which generally occurs within 1 week but may take several months.[44] Lowering saddle height and reducing saddle tilt may help prevent recurrence, as may switching to a wider saddle[35] or, for men, a saddle with an open midline section.[44]

Stress Fractures (Running)

Introduction

Stress fractures are common in runners. They are categorized as low or high risk based on healing potential (**Box 4**).

Box 4	
Low-risk and high-risk stress fractures in runners	
Low Risk	**High Risk**
• Sacrum	• Femoral neck
• Pubic ramus	• Anterior tibia
• Femoral shaft	• Medial malleolus
• Tibia (except anterior)	• Navicular
• Fibula	• Proximal fifth metatarsal
• Metatarsal shaft	• Sesamoids

Tibial stress fractures are the most common fractures in runners, accounting for 50% of stress fractures.[64]

Cause
Ordinarily, bone remodels to match demands, but if bone is under repetitive stress and deprived of sufficient time to remodel, stress fractures can result. Most stress fractures occur in cortical bone and result from fatigue; cortical bone is found in the diaphysis of long bones and the shell of square bones. When the active remodeling of cancellous bone is limited, such as with the female athlete triad, metabolic bone disease, or osteoporosis, it becomes susceptible to insufficiency fractures.[65] Risk factors for stress fracture are shown in **Box 5**.[18,66]

Clinical presentation
Runners with stress fractures commonly present with localized pain of insidious onset. Patients often report increasing amounts of pain earlier in their runs and occasionally during activities of daily living.

Physical examination
The hallmark of the examination is focal bone tenderness. Swelling, erythema, or warmth may be evident over the stress fracture. Biomechanical factors that may

Box 5	
Risk factors for stress fractures	
Intrinsic Risk Factors	**Extrinsic Risk Factors**
• Poor preparticipation conditioning	• Rapid increase in training program
	• High weekly training mileage
• Female gender	• Irregular or angled surface
• Menstrual imbalance	• Poor footwear
• Decreased bone mineral density	• Running shoes >6 months old
• Genu valgus/varum	• Low fat diet
• Leg length discrepancy	• Decreased calcium and vitamin D intake
	• Tobacco use

predispose to stress fracture should be noted, including muscle imbalances, leg length discrepancy, extreme foot types (high longitudinal arch or excessive forefoot varus), genu valgus/varum, and femoral anteversion.[64,67,68] Imaging is used in times of uncertainty or when counseling a runner who desires ongoing training. Radiographs have low sensitivity during the first 2 to 3 weeks. Periosteal bone formation and callus formation can be detected on radiographs. Bone scans are used less frequently because of radiation exposure, time constraints, and lack of specificity. MRI may be helpful in grading stress fractures and providing prognostic information, but false-positive results can occur.[69]

Treatment
Low-risk stress fractures have adequate vascularity and less strain than high-risk stress fractures. Activity modification and relative rest are frequently recommended. The runner must be pain free with ambulation before advancement. If pain occurs with walking, crutches or non–weight bearing may be indicated until pain free. Non–weight-bearing activities can be continued in most runners to preserve some conditioning, including biking, swimming, aqua running, and upper body cross-training. Once asymptomatic, runners can begin a slow transition back to running, beginning at 50% duration and intensity, increasing no more than 10% weekly. In our experience, healing commonly takes 4 to 8 weeks.

High-risk stress fractures require strict immobilization, non–weight bearing, and consideration for early surgical intervention (especially for tension-sided stress fractures). Sports medicine referral should be considered for all high-risk stress fractures.

Ulnar Compression Neuropathy (Cyclist's Palsy) (Biking)

Introduction
Ulnar compression symptoms are the most common upper extremity complaint in cyclists, occurring significantly more frequently than median nerve symptoms. There may be sensory involvement, motor involvement, or both.

Cause
Excessive and sustained pressure on the handlebars, with more of the force on the lateral (ulnar) aspect of the hand, compresses the ulnar tunnel and the ulnar nerve within it. The addition of vibration (eg, with riding on uneven or rough surfaces) may exacerbate symptoms. The more superficial location of the ulnar tunnel makes these symptoms significantly more common among cyclists than symptoms of compression from the deeper median nerve.[39] Lower hand positions increase pressure on the handlebars, whether related to drop-style handlebars, a stem too short or too low, or a saddle positioned too far forward or tilted downward.[35]

Clinical presentation
Patients typically complain of paresthesias of the fourth and fifth fingers, and may experience weakness of the hand as well. Symptoms may be progressive over the course of a sustained training program, or they may begin acutely, most often after a prolonged ride.[39] A careful history should include type of handlebars, preferred hand location, seating position, type of terrain, and the use of any gloves or padding.

Physical examination
On inspection, atrophy of the hypothenar eminence is consistent with motor involvement. Sensory assessment should include the hypothenar eminence and both the palmar and volar aspects of the fourth and fifth fingers. Motor assessment should

focus on identifying areas of hand weakness, especially finger adduction and abduction, and thumb adduction.[44]

Treatment

Most symptoms resolve promptly on cessation of the compressive activity, although they sometimes persist for months. Suggestions to alleviate symptoms and prevent recurrence include:[35,39,44]

- Addition of handlebar padding
- Use of padded cycling gloves
- Raising handlebars
- Changing hand position frequently
- Adopting a more upright cycling position
- Leveling seat if tilted forward
- Repositioning saddle if too far forward

REFERENCES

1. Heckman GA, McKelvie RJ. Cardiovascular aging and exercise in healthy older adults. Clin J Sport Med 2008;18(6):479–85.
2. Centers for Disease Control and Prevention. Prevalence of obesity in the United States, 2009-1010. Available at: http://www.cdc.gov/nchs/fastats/overwt.htm. Accessed February 18, 2013.
3. Council on Sports Medicine and Fitness, Council on School Health. Active healthy living: prevention of childhood obesity through increased physical activity. Pediatrics 2006;117(5):1834–42.
4. Haskell W, Lee I, Pate R, et al. Physical activity and public health: updated recommendation for adults from the American College of Sports Medicine and the American Heart Association. Med Sci Sports Exerc 2007;39(8): 1423–34.
5. Nelson M, Rejeski W, Blair S, et al. Physical activity and public health in older adults: recommendations from the American College of Sports Medicine and the American Heart Association. Med Sci Sports Exerc 2007; 39(8):1435–45.
6. Chalufour M. How demographics are affecting the racing scene. Running Times, October 14, 2010. Available at: http://www.runnersworld.com/rt-columns/how-demographics-are-affecting-racing-scene?page. Accessed February 19, 2013.
7. Fields KB, Sykes J, Walker K, et al. Prevention of running injuries. Curr Sports Med Rep 2012;9:176–82.
8. Cooper KH. Aerobics. New York: Bantam Books: Random House; 1968.
9. Fixx J. The complete book of running. New York: Random House; 1977.
10. Bloom M. Running: the numbers. Running Times 2011;71–2.
11. Larson P, Katovsky B. Tread lightly: form, footwear, and the quest for injury-free running. New York: Skyhorse; 2012.
12. Chakravarty E, Hubert H, Lingala V, et al. Reduced disability and mortality among aging runners: a 21 year longitudinal study. Arch Intern Med 2008; 168(15):1638–46.
13. van Mechelen W. Running injuries: a review of the epidemiological literature. Sports Med 1992;14:320–35.
14. Hootman JM, Macera CA, Ainsworth BE, et al. Predictors of lower extremity injury among recreationally active adults. Clin J Sport Med 2002;12:99–106.

15. Jacobs SJ, Berson BL. Injuries to runners: a study of entrants to a 10,000 meter race. Am J Sports Med 1986;14:151–5.
16. Walter SD, Hart LE, McIntosh JM, et al. The Ontario study of running related injuries. Arch Intern Med 1989;149:2561–4.
17. van Gent RN, Siem D, van Middelkoop M, et al. Incidence and determinants of lower extremity running injuries in long distance runners: a systematic review. Br J Sports Med 2007;41:469–80.
18. Gallo R, Plakke M, Silvis M. Common leg injuries of long-distance runners: anatomical and biomechanical approach. Sports Health 2012;4(6):485–95.
19. Taunton JE, Ryan MB, Clement DB, et al. A retrospective case-control analysis of 2002 running injuries. Br J Sports Med 2002;36:95–101.
20. Plastaras CT, Rittenberg JD, Rittenberg KE, et al. Comprehensive functional evaluation of the injured runner. Phys Med Rehabil Clin N Am 2005;16:623–49.
21. Dugan SA, Bhat KP. Biomechanics and analysis of running gait. Phys Med Rehabil Clin N Am 2005;16:603–21.
22. Fields KB, Bloom OJ, Priebe D, et al. Basic biomechanics of the lower extremity. Prim Care 2005;32:245–51.
23. Lieberman DE, Venkadesan M, Werbel WA, et al. Foot strike patterns and collision forces in habitually barefoot versus shod runners. Nature 2010;463:531–5.
24. Knapik JJ, Trone DW, Swedler DI, et al. Injury reduction effectiveness of assigning running shoes based on plantar shape in Marine Corps basic training. Am J Sports Med 2010;38:1759–67.
25. Knapik JJ, Brosch LC, Venuto M, et al. Effect on injuries of assigning shoes based on foot shape in Air Force basic training. Am J Prev Med 2010;38: S197–211.
26. Richards CE, Magin PJ, Callister R. Is your prescription of distance running shoes evidence based? Br J Sports Med 2009;43:159–62.
27. Ryan MB, Valiant GA, McDonald K, et al. The effect of three different levels of footwear stability on pain outcomes in women runners: a randomized control trial. Br J Sports Med 2011;45:715–21.
28. McDougall C. Born to run: a hidden tribe, superathletes, and the greatest race the world has never seen. New York: Vintage Books; 2009.
29. Rixe JA, Gallo RA, Silvis ML. The barefoot debate: can minimalist shoes reduce running related injuries. Curr Sports Med Rep 2012;11(3):160–5.
30. Altman AR, Davis IS. Barefoot running: biomechanics and implications for running injuries. Curr Sports Med Rep 2012;11(5):244–50.
31. Lieberman DE. What we can learn about running from barefoot running: an evolutionary medical perspective. Exerc Sport Sci Rev 2012;40(2):63–72.
32. Bresler M, Mar W, Toman J. Diagnostic imaging in the evaluation of leg pain in athletes. Clin Sports Med 2012;31:217–45.
33. Outdoor Foundation. Outdoor recreation participation topline report 2011. Available at: http://www.outdoorindustry.org/research/participation.php?action=detail&research_id=133. Accessed February 20, 2013.
34. Cosca D, Navazio F. Common problems in endurance athletes. Am Fam Physician 2007;76(2):237–44.
35. Silberman MR, Webner D, Collina S, et al. Road bicycle fit. Clin J Sport Med 2005;15(4):271–6.
36. Strock GA, Cottrell ER, Lohman JM. Triathlon. Phys Med Rehabil Clin N Am 2006;17(3):553–64.
37. Asplund C, Webb C, Barkdull T. Neck and back pain in bicycling. Curr Sports Med Rep 2005;4:271–4.

38. Dettori NJ, Norvell DC. Non-traumatic bicycle injuries: a review of the literature. Sports Med 2006;36(1):7–18.
39. Richmond D. Handlebar problems in bicycling. Clin Sports Med 1994;13(1): 165–73.
40. Attewell R, Glase K, McFadden M. Bicycle helmet safety: a meta-analysis. Accid Anal Prev 2001;33(3):345–52.
41. Macpherson A, Spinks A. Bicycle helmet legislation for the uptake of helmet use and prevention of head injuries. Cochrane Database Syst Rev 2008;(3):CD005401. http://dx.doi.org/10.1002/14651858.CD005401.pub3.
42. Lopes A, Junior L, Yeung S, et al. What are the main running related musculo-skeletal injuries? Sports Med 2012;42(10):891–905.
43. Wanich T, Hodgkins C, Columbier JA, et al. Cycling injuries of the lower extremity. J Am Acad Orthop Surg 2007;15(12):748–56.
44. Thompson M, Rivara F. Bicycle-related injuries. Am Fam Physician 2001;63(10): 2007–14.
45. Ohberg L, Lorentzon R, Alfredson H. Eccentric training in patient with chronic Achilles tendinosis: normalized tendon structure and decreased thickening at follow-up. Br J Sports Med 2004;38:8–11.
46. Clanton T, Solcher B. Chronic leg pain in the athlete. Clin Sports Med 1994; 13(4):743–59.
47. Styf J. Diagnosis of exercise-induced pain in the anterior aspect of the lower leg. Am J Sports Med 1988;16(2):165–9.
48. George C, Hutchinson M. Chronic exertional compartment syndrome. Clin Sports Med 2012;31:307–19.
49. Pedowitz R, Hargens A, Mubarak S, et al. Modified criteria for the objective diagnosis of chronic compartment syndrome of the leg. Am J Sports Med 1990;18(1):35–40.
50. Hislop M, Batt M. Chronic exertional compartment syndrome testing: a minimalist approach. Br J Sports Med 2011;45:954–5.
51. Diebal A, Gregory R, Alitz C, et al. Forefoot running improves pain and disability associated with chronic exertional compartment syndrome. Am J Sports Med 2012;40:1060–7.
52. Khaund R, Flynn S. Iliotibial band syndrome: a common source of knee pain. Am Fam Physician 2005;71(8):1545–50.
53. van der Worp MP, van der Horst N, de Wijer A, et al. Iliotibial band syndrome in runners: a systematic review. Sports Med 2012;42(11):969–92.
54. Paluska S. An overview of hip injuries in runners. Sports Med 2005;35(11): 991–1014.
55. Fredericson M, White J, MacMahon J, et al. Quantitative analysis of the relative effectiveness of 3 iliotibial band stretches. Arch Phys Med Rehabil 2002;83: 589–92.
56. Moen M, Tol J, Weir A, et al. Medial tibial stress syndrome: a critical review. Sports Med 2009;39(7):523–46.
57. Detmer D. Chronic shin splints: classification and management of medial tibial stress syndrome. Sports Med 1986;3:436–46.
58. Rashef N, Guelich D. Medial tibial stress syndrome. Clin Sports Med 2012;31: 273–90.
59. Collado H, Fredericson M. Patellofemoral pain syndrome. Clin Sports Med 2010; 29(3):377–98.
60. Juhn M. Patellofemoral pain syndrome: a review and guidelines for treatment. Am Fam Physician 1999;60(7):2012–22.

61. Goff J, Crawford R. Diagnosis and treatment of plantar fasciitis. Am Fam Physician 2011;84(6):676–82.

62. Neufeld S, Cerrato R. Plantar fasciitis: evaluation and treatment. J Am Acad Orthop Surg 2008;16:338–46.

63. Cole C, Seto C, Gazewood J. Plantar fasciitis: evidence-based review of diagnosis and therapy. Am Fam Physician 2005;72(11):2237–42.

64. Matheson G, Clement D, McKenzie D, et al. Stress fractures in athletes: a study of 320 cases. Am J Sports Med 1987;15(1):46–58.

65. Harrast M, Colonno D. Stress fractures in runners. Clin Sports Med 2010;29: 399–416.

66. McCormick F, Nwachukwu B, Provencher M. Stress fractures in runners. Clin Sports Med 2012;31:291–306.

67. Barnes A, Wheat J, Milner C. Association between foot type and tibial stress injuries: a systematic review. Br J Sports Med 2008;42:93–8.

68. Jones B, Bovee M, Harris J, et al. Intrinsic risk factors for exercise-related injuries among male and female army trainees. Am J Sports Med 1993;2(5): 705–10.

69. Bergman A, Fredericson M, Ho C, et al. Asymptomatic tibial stress reactions: MRI detection and clinical follow-up in distance runners. AJR Am J Roentgenol 2004;183:635–8.

Common Injections in Musculoskeletal Medicine

Aaron J. Monseau, MD[a,b,*], Parminder Singh Nizran, MD[c]

KEYWORDS

- Joint injection • Osteoarthritis • Corticosteroid injection • Arthrocentesis • Bursitis
- Adhesive capsulitis • Lateral epicondylalgia

KEY POINTS

- When performed for the correct indication and using proper technique, musculoskeletal injections can be beneficial for patients and rewarding for physicians.
- Although the most current evidence suggests that steroids only relieve pain and improve function for a short period, this time can be very meaningful for patients who have been experiencing chronic pain.
- Recent evidence suggests that steroid injections for lateral epicondylalgia can actually worsen the outcome.
- More high-quality trials are needed to delineate the usefulness of injection therapy for each indication and location.

INTRODUCTION

Musculoskeletal injections are a common procedure in many offices but can pose a daunting task for some providers, even those who are experienced. Some physicians choose to attempt only a couple types of musculoskeletal injections, whereas others will attempt to inject just about any anatomically feasible target. The available evidence for musculoskeletal injections is not as robust as that for other topics, and is fraught with differences in injection technique, variability of substance injected, debate over meaningfulness of end points, and more than occasional pharmaceutical industry influence.

Taking all of this into account, most still believe that corticosteroid injections can offer some form of pain control or increased function for certain patients with certain

[a] Department of Emergency Medicine, Robert C. Byrd Health Sciences Center, School of Medicine, West Virginia University, PO Box 9149, Morgantown, WV 26506, USA; [b] Department of Orthopaedics, Robert C. Byrd Health Sciences Center, School of Medicine, West Virginia University, PO Box 9196, Morgantown, WV 26506, USA; [c] Department of Family and Community Medicine, Penn State Milton S. Hershey Medical Center, Penn State College of Medicine, 500 University Drive, H154, Hershey, PA 17033, USA
* Corresponding author. Department of Emergency Medicine, Robert C. Byrd Health Sciences Center, School of Medicine, West Virginia University, PO Box 9149, Morgantown, WV 26506.
E-mail address: amonseau@gmail.com

Prim Care Clin Office Pract 40 (2013) 987–1000
http://dx.doi.org/10.1016/j.pop.2013.08.012
0095-4543/13/$ – see front matter © 2013 Elsevier Inc. All rights reserved.
primarycare.theclinics.com

musculoskeletal conditions. This article briefly addresses the basic preparation for an injection, indications for the procedure, and some points on substances injected. However, this article focuses more on the actual procedural techniques for the different injections. Some controversies and currently evolving techniques are also addressed. Because of space limitations and consideration for injections believed to be high-yield, this article covers injections of the knee joint, subacromial bursa, glenohumeral joint, lateral epicondyle, de Quervain tenosynovitis, and greater trochanteric bursitis.

PREPARATION

Every procedure begins with collecting the appropriate equipment, and joint injections are no different. **Box 1** lists the suggested equipment.

Full sterile technique is not required for musculoskeletal injections as long as the area of skin is not touched after it is cleaned and the needle is not touched. Creamer and colleagues[1] investigated the infectious risk of sterile versus clean gloves in a study published in the The American Journal of Surgery in December of 2012. After comparing cultures obtained from clean gloves donned by the subject alone, sterile gloves donned by the subject alone, and sterile gloves donned with the assistance of a surgical technician, the authors reported a statistically significant larger number of organisms on the clean gloves compared with the sterile gloves. However, they also noted that the number of organisms on all the gloves were below what is generally considered sufficient to cause an infection. Therefore, although clean gloves had more bacteria than sterile gloves, the investigators concluded that it may not be a clinically relevant number of bacteria, but one may argue that this was not a proper study design to make that conclusion.

Povidone-iodine is the typical skin cleanser used in most clinics, but chlorhexidine and isopropyl alcohol are also acceptable. All should be applied in a circular pattern starting at the injection site and working outward. This technique may reduce the probability of dragging bacteria into the injection field. Each cleanser should not be

---

Box 1
List of suggested equipment for musculoskeletal injections

- Gloves
- Skin cleanser
- Ethyl chloride
- Needle
- Syringe
- Injectable substances
- Gauze
- Band-Aid
- Epinephrine autoinjector

If joint aspiration is planned along with injection, a larger-bore needle is needed and the following should be added:

- Large syringe for aspiration
- Hemostat to hold needle steady while changing syringe

permitted to pool on the skin but rather be allowed to air-dry before placing the needle onto the skin.

Many clinicians use ethyl chloride spray to cool the skin and decrease the pain of needle insertion. Other techniques, such as stretching the skin tight, briefly shaking the skin, and having the patient cough can also decrease the pain of needle insertion.[2]

Needle size is another important consideration in the success of the procedure and the pain experienced by the patient. Needle length is of paramount importance because it is directly related to the success of the procedure. Once the required needle length is determined, then the smallest bore of needle available should be used. If aspiration of the joint is planned or even considered, then an 18-gauge or 20-gauge needle will likely be required, because smaller needles may lead to difficulty aspirating thick joint fluid.[2–5] **Table 1** summarizes common needle choices.[2,5,6]

As the final point on preparation, an epinephrine autoinjector should be accessible in any clinic where injections are being performed. This intervention is potentially life-saving in the rare event of anaphylaxis.

INJECTABLE SUBSTANCES
Corticosteroids

The mode of action of corticosteroids is still at least partially unknown. Therefore, the usefulness and degree of therapeutic effect are debated by experts in the field on both sides. Despite this, steroids remain a mainstay of treatment for myriad musculoskeletal complaints. For joint injections, widespread support remains for using corticosteroid injections to reduce pain, especially from osteoarthritis, for a short period, such as less than 4 to 6 weeks.[7–9] After 6 weeks, most studies find no difference in pain or function between steroid and placebo.[7,9–11]

Steroid injections performed for tendon pain or tendinopathy are even more complicated. Coombes and colleagues[12] found that steroids actually worsened the course of lateral epicondylalgia, commonly called *tennis elbow*. A review of the efficacy and safety of corticosteroids in tendinopathy showed that their efficacy for rotator cuff tendinopathy was unclear.[13] **Table 2** provides a summary of different steroids that may be used. Steroid injections should be limited to 3 to 4 injections per 12 months at the most.

Local Anesthetics

The other mainstay of injection therapy is a local anesthetic such as lidocaine. The addition of lidocaine can provide temporary pain relief and improve the accuracy of

Table 1
Needle sizes for common musculoskeletal injections

Injection Site or Disorder	Needle Gauge	Minimum Needle Length[a]	Typical Total Volume
Knee	20–22 G	1.5 inches (40 mm)	5–10 mL
Subacromial bursa	21–25 G	1.5–2 inches (40–50 mm)	5–8 mL
Glenohumeral joint	20–22 G	1.5–2 inches (40–50 mm)	5–8 mL
Lateral epicondyle	22–25 G	0.5 inch (16 mm)	1–2 mL
de Quervain tenosynovitis	22–25 G	0.5 inch (16 mm)	1–2 mL
Greater trochanteric bursitis	22–25 G	1.5–2 inches (40–50 mm)	4–6 mL

[a] A longer needle may be needed for obese patients.
Data from Refs.[2,3,5,6]

Table 2 Summary of commonly used steroids				
	Methylprednisolone Acetate	Triamcinolone Acetonide[a]	Betamethasone Acetate and Disodium Phosphate	Dexamethasone
Potency[b]	5	5	25	25
Duration	Intermediate	Long	Long	Long
Knee joint	40.0 mg	40.0 mg	12.0 mg	6.0 mg
Subacromial bursa	40.0 mg	40.0 mg	12.0 mg	6.0 mg
Glenohumeral joint	40.0 mg	40.0 mg	12.0 mg	6.0 mg
Lateral epicondyle[c]	10.0 mg[c]	10.0 mg[c]	3.0 mg[c]	1.5 mg[c]
de Quervain tenosynovitis	10.0 mg	10.0 mg	3.0 mg	1.5 mg
Greater trochanter bursitis	20.0 mg	20.0 mg	6.0 mg	3.0 mg

[a] Typically considered the best compound for intra-articular injection.
[b] Hydrocortisone equivalents (per mg).
[c] Recent evidence suggests that steroids can actually worsen the course of lateral epicondylalgia.
Data from Refs.[2,3,5,6]

injection placement. Short-acting local anesthetics are the most commonly used agents and should be used without epinephrine.[2,5] Some clinicians advocate using long-acting agents, such as bupivacaine, whereas others will mix lidocaine and bupivacaine. On average, lidocaine will last approximately 1 hour, but bupivacaine will last approximately 8 hours.[5] Generally, 0.5% or 1% lidocaine or 0.25% or 0.5% bupivacaine are recommended. The overall volume of local anesthetic plus corticosteroid that is suggested for each injection can be found in **Table 1**.

Over the past few years, questions have been raised regarding chondrotoxicity caused by local anesthetics. Bupivacaine is probably the most investigated and has been found to cause more chondrocyte death than lidocaine in some studies.[14] Dragoo and colleagues[15] found a statistically significant increase in chondrotoxicity with a single dose of 1% lidocaine versus control, whereas no statistical difference was found between bupivacaine and ropivacaine. To even make this issue more confusing, Braun and colleagues[16] found that the addition of betamethasone sodium phosphate/betamethasone acetate, methylprednisolone acetate, or triamcinolone acetonide to 1% lidocaine actually increased chondrotoxicity over lidocaine alone, whereas only the betamethasone compound with bupivacaine resulted in increased chondrotoxicity over bupivacaine alone. Considering all of the current evidence, growing concern exists about intra-articular injection of local anesthetics, but the clinical relevance of in vitro studies and animal studies is still unknown. Many believe that the in vitro nature of the available studies does not account for the complicated composition of in vivo articular cartilage. Therefore, the damage caused by local anesthetics may just be mild and only cause subtle, possibly undetectable, clinical effects.[17]

Hyaluronic Acid

The term *viscosupplementation* has become synonymous with injecting hyaluronic acid or hyaluronan to improve the lubrication of a joint, which is nearly always the knee. Other joints are being studied,[18] but most of the data available pertain to treating osteoarthritis of the knee. Because the compounds only stay in the knee for a couple days, other actions have also been hypothesized, such as stimulation of endogenous hyaluronic acid production and a local anti-inflammatory effect.[2]

Multiple studies have shown decrease in pain and increase in function as early as 2 weeks after beginning treatment and continuing for several months, but when tested against steroid or conservative management with nonsteroidal anti-inflammatory drugs, hyaluronic acid injections have shown no benefit and an exponentially higher cost.[2,4,19,20] Any benefit found is more reliable in milder cases of osteoarthritis. Hyaluronic acid injections are not without risk, though, as Evanich and colleagues[21] reported a 15% adverse reaction rate, including one case of septic arthritis. Many clinicians will only consider hyaluronic acid injections after failure of conservative management and either failure or intolerance of corticosteroid injection in patients with mild to moderate osteoarthritis.

ULTRASOUND GUIDANCE

Bedside ultrasound can be very useful for diagnosing musculoskeletal conditions and guiding procedures such as injections.[22,23] As physicians in the United States become more comfortable with ultrasound, many other parts of the worldwide medical community have been using ultrasound for years and are adept at using ultrasound for musculoskeletal purposes. Numerous studies have shown improved injection accuracy and decreased injection pain with ultrasound guidance.[24–28] With increasing access to ultrasound machines and increasing comfort with the technology, sonographic guidance for musculoskeletal injections will also likely increase. This article discusses only landmark-guided procedures.

CONTRAINDICATIONS TO INJECTIONS

Each injection has a separate list of indications, but contraindications to injections are rather consistent. Some absolute contraindications are covered here, and **Box 2** provides a summary of absolute and relative contraindications. Any infection of skin overlying the injection site, bursa, joint, or bone and any systemic infection (ie, febrile illness) should be viewed as absolute contraindications. An unstable joint, a prosthetic joint, or an intra-articular fracture should also prompt a different course of action.[2,5,6]

Knee

Indications
The main indication for steroid injection of the knee is osteoarthritis. Corticosteroid injections are also commonly used in a conservative treatment plan when attempting to avoid surgery for a meniscus tear without mechanical symptoms such as locking. Other knee pain conditions that have not responded to physical therapy may prompt an attempt at a steroid injection.

Techniques
Medial mid-patellar For the medial mid-patellar approach, the patient should have the leg fully extended, which will allow the quadriceps to relax and cause the space between the patella and distal femur to open (**Fig. 1**). Patients should be encouraged to lie down flat on their back, because this will typically allow them to relax the quadriceps more easily and will prevent the apprehension associated with watching the needle enter the joint. Identifying the mid-point of the patella on the medial border, the skin is entered about one finger-breadth posterior to the patellar border. The patella is shaped like a triangle, so the needle and syringe should be at a 30° to 45° angle

---

Box 2
Contraindications to musculoskeletal injections

Absolute

- Corticosteroid or injectable substance hypersensitivity
- Infection (systemic, overlying cellulitis, septic arthritis/bursitis, osteomyelitis)
- Uncontrolled bleeding disorder
- Prosthetic or unstable joint
- Intra-articular fracture

Relative

- Corrected bleeding disorder
- Anticoagulated patient
- Hemarthrosis
- Immunosuppressed patient
- Diabetes
- High risk of tendon rupture
- Psychogenic pain

Data from Refs.[2,5,6]

---

to the bed to allow the needle to pass between the patella and the medial femoral condyle. An assistant may help by pushing on the lateral aspect of the patella, making it easier to enter the space between the patella and the distal femur.

Superolateral The superolateral approach is excellent for aspirating large joint effusions (**Fig. 2**). With the patient lying supine and the knee fully extended and supported, the superolateral corner of the patella should be identified. The skin is then entered one finger-breath proximal and one finger-breadth posterior to the superolateral corner of the patella. The triangular shape of the patella tapers off in the superior third, so a steep angle of approach is not needed. The needle and syringe should be at a 15° to 30° angle to the bed and directed medially and distally to slip under the superior border of the patella.

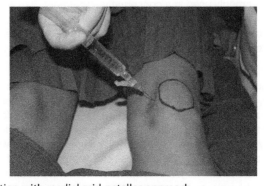

Fig. 1. Knee injection with medial mid-patellar approach.

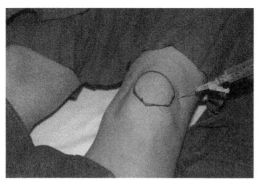

Fig. 2. Knee injection with superolateral approach.

Anterior joint line With the patient seated, knees flexed at 90°, and feet dangling off the table, the patellar tendon is identified, and then the skin entered either on the medial or lateral border of the tendon while directing the needle toward the center of the knee and slightly cephalad (**Fig. 3**). If the injection does not flow freely, repositioning of the needle is required to avoid injecting the anterior cruciate ligament. If attempting aspiration, another approach is recommended, because the anterior approach is notorious for dry taps. When performing any injection in the seated position, the physician should exercise caution, because syncopal episodes are not uncommon with joint injections.

Subacromial Bursa

Indications
Rotator cuff tendinosis and impingement syndrome are common diagnoses that are often treated with a steroid injection into the subacromial bursa.[2,5,6,29] Some studies have questioned the accuracy of injection placement, whereas others even question the effectiveness of steroid injections for rotator cuff tendinopathy.[10,30,31] The Cochrane Collaboration summarized the evidence in a 2003 review published online in 2009 still indicated that subacromial injection for rotator cuff disease may have some benefit.[29]

Techniques
All 3 of the techniques discussed are performed with the patient seated and the arm distracted by gravity.

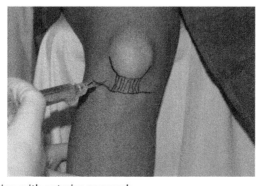

Fig. 3. Knee injection with anterior approach.

Posterior The posterolateral corner of the acromion should be identified (**Fig. 4**). The skin is entered one finger-breadth inferior to this with the needle directed slightly medially and cephalad to follow the undersurface of the acromion.

Lateral The lateral border of the acromion should be identified (**Fig. 5**). The skin is entered one finger-breadth inferior to the midway point of the lateral border of the acromion with the needle directed perpendicular to the border of the acromion and slightly cephalad to follow the undersurface of the acromion. A similar technique is also described as anterolateral when entering the skin anterior to the midway point of the lateral border and directing the needle slightly posterior in addition to slightly cephalad.

Glenohumeral Joint

Indications
Osteoarthritis of the glenohumeral joint can be painful and is a common indication for injection. Trauma to the shoulder and chronic rotator cuff tendinosis, in addition to or in combination with osteoarthritis, can lead to the debilitating condition known as *adhesive capsulitis* or *frozen shoulder*. Adhesive capsulitis may also be improved with a glenohumeral steroid injection, and some evidence shows that multiple injections, up to 3 in 16 weeks, may actually be more helpful.[2,3,5,32,33] As with other conditions, steroids seem to provide an advantage with respect to initial improvement, but in the long-term, outcomes in the steroid groups were no different than in the controls.[7] The Cochrane Collaboration once again supports steroid injections for short-term improvement in pain but admits that the evidence is equivocal.[28]

Techniques
Posterior The patient should be in a seated position with arms folded across the abdomen to open up the posterior joint space (**Fig. 6**). The posterolateral corner of the acromion and the coracoid process should be identified. The easiest technique is to hold the acromion with the thumb and the coracoid with the index finger of the nondominant hand. The skin is entered 2 finger-breadths inferior to the posterolateral corner of the acromion. The needle is directed at the coracoid. If the needle strikes bone, it should be pulled back slightly, then the injection performed.

Anterior With the patient seated and the arm in slight external rotation, the coracoid process and the spine of the scapula should be identified (**Fig. 7**). The skin is entered one finger-breadth inferior and one finger-breadth lateral to the coracoid while

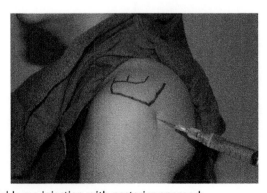

Fig. 4. Subacromial bursa injection with posterior approach.

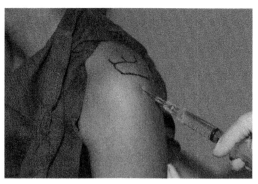

Fig. 5. Subacromial bursa injection with lateral approach.

directing the needle slightly medially and at the spine of the scapula. If the needle strikes bone, it should be pulled back slightly, then the injection performed.

Lateral Epicondyle

Indications

Historically, steroid injections for lateral epicondylalgia (formerly epicondylitis) are a very common procedure. A recently published and methodologically excellent randomized controlled trial and review article showed worse clinical outcomes with steroid injections compared with placebo and showed no difference with physical therapy.[12,13] Other substances, such as platelet-rich plasma, are still being tested, and the evidence is promising but still inconclusive at this point, because the highest-quality studies compared platelet-rich plasma with steroid injection, which has now been called into question.[34]

Techniques

The patient should be seated with the arm supported and with the elbow flexed to 90° (**Fig. 8**). The lateral epicondyle and the radial head should be identified. The injection should be performed into the area just anterior to the lateral epicondyle and at the point of maximal tenderness. The needle should be advanced down to bone and the tendon enthesis repeatedly peppered with the solution being injected. Another technique is to deposit the solution around the tendon and then pepper the tendon enthesis with the needle alone.

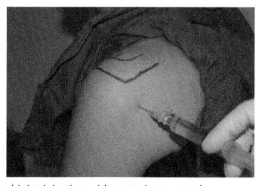

Fig. 6. Glenohumeral joint injection with posterior approach.

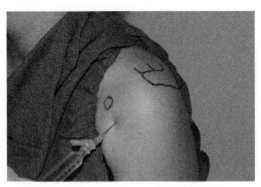

Fig. 7. Glenohumeral joint injection with anterior approach.

de Quervain Tenosynovitis

Indications

The syndrome of overuse and pain of the abductor pollicis longus and extensor pollicis brevis is known as *de Quervain disease* or *tenosynovitis*. The typical sign of this is pain with ulnar deviation of the wrist while the thumb is flexed across the palm (Finkelstein's test).[2] A Cochrane review in 2009 was only able to find one controlled clinical trial, which only enrolled pregnant or lactating women, but it did show significantly better outcomes with steroid injection versus thumb spica splint.[35] Obviously, this presents a problem with generalizability, but at least the available evidence indicates a benefit with steroid injection.

Techniques

The patient should be seated or supine with the forearm pronated 90° so the thumb is up (**Fig. 9**). The patient is asked to extend the thumb against resistance to identify the anatomic snuffbox. The radial or volar border of the snuffbox consists of the abductor pollicis longus and extensor pollicis brevis. These tendons are then followed proximally to the level of the radial styloid where the typical area of maximal tenderness is located. The goal is to inject into the tendon sheath but not into the tendon itself. If a division is felt between the 2 tendons, the injection should be performed here, directing the needle proximally. After entering the skin over the point of maximal tenderness, if the needle is felt to be in the tendon sheath, the patient should be asked

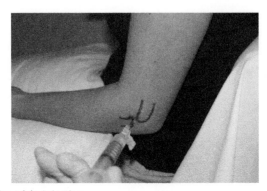

Fig. 8. Lateral epicondyle injection.

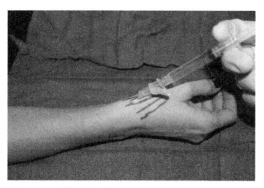

Fig. 9. de Quervain's tenosynovitis injection.

to extend and flex the thumb. If the needle moves forcefully with each movement, it is likely in the tendon and should be pulled back slightly. If the needle does not move with each movement, the injection should be performed slowly and the needle pulled back slightly whenever any resistance is felt. On the contrary, a very superficial injection may result in skin atrophy and discoloration, so this should also be avoided.

Greater Trochanteric Bursa

Indications
Pain over the greater trochanter is a common complaint, especially in the elderly. Many patients present complaining of hip pain but point to the greater trochanter when asked to indicate the location of their pain. This discomfort may originate from a direct blow or fall, chronic overuse, or chronic irritation (possibly sleeping on the same side every night).[2] It may also originate from gluteal tendinopathy or weakness that is often described as core weakness.[36] A randomized controlled trial published in 2011 indicated significant improvement in the steroid injection group at 3 months compared with the oral analgesic group. At 12 months, this advantage disappeared. No placebo or blinding was used in this trial, and therefore some bias may be attributable to the mere fact that the treatment group received an injection. However, the results are compatible with those of other studies noting short-term pain relief with steroid injections.[37]

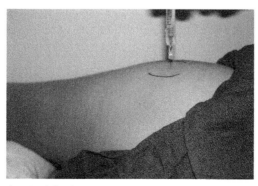

Fig. 10. Greater trochanter injection.

Techniques

The patient should lie down on the contralateral side so the affected greater trochanter is up (**Fig. 10**). The greater trochanter and the point of maximal tenderness, which are typically the same, should be identified. The skin should be entered perpendicular to the table and an attempt made to hit the point of maximal tenderness. After striking bone, the needle should be withdrawn slowly while carefully injecting. Once the fluid flows freely from the syringe, the withdrawing motion should be stopped and the fluid injected as a bolus. Another technique instructs the physician to inject 1 mL at a time starting at the point of maximum tenderness and moving outward in a fan pattern until all of the substance has been injected.[37]

SUMMARY

When performed for the correct indication and using proper technique, musculoskeletal injections can be beneficial for patients and rewarding for physicians. Although the most current evidence suggests that steroids only relieve pain and improve function for a short period, this time can be very meaningful for patients who have been experiencing chronic pain. Finally, more high-quality trials are needed to delineate the usefulness of injection therapy for each indication, because some recent literature suggests that steroids can actually be detrimental for some conditions.

REFERENCES

1. Creamer J, Davis K, Rice W. Sterile gloves: do they make a difference? Am J Surg 2012;204(6):976–9.
2. Saunders S, Longworth S. Injections techniques in orthopaedics and sports medicine: a practical manual for doctors and physiotherapists. 3rd edition. Edinburgh (United Kingdom): Elsevier; 2006.
3. Parrillo SJ, Morrison DS, Panacek EA. Arthrocentesis. In: Roberts JR, Hedges JR, editors. Clinical procedures in emergency medicine. 5th edition. Philadelphia: Saunders Elsevier; 2010. p. 971–85.
4. Courtney P, Doherty M. Joint aspiration and injection and synovial fluid analysis. Best Pract Res Clin Rheumatol 2009;23:161–92.
5. Howard TM, Rassner LH. Therapeutic and diagnostic injection and aspirations. In: Seidenberg PH, Beutler A, editors. The sports medicine resource manual. Philadelphia: Saunders; 2008. p. 574–97.
6. Foley BA, Christopher TA. Injection therapy of bursitis and tendinitis. In: Roberts JR, Hedges JR, editors. Clinical procedures in emergency medicine. 5th edition. Philadelphia: Saunders Elsevier; 2010. p. 944–70.
7. Ryans I, Montgomery A, Galway R, et al. A randomized controlled trial of intra-articular triamcinolone and/or physiotherapy in shoulder capsulitis. Rheumatology 2005;44:529–35.
8. Lambert RG, Hutchings EJ, Grace MG, et al. Steroid injections for osteoarthritis of the hip: a randomized, double-blind, placebo-controlled trial. Arthritis Rheum 2007;56(7):2278–87.
9. Bellamy N, Campbell J, Welch V, et al. Intraarticular corticosteroid for treatment of osteoarthritis of the knee [review]. Cochrane Database Syst Rev 2006;(2): CD005328.
10. Alvarez CM, Litchfield R, Jackowski D, et al. A prospective, double-blind, randomized clinical trial comparing subacromial injection of betamethasone and xylocaine to xylocaine alone in chronic rotator cuff tendinosis. Am J Sports Med 2005;33(2):255–62.

11. Lindenhovius A, Henket M, Gilligan BP, et al. Injection of dexamethasone versus placebo for lateral elbow pain: a prospective, double-blind, randomized clinical trial. J Hand Surg Am 2008;33:909–19.
12. Coombes BK, Bisset L, Brooks P, et al. Effect of corticosteroid injection, physiotherapy, or both on clinical outcomes in patients with unilateral lateral epicondylalgia: a randomized controlled trial. JAMA 2013;309(5):461–9.
13. Coombes BK, Bisset L, Vicenzino B. Efficacy and safety of corticosteroid injections and other injections for management of tendinopathy: a systematic review of randomized controlled trials. Lancet 2010;376:1751–67.
14. Park J, Sutradhar BC, Hong G, et al. Comparison of the cytotoxic effects of bupivacaine, lidocaine, and mepivacaine in equine articular chondrocytes. Vet Anaesth Analg 2011;38(2):127–33.
15. Dragoo JL, Braun HJ, Kim HJ, et al. The in vitro chondrotoxicity of single-dose local anesthetics. Am J Sports Med 2012;40(4):794–9.
16. Braun HJ, Wilcox-Fogel N, Kim HJ, et al. The effect of local anesthetic and corticosteroid combinations on chondrocyte viability. Knee surgery, sports traumatology. Arthroscopy 2012;20(9):1689–95.
17. Hepburn J, Walsh P, Mulhall KJ. The chondrotoxicity of local anaesthetics: any clinical impact? Joint Bone Spine 2011;78(5):438–40.
18. Heyworth BE, Lee JH, Kim PD, et al. Hylan versus corticosteroid versus placebo for treatment of basal joint arthritis: a prospective, randomized, double-blind clinical trial. J Hand Surg Am 2008;33:40–8.
19. Bellamy N, Campbell J, Robinson V, et al. Viscosupplementation for the treatment of osteoarthritis of the knee. Cochrane Database Syst Rev 2006;(2):CD005321.
20. Housman L, Arden N, Schnitzer TJ, et al. Intra-articular hylastan versus steroid for knee osteoarthritis. Knee Surg Sports Traumatol Arthrosc 2013. [Epub ahead of print].
21. Evanich JD, Evanich CJ, Wright MB, et al. Efficacy of intraarticular hyaluronic acid injections in knee osteoarthritis. Clin Orthop Relat Res 2001;390:173–81.
22. Bloom JE, Rischin A, Johnston RV, et al. Image-guided versus blind glucocorticoid injection for shoulder pain. Cochrane Database Syst Rev 2012;(8):CD009147.
23. Molini L, Mariacher S, Bianchi S. US guided corticosteroid injection into the subacromial-subdeltoid bursa: technique and approach. J Ultrasound 2012;15:61–8.
24. Sibbitt WL, Kettwich LG, Band PA, et al. Does ultrasound guidance improve the outcomes of arthrocentesis and corticosteroid injection of the knee? Scand J Rheumatol 2012;41:66–72.
25. Raza K, Lee CY, Pilling D, et al. Ultrasound guidance allows accurate needle placement and aspiration from small joints in patients with early inflammatory arthritis. Rheumatology 2003;42(8):976–9.
26. Punzi L, Oliviero F. Arthrocentesis and synovial fluid analysis in clinical practice: value of sonography in difficult cases. Ann N Y Acad Sci 2009;1154:152–8.
27. Tsung JW, Blaivas M. Emergency department diagnosis of pediatric hip effusion and guided arthrocentesis using point-of-care ultrasound. J Emerg Med 2008; 35(4):393–9.
28. Cunnington J, Marshall N, Hide G, et al. A randomized, double-blind, controlled study of ultrasound-guided corticosteroid injection into the joint of patients with inflammatory arthritis. Arthritis Rheum 2010;62(7):1862–9.
29. Buchbinder R, Green S, Youd JM. Corticosteroid injections for shoulder pain. Cochrane Database Syst Rev 2003;(1):CD004016.
30. Marder RA, Kim SH, Labson JD, et al. Injection of the subacromial bursa in patients with rotator cuff syndrome: a prospective, randomized study comparing the effectiveness of different routes. J Bone Joint Surg Am 2012;94:1442–7.

31. Mathews PV, Glousman RE. Accuracy of subacromial injection: anterolateral versus posterior approach. J Shoulder Elbow Surg 2005;14:145–8.
32. Bettencourt RB, Linder MM. Arthrocentesis and therapeutic joint injection: an overview for the primary care physician. Prim Care 2010;37:691–702.
33. Shah N, Lewis M. Shoulder adhesive capsulitis: systematic review of randomized trials using multiple corticosteroid injections. Br J Gen Pract 2007;57:662–7.
34. Gosens T, Peerbooms JL, van Laar W, et al. Ongoing positive effect of platelet-rich plasma versus corticosteroid injection in lateral epicondylitis: a double-blind randomized controlled trial with 2-year follow-up. Am J Sports Med 2011; 39(6):1200–8.
35. Peters-Veluthamaningal C, van der Windt DA, Winters JC, et al. Corticosteroid injection for de Quervain's tenosynovitis. Cochrane Database Syst Rev 2009;(3): CD005616.
36. Klauser AS, Martinoli C, Tagliafico A, et al. Greater trochanteric pain syndrome. Semin Musculoskelet Radiol 2013;17(1):43–8.
37. Brinks A, van Rijn RM, Willemsen SP, et al. Corticosteroid injections for greater trochanteric pain syndrome: a randomized controlled trial in primary care. Ann Fam Med 2011;9(3):226–34.

Considerations in Footwear and Orthotics

Muhammad Nausherwan Khan, MD[a],*, Bret C. Jacobs, DO, MA[b,c],
Stephanie Ashbaugh, MD[a]

KEYWORDS

- Footwear • Foot orthosis • Patella-femoral syndrome • Plantar fasciitis • Flat foot
- Tarsal tunnel syndrome • Medial tibial stress syndrome • Pes cavus

KEY POINTS

- Understanding the history of footwear and orthotics makes one reason why it plays such an important part in one's daily life.
- Anatomy of the running shoe helps one understand why it is paramount toward diagnosis and management of shoe-related problems.
- Barefoot running and minimalist footwear is an area of significant interest among physicians and people from various walks of life.
- Description, diagnosis, and management of various clinical conditions are highlighted at the end of the article.

TRADITIONAL FOOTWEAR
Discovery of the Oldest Footwear

Luther Cressman, a well-known anthropologist from the United States, discovered the oldest dated footwear in 1938, inside Fort Rock Cave in Oregon. It was radiocarbon dated to about 10,000 years old. The simple construction of this footwear incorporated sagebrush bark knotted together, creating an outsole with ridges for traction, a covering for the forefoot and straps to go around the heel.[1,2]

Ancient History and Footwear

Ancient Greeks started using race sandals in the Olympics to improve traction and enhance their performance in competitive running events. They excelled in footwear design, designing anything from sandals to boots, to moccasins.[2,3]

[a] Department of Family and Community Medicine, Penn State Milton S. Hershey Medical Center, Penn State Hershey Medical Group, 121 Nyes Road, Suite A, Family Medicine Offices, Harrisburg, PA 17112, USA; [b] Department of Family and Community Medicine, Penn State Milton S. Hershey Medical Center, 500 University Drive, Hershey, PA 17033, USA; [c] Department of Orthopaedics and Rehabilitation, Penn State Milton S. Hershey Medical Center, 500 University Drive, Hershey, PA 17033, USA
* Corresponding author.
E-mail address: mkhan5@hmc.psu.edu

Prim Care Clin Office Pract 40 (2013) 1001–1012
http://dx.doi.org/10.1016/j.pop.2013.08.013   primarycare.theclinics.com
0095-4543/13/$ – see front matter © 2013 Elsevier Inc. All rights reserved.

The first sports-specific shoe was designed for playing cricket in Britain in the seventeenth century.[1] This shoe was constructed using low-cut design, leather uppers, and spikes on the outsoles. The spiked shoes also became a norm among runners participating in track and field. In early modern Olympic Games, marathon runners competed in heavy boots or shoes with leather uppers and soles, allowing for little plasticity, decreasing their performance and causing multiple running injuries, which led to another race in the world as manufacturers tried to make running shoes that were more comfortable and lighter and increased athletic performance.[1,2]

Today's Casual and Running Shoes

A multitude of shoes started to evolve in the 1800s. The evolution of footwear was taking place across the world in many different countries, including the United Kingdom, Germany, Japan, and the United States, to name a few. This evolution ultimately led to the creation of many of the modern athletic shoe companies that are known today.[2]

Multiple podiatrists, sports medicine physicians, orthopedic surgeons, scientists, athletic trainers, and physical therapists have played a role in improving the footwear and orthotic industry.

RUNNING SHOE ANATOMY

An understanding of the anatomy of a running shoe can be helpful to prevent and treat lower extremity shoe-related problems and enhance athletic performance.

Upper

The upper is the part of a shoe that covers the top and sides of the foot. The construction uses a highly breathable fabric that can prevent heat buildup, at the same time enhancing durability and providing water resistance, hence making it washable. The typical material used is nylon. Reinforcements are added as leather or synthetic leatherlike materials.

Different lacing techniques are available and increase stability and tension on the feet. The tongue is a padded piece that lies immediately beneath the lacing to provide cushioning to the top of the foot. The collar covers the ankle and has a projection that comes up above the heel to help protect the Achilles tendon from friction and irritation. This projection is called the heel counter and has a pocket for a stiffener to help control the rear foot during motion and to hold the foot in place.[1,2,4,5]

Bottom

The bottom of the athletic shoe is made up of the following components: midsole, wedge, outsole, insole, and sock liner.

Midsole

The midsole is an important part of the bottom of the shoe. It helps in providing cushioning and stability to the feet. The more cushioned the midsole, the less stability it provides to the feet; therefore, a balance between cushioning and stability to the feet is vital in a shoe. A runner often purchases a new shoe based on the "soft, cushy feel," only to develop excessive pronation and associated injuries that are directly related to the shoe selection. Purchasing the wrong type of shoe could lead to altered gait mechanics and cause injury.[2]

The midsole is commonly made of a mixture of polymer materials, including ethylene vinyl acetate (EVA) and polyurethane (PU).[4] EVA is a type of foam polymer that is light and available in multiple densities. It provides cushioning, increases shock absorption, decreases shearing, and is not as heavy as other materials. PU is a polymer that is heavier and harder than EVA. Because of this, it improves compression and durability of the shoe. Most companies use EVA in the forefoot and PU in the rear foot.[4] Increased-density materials are also common along the medial aspect of the shoes to help control pronation. Multidensity materials might also be used depending on athletes' requirements. Gel, air, and rubber have been used in varying amounts to improve compressibility and durability and to quicken rebound of an athletic shoe.[1,2,4,5]

Wedges

Wedges are also known as the medial post of a shoe. They lie between the midsole and outsole at the rear of a shoe. They provide shock attenuation and absorption on foot impact and also provide a heel lift. They are designed by tapering the midsole so that the medial side is thicker than the outside, which increases stability and reduces chances of overpronation during running.[1,2]

Wedges are often made from a material with higher density foam or thermal plastic, which creates stiffness in the midsole and makes the shoe lighter, while also preventing the medial arch from collapsing.[1,2]

Outsole

The outsole is the layer of the shoe that comes in contact with the ground. Different forms of rubber have been the material of choice for the outsole. The outsole not only helps in maintaining traction but also provides durability, shock absorption, torsional rigidity, and flexibility. It ranges in shape from curved to straight. Curved ones are less stable and mainly used for supinators and neutral runners. Straight ones are more rigid and primarily used by overpronators.[2,5]

Insole

The insole lies on top of the midsole. It is a thin layer of cushion material and helps to smooth the surface of the foot. It serves as a base for the shoe and is flexible enough to allow foot movement in the shoe. Because the insole is exposed to sweat from the feet, better materials include components to inhibit bacterial and fungal growth from the moisture in the shoe. The insole can be removed to accommodate over-the-counter (OTC) shoe inserts or custom orthotics.[2,4]

Sock Liner

The sock liner is a layer that lies between the foot and the insole board. Its principal functions are to absorb perspiration and energy, generate enough friction to prevent sliding of the feet inside the shoe, and provide some comfort.[2,4]

Final Construction of the Shoe

The final construction of the running shoe uses attachment of the upper to the bottom through any of these 3 options: board lasting, slip (or California) lasting, or combination lasting. It is either glued or stitched, depending on the stability requirements. Board lasting is mainly made up of fibers. It runs all the way from the forefoot to the rear foot. Shoes with this type of lasting have the most stability and increase torsional rigidity for a runner. Slip (or California) lasting has no board at all. It mainly provides cushioning and flexibility, improving shoe comfort. A combination of lasting uses board lasting at the rear foot for stability and slip lasting in the forefoot for flexibility and comfort.[2,4]

FOOT ORTHOSES

Physicians often use foot orthoses (whether custom-made or prefabricated) to manage lower limb injuries. Some specific patients who benefit from foot orthoses include athletes of all levels with specific injuries and military personnel.

Basics and Definition

A foot orthosis is defined as an orthopedic appliance or apparatus used as an in-shoe medical device that may help support, align, correct deformity, alter, or improve the moving parts of the body.

Evolution of Foot Orthoses

Around 1845, the English chiropodist, Durlacher, and many others of that era described the importance of using in-shoe leather materials.[1] Since then, the medical literature has given incredible importance to foot orthoses as being invaluable in treating and preventing injuries of the feet and lower limbs. In 1958, the era of modern foot orthoses therapy began. It was at this time that a California podiatrist, Merton Root, began to fabricate thermoplastic foot orthoses.[2]

Computerized and technological advancements have enabled clinicians and scientists to further enhance biomechanical uses of foot orthoses in the modern day. Foot orthoses alter the contractile activities of lower extremity musculature, improve postural stability, and reduce plantar pressures and forces.[2]

Indications and Effectiveness

Foot orthoses have been used for more than 150 years by physicians to treat lower limb and foot injuries, prevent new injuries, and optimize biomechanics of the lower limb. They are made from a multitude of synthetic and natural materials. Orthoses alter the location, magnitude, and temporal patterns of the reaction forces on the foot (especially on the plantar aspect) and lower extremity, hence allowing normal functionality. They have a role in supporting the medial longitudinal arch, reducing pathologic loading on the foot and lower extremity during weight-bearing activities.[2,6]

Foot orthoses might be helpful in bringing greater balance to the foot and lower extremity, preventing falls in elderly patients.[7] Preliminary research in certain muscular dystrophies suggests that using orthoses might be of benefit in reducing pain due to contractures. Orthoses also help in reducing pain and forefoot plantar pressures in patients affected with rheumatoid arthritis of the foot and ankle.[8] Orthoses are also frequently used to treat patients with anterior knee pain,[9] plantar foot types, excessive knee flexion leading to gait abnormality in spastic cerebral palsy, and Charcot-Marie-Tooth disease.[10] More studies are recommended by most investigators to highlight the uses of orthoses in different medical conditions affecting the feet and lower extremities.

In general, most foot orthoses are divided into (1) OTC or prefabricated orthoses and (2) custom foot orthoses (CFO).

OTC foot orthoses are used by most physicians as initial treatment of various clinical conditions, highlighted in this article in another section. They are not individual specific and are less durable, but they are much cheaper. CFO are used for patients who continue to experience problems and take into account the plantar pressures of the foot. They allow the physician to prescribe individual-specific orthoses, which can help treat the pathologic condition of the foot and/or lower extremity. They are more durable but are expensive.

BAREFOOT RUNNING AND MINIMALIST FOOTWEAR

Barefoot running and minimalist footwear has become a topic of great interest nowadays among physicians, athletes, recreational runners, and the society in general. The literature has shown considerable difference in the running mechanics of the feet and lower extremities when being barefoot compared with being in all shod conditions.[11] There is an ongoing debate about the benefits of barefoot running and minimalist footwear running versus shod running. It has been suggested through various biomechanical studies that there may be an injury reduction of the lower extremities and feet when using minimalist footwear and gait retraining.[12] It has been noted that minimalist runners, when compared with traditional footwear runners experience certain injuries more commonly because of an altered gait pattern. These injuries include stress fractures of the feet and plantar fascia rupture.[13] Even though there is literature indicating that biomechanical studies favor barefoot-style running, more randomized controlled trials are needed to establish the benefits and injury patterns seen in runners transitioning from traditional shod running to barefoot or minimalist running.

Barefoot-style running (barefoot and minimalist footwear use) uses running mechanics different from those of shod running. Barefoot-style running results in a shorter stride length, more plantar flexion of the ankle at contact and reduced joint torques. It is hypothesized that minimalist shoes can accomplish this goal and lead to a gait style similar to barefoot running.[4] With the use of traditional shoes, rearfoot elevation is noted, resulting in an initial heel strike. The ensuing loading toward the forefoot creates a firing pattern of the quadriceps above the gluteus maximus and alters normal walking and running postures.[4]

CLINICAL CONDITIONS
Patellofemoral Pain Syndrome

Patellofemoral pain syndrome is a common problem among athletes. Predisposing factors include bony abnormalities, lower extremity misalignment, and muscle and soft-tissue imbalances. A good history and examination are paramount to a clearer diagnosis. Radiologic studies can be used to assist in the diagnosis as well. Soft-tissue and quadriceps muscle strengthening exercises, physical therapy, patellar bracing, and use of CFO can aid in management.[14]

Multiple research studies have identified individuals at risk of developing patellofemoral pain syndrome due to abnormal lower extremity kinematics. A prospective trial done recently focused on the gait-related risk factors such as a disturbance of the normal dynamic foot alignment, contributing to patellofemoral pain syndrome.[15]

Another prospective study has identified a pronated foot type (measured as navicular drop) as being a risk factor for the development of patellofemoral pain syndrome.[16]

A recent systematic review found limited evidence that prefabricated foot orthoses provide greater short-term improvements in individuals with patellofemoral pain syndrome compared with flat inserts. Combining foot orthotics with physical therapy may be superior to prefabricated foot orthoses alone.[17,18] It is hypothesized that patients who have pronated foot types benefit more from foot orthotics than patients with normal foot posture.[17,18]

Plantar Fasciitis

The plantar fascia is a tight band of connective tissue that supports the arch of the foot. Plantar fasciitis is a degenerative pathologic condition that, in most cases, resolves over time with minimally invasive management. Multiple treatments have been recommended with moderate levels of evidence. Prefabricated orthotics and low-dye taping can be used initially. If helpful, more expensive treatments such as custom-made orthotics can be used. Footwear modification, particularly rocker-sole shoes, can be used. Physical therapy can be tried with stretching exercises of the feet. The use of night-splints may be helpful in some cases. Extracorporeal shock wave therapy can be tried. Cortisone injections have been used at times with success, with preference given to ultrasound-guided injections.[19,20] Some trials have shown botulinum toxin injections to be helpful as well. Surgery remains the last resort for long-standing plantar fasciitis.[19,20]

The literature describes successful methods of orthoses casting and prescription writing for custom-molded orthoses for multiple medical conditions, including but not limited to plantar fasciitis.[21]

Studies done in the past have shown that mechanical treatment with taping and orthoses is more effective than either antiinflammatory or accommodative modalities.[22]

A wide variety of plantar fasciitis treatments use prefabricated and custom-made orthoses, including heel pads and cups. These orthoses have been used to elevate and cushion the heel, as well as provide medial arch support. Conflicting evidence exists regarding the use of prefabricated or custom-made orthotic devices used with and without physical therapy or exercises in the management of plantar fasciitis.[23]

Tarsal Tunnel Syndrome

Tarsal tunnel syndrome is a neuropathic condition that results from entrapment of the posterior tibial nerve or its branches within the tarsal tunnel, a fibro-osseous tunnel beneath the flexor retinaculum on the medial malleolus side of the ankle. It is a rare but important condition that is regularly underdiagnosed, leading to a range of symptoms affecting the plantar aspect of the foot. Early management such as surgical decompression can prevent further problems and future complications.[24]

Patients with tarsal tunnel syndrome usually exhibit symptoms of numbness and tingling in the toes and base of the foot or heel, along with burning and electrical sensations. If the entrapment is high in the tarsal tunnel, the foot can be affected, as varying branches of the tibial nerve become involved. Ankle pain is also present in patients who have high-level entrapments.

CFO may be used for the initial conservative treatment of tarsal tunnel syndrome. For patients exhibiting chronic plantar fasciitis, custom-foot orthoses coupled with stretching exercises can be helpful.[25]

Posterior Tibial Tendon Dysfunction

Posterior tibial tendon dysfunction is a progressive deformity that can significantly affect the quality of life for patients and is the most common cause of adult-acquired pathologic flatfoot deformity. Early diagnosis and initiation of conservative management can improve patient's condition dramatically and prevent possible surgery.[26]

Risk factors associated with the development of posterior tibial tendon dysfunction include age-related degeneration, inflammatory arthritides, diabetes mellitus, hypertension, obesity, and acute traumatic rupture.[27]

There are 4 stages of posterior tibial tendon dysfunction. These stages are based on the dysfunction of the posterior tibial tendon, reducibility of the deformity, and condition of the hind foot joints. Approximately 80% of early disease (stage I and IIA/B) respond well to nonoperative management. Immobilization of the foot for a longer period, use of nonsteroidal antiinflammatories, custom-made orthotic use in stages I and II (specifically ankle foot orthoses in stage III), and a regular exercise program can be helpful.[28,29] Operative management is used to bring functional mobility in early stages of the disease and to achieve rigid stabilization of the hind foot in the late stages.[28,29]

Stress Fractures

Stress fractures are a common occurrence in avid runners, athletes, and military personnel, the usual fracture types being tibial, metatarsal, femoral, sacral, or spondylolysis. Risk factors include moderate to severe alcohol consumption, smoking, excessive and sudden increase in physical activity, female athlete triad, female gender, low vitamin D levels, significant recreational running, and participation in track and field. Radiologic testing should be used early on if there is significant clinical suspicion.[30]

There is weak evidence for the use of orthotics to decrease risk of stress fractures. There is no clear evidence that they will decrease the risk of those athletes with leg length inequality or cavus feet.[31]

The use of shock-absorbing inserts in footwear probably reduces the incidence of stress fractures in military personnel. Comfort and tolerability should be considered when using these inserts. Insufficient evidence exists regarding the best design of such inserts. There is insufficient evidence regarding the use of pneumatic bracing for aiding rehabilitation after tibial stress fractures.[32]

Medial Tibial Stress Syndrome

Medial tibial stress syndrome is a common and painful clinical condition prevalent among military personnel, avid runners, and dancers. Common names for this problem include shin splints, soleus syndrome, tibial stress syndrome, and periostitis. The exact cause of this condition is unknown. Risk factors include hyperpronation of the foot, female gender, and past history of medial tibial stress syndrome. Diagnosis is clinical, but imaging can be helpful in select cases. Conservative treatment is almost always successful. If it fails, surgery is performed in some cases with good results.[33]

There is limited evidence for prevention strategies regarding medial tibial stress syndrome. There is some evidence for the use of shock-absorbing insoles as possible prevention for lower limb soft-tissue injuries. There was a trial completed on army recruits that showed that custom-made biomechanical shoe orthoses are effective in the reduction of incidence of shin splints. Another study with a high risk of bias was completed on soccer referees, and this showed that wearing shock-absorbing heel inserts can significantly lessen soreness on subsequent days of a tournament. Using a knee brace might also be helpful. Stretching can be used with benefit in some select cases. Prescription of running shoes, however, does not reduce lower limb soft-tissue injuries.[34]

The American College of Foot and Ankle Orthopedics and Medicine has a position statement on CFO, which states that the latter can treat the symptoms of shin splints and stabilize the cause of the condition.[4]

Pes Cavus

Pes cavus is a multiplanar foot deformity that results because of an abnormally high medial longitudinal arch of the foot. It may result secondary to Charcot-Marie-Tooth disease, poliomyelitis, and other neuromuscular medical conditions, or it may be idiopathic in nature. Chronic foot pain, pain in other parts of the lower extremities, and subsequent disability are known complications. There is significant evidence to suggest that custom-foot orthoses can be helpful in painful pes cavus unlike prefabricated foot orthoses, which are not as helpful. Some secondary biomechanical outcomes can be improved using custom-made orthoses and specialized footwear cushioning.

Physical therapy and medications may be tried. Surgery can be used in select refractory cases.[35,36]

Adult-Acquired Flatfoot Deformity

The most common factor associated with the development of adult-acquired flatfoot deformity is posterior tibial tendon dysfunction. Due to multifactorial reasons, failure of the tendon and ligaments supporting the arch of the foot leads to progressive flatfoot deformity. There are 4 clinical stages of this problem and symptoms vary with each stage of the disease process. The clinical presentation of adult flatfoot can range from a flexible deformity with normal joint integrity to a rigid, arthritic foot. Pain and swelling along the medial aspect of the foot are common initial presentations. Subsequently, the lateral aspect of the foot gets involved as well. Conservative treatment may be helpful initially in alleviating symptoms. Immobilization followed by support may be tried. Nonsteroidal antiinflammatory medications may be helpful. Immobilization is achieved for highly symptomatic patients by a removable boot or cast. Support may be achieved with customized ankle brace or foot orthoses (with a medial longitudinal arch support and medial heel wedge). Foot orthoses are typically used for less severe deformities, especially when the initial symptoms subside. Orthoses have been noted to be most helpful for providing some support to the arch of the foot and for hyperpronated feet. Surgery may be used early on with good results to prevent significant deformity.[37,38]

Pediatric Flatfoot

Pediatric flatfoot is a common presentation in clinical practice and is mostly of the flexible type. Joint hypermobility and increased weight are risk factors. Clinical parameters and imaging studies can help identify severity of the problem. Prefabricated foot orthoses suffice for management in most children. However, CFO can be used in children with significant symptoms, risk of developing arthritis, unusual morphology, or those unresponsive to prefabricated orthoses. Surgery is used for cases refractory to conservative management and if rigidity of the flatfeet is noted.[39]

Hallux Valgus

Hallux valgus is deviation of the great toe (hallux) toward the other toes or midline of the foot. This deviation can result in joint pain and deformity, swelling (a bunion), or formation of a fluid-filled sac (bursa). Genetic predisposition may play a role in causation. Different shoe styles can potentially aggravate the condition. Conservative treatment includes using foot orthoses, night splints, and foot exercises. Surgery (chevron osteotomy) can be helpful, but no one technique is superior to the other.[40]

In hallux valgus, custom orthoses can help in the redistribution of weight, prevent excessive dorsiflexion, and improve gait transition. There is silver-level evidence for the use of custom orthotics with painful hallux valgus.[36]

Hallux Rigidus (or Limitus)

Hallux rigidus (or limitus) results from osteoarthritis of the big toe joint (or first metatarsophalangeal joint). It is a common and painful condition that causes significant deformity in the aging population. Multiple risk factors have been identified in leading to this problem. Patients present with pain, stiffness, and enlargement of the big toe joint. Conservative interventions include mobilization (vs immobilization in some cases), physical therapy with specific exercises and procedures, alternative medicine techniques such as acupuncture, accommodative insoles and CFO, use of nonsteroidal antiinflammatory medications, selective joint injections, and use of topical prepara- tions. Surgery is used if conservative treatments fail.[41,42]

Conservative management with orthotics and shoe modifications is successful in many cases. Focus should be on being realistic, trying to identify the mechanical issues with a patient's foot causing pain and discomfort and then incorporating the specific design features into the orthotic.[43]

Chronic Ankle Instability/Recurrent Ankle Sprains

Chronic ankle instability can result due to multiple factors resulting in recurrent ankle sprains in athletes, avid runners, military personnel, and the general population. It imposes a significant burden on the health care costs of any nation. Early treatment and prevention of recurring injuries can be helpful.

Lateral ligament injuries are the most common and are divided into grades 1, 2, and 3.

The American College of Sports Medicine recommends ankle injury rehabilitation byphysical therapy and exercises with guided stretching and balance training to enable ankle strengthening and prevention of future injuries. The American Orthopedic Society for Sports Medicine and American College of Sports Medicine both recom- mend external ankle supports, such as semirigid orthotics or air cast braces, instead of taping, to prevent ankle reinjury.[44]

Neuromuscular training alone seems effective in short-term management. Surgery may be considered for select cases where conservative treatment fails or early improvement is a priority.[45]

External ankle supports, such as ankle tapes, braces, or orthosis, seem equally effective in the prevention of recurrent ankle sprains.[46]

Low Back Pain

Low back pain is one of the most common problems encountered in a primary care physician's office. Reasons for low back pain can be multifactorial. Treating musculo- skeletal low back pain poses a significant challenge not only to primary care physi- cians but also to sports physicians, orthopedic physicians, physical therapists, and other involved health care workers.

The most promising approach for preventing low back pain is to combine physical activity and exercise with appropriate (biopsychosocial) education, at least for adults. No single intervention can alone solve the back pain problem, and the likely benefit is from using all the possible factors that could be playing a role in the cause of back pain.[47]

There is no significant evidence that lumbar supports, foot orthotics, or insoles help in prevention of low back pain.[48,49]

SUMMARY

Man has been in the quest to make better footwear for centuries. Significant improve- ments have been made on footwear and the development of foot orthoses, and these have been used by the general population, athletes, and military personnel. Many studies during the last few decades have compared the possible benefits and harms of traditional footwear and orthoses with those of barefoot-style running and mini- malist footwear. A multitude of clinical conditions may benefit from using the right kind of footwear and orthoses. More randomized controlled trials will be helpful in highlighting the pros and cons of using specific footwear and orthoses in different con- ditions. Selection of particular footwear and orthoses for patients should be individual specific and tailored toward prevention and treatment of running injuries and maintaining comfort and better quality of life.

REFERENCES

1. Peter C. The running shoe book. Mountain View (CA): Anderson World Inc; 1980.
2. Werd MB, Knight EL. Athletic footwear and orthoses in sports medicine. 2010.
3. Kippen C. The history of sports shoes. 2007.
4. O'Connor FG. ACSM's sports medicine: a comprehensive review. 2012.
5. Deconstructing shoes: running warehouse. Available at: http://www.running warehouse.com/LearningCenter/ShoePhD.html. Accessed February 2013.
6. Kirby KA. Foot and lower extremity biomechanics II: Precision Intricast newsletters, 1997–2002. Payson (AZ): Precision Intricast, Inc; 2002.
7. Gross MT, Mercer VS, Lin FC. Effects of foot orthoses on balance in older adults. J Orthop Sports Phys Ther 2012;42(7):649–57.
8. Hennessy K, Woodburn J, Steultjens MP. Custom foot orthoses for rheumatoid arthritis: a systematic review. Arthritis Care Res (Hoboken) 2012;64(3):311–20.
9. Mills K, Blanch P, Dev P, et al. A randomised control trial of short term efficacy of in-shoe foot orthoses compared with a wait and see policy for anterior knee pain and the role of foot mobility. Br J Sports Med 2012;46(4):247–52.
10. Phillips MF, Robertson Z, Killen B. A pilot study of a crossover trial with randomized use of ankle-foot orthoses for people with Charcot-Marie-Tooth disease. Clin Rehabil 2012;26(6):534–44.
11. Bonacci J, Saunders PU, Hicks A, et al. Running in a minimalist and lightweight shoe is not the same as running barefoot: a biomechanical study. Br J Sports Med 2013;47(6):387–92.
12. Rixe JA, Gallo RA, Silvis ML. The barefoot debate: can minimalist shoes reduce running-related injuries? Curr Sports Med Rep 2012;11(3):160–5.
13. Salzler MJ, Bluman EM, Noonan S, et al. Injuries observed in minimalist runners. Foot Ankle Int 2012;33(4):262–6.
14. Collado H, Fredericson M. Patellofemoral pain syndrome. Clin Sports Med 2010; 29(3):379–98.
15. Thijs Y, Van Tiggelen D, Roosen P, et al. A prospective study on gait-related intrinsic risk factors for patellofemoral pain. Clin J Sport Med 2007;17(6):437–45.
16. Boling MC, Padua DA, Marshall SW, et al. A prospective investigation of biomechanical risk factors for patellofemoral pain syndrome: the Joint Undertaking to Monitor and Prevent ACL Injury (JUMP–ACL) cohort. Am J Sports Med 2009; 37:2108–16.
17. Barton CJ, Munteanu SE, Menz HB, et al. The efficacy of foot orthoses in the treatment of individuals with patellofemoral pain syndrome: a systematic review. Sports Med 2010;40(5):377–95.
18. Swart NM, van Linschoten R, Bierma-Zeinstra SM, et al. The additional effect of orthotic devices on exercise therapy for patients with patellofemoral pain syndrome: a systematic review. Br J Sports Med 2012;46(8):570–7.
19. Orchard J. Plantar fasciitis. BMJ 2012;345:e6603.
20. Kaikkonen M, Joukainen A, Sahlman J. Treatment of plantar fasciopathy [Abstract in English, article in Finnish]. Duodecim 2012;128(17):1777–85.
21. Rosenbloom KB. Pathology-designed custom molded foot orthoses. Clin Podiatr Med Surg 2011;28(1):171–87.
22. Lynch DM, Goforth WP, Martin JE, et al. Conservative treatment of plantar fasciitis. A prospective study. J Am Podiatr Med Assoc 1998;88(8):375–80.

23. Buchbinder R. Clinical practice. Plantar fasciitis. N Engl J Med 2004;350(21): 2159–66.
24. Ahmad M, Tsang K, Mackenney PJ, et al. Tarsal tunnel syndrome: a literature review. Foot Ankle Surg 2012;18(3):149–52.
25. Gould JS. Tarsal tunnel syndrome. Foot Ankle Clin 2011;16(2):275–86.
26. Durrant B, Chockalingam N, Hashmi F. Posterior tibial tendon dysfunction: a review. J Am Podiatr Med Assoc 2011;101(2):176–86.
27. Kulig K, Pomrantz AB, Burnfield JM, et al. Non-operative management of posterior tibialis tendon dysfunction: design of a randomized clinical trial. BMC Musculoskelet Disord 2006;7:49.
28. Zaw H, Calder JD. Operative management options for symptomatic flexible adult acquired flatfoot deformity: a review. Knee Surg Sports Traumatol Arthrosc 2010; 18(2):135–42.
29. Crevoisier X, Assal M. Acquired adult flatfoot deformity: a pragmatic approach. Rev Med Suisse 2007;3(138):2892–4, 2896–8. [in French].
30. Patel DS, Roth M, Kapil N. Stress fractures: diagnosis, treatment, and prevention. Am Fam Physician 2011;83(1):39–46.
31. Fields KB, Sykes JC, Walker KM, et al. Prevention of running injuries. Curr Sports Med Rep 2010;9(3):176–82.
32. Rome K, Handoll HH, Ashford R. Interventions for preventing and treating stress fractures and stress reactions of bone of the lower limbs in young adults. Cochrane Database Syst Rev 2005;(2):CD000450.
33. Reshef N, Guelich DR. Medial tibial stress syndrome. Clin Sports Med 2012; 31(2):273–90.
34. Yeung SS, Yeung EW, Gillespie LD. Interventions for preventing lower limb soft-tissue running injuries. Cochrane Database Syst Rev 2011;(7):CD001256.
35. Burns J, Landorf KB, Ryan MM, et al. Interventions for the prevention and treatment of pes cavus. Cochrane Database Syst Rev 2007;(4):CD006154.
36. Hawke F, Burns J, Radford JA, et al. Custom-made foot orthoses for the treatment of foot pain. Cochrane Database Syst Rev 2008;(3):CD006801.
37. Deland JT. Adult-acquired flatfoot deformity. J Am Acad Orthop Surg 2008;16(7): 399–406.
38. Giza E, Cush G, Schon LC. The flexible flatfoot in the adult. Foot Ankle Clin 2007; 12(2):251–71, vi.
39. Evans AM, Rome KA. Cochrane review of the evidence for non-surgical interventions for flexible pediatric flat feet. Eur J Phys Rehabil Med 2011;47(1):69–89.
40. Ferrari J, Higgins JP, Prior TD. Interventions for treating hallux valgus (abducto-valgus) and bunions. Cochrane Database Syst Rev 2004;(1):CD000964.
41. Zammit GV, Menz HB, Munteanu SE, et al. Interventions for treating osteoarthritis of the big toe joint. Cochrane Database Syst Rev 2010;(9):CD007809.
42. Shurnas PS. Hallux rigidus: etiology, biomechanics, and nonoperative treatment. Foot Ankle Clin 2009;14(1):1–8.
43. Sammarco VJ, Nichols R. Orthotic management for disorders of the hallux. Foot Ankle Clin 2005;10(1):191–209.
44. Hemphill B, Whitworth JD, Smith RF. Clinical inquiry: how can we minimize recurrent ankle sprains? J Fam Pract 2011;60(12):759–60.
45. De Vries JS, Krips R, Sierevelt IN, et al. Interventions for treating chronic ankle instability. Cochrane Database Syst Rev 2011;(8):CD004124.
46. Dizon JM, Reyes JJ. A systematic review on the effectiveness of external ankle supports in the prevention of inversion ankle sprains among elite and recreational players. J Sci Med Sport 2010;13(3):309–17.

47. Burton AK, Balagué F, Cardon G, et al. How to prevent low back pain. Best Pract Res Clin Rheumatol 2005;19(4):541–55.
48. Mattila VM, Sillanpää P, Salo T, et al. Orthotic insoles do not prevent physical stress-induced low back pain. Eur Spine J 2011;20(1):100–4.
49. Van Duijvenbode IC, Jellema P, van Poppel MN, et al. Lumbar supports for prevention and treatment of low back pain. Cochrane Database Syst Rev 2008;(2):CD001823.

Index

Note: Page numbers of article titles are in **boldface** type.

Moving?

Make sure your subscription moves with you!

To notify us of your new address, find your **Clinics Account Number** (located on your mailing label above your name), and contact customer service at:

Email: journalscustomerservice-usa@elsevier.com

800-654-2452 (subscribers in the U.S. & Canada)
314-447-8871 (subscribers outside of the U.S. & Canada)

Fax number: 314-447-8029

Elsevier Health Sciences Division
Subscription Customer Service
3251 Riverport Lane
Maryland Heights, MO 63043

*To ensure uninterrupted delivery of your subscription,
please notify us at least 4 weeks in advance of move.

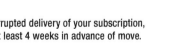
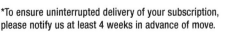

Printed and bound by CPI Group (UK) Ltd, Croydon, CR0 4YY

03/10/2024

01040478-0005